# Indian Sisters

# South Asian History and Culture

Series Editors: **David Washbrook,** University of Cambridge, UK
**Boria Majumdar,** University of Central Lancashire, UK
**Sharmistha Gooptu,** South Asia Research Foundation, India
**Nalin Mehta,** Institute of South Asian Studies, National University of Singapore

This series brings together research on South Asia in the humanities and social sciences, and provides scholars with a platform covering, but not restricted to, their particular fields of interest and specialisation.

A significant concern for the series is to focus across the whole of the region known as South Asia, and not simply on India, as is often the case. There will be a conscious attempt to publish regional studies and bring together scholarship on and from Pakistan, Bangladesh, Sri Lanka, Nepal and other parts of South Asia.

This series will consciously initiate synergy between research from within academia and that from outside the formal academy. A focus will be to bring into the mainstream more recently developed disciplines in South Asian studies which have till date remained in the nature of specialised fields: for instance, research on film, media, photography, sport, medicine, environment, to mention a few. The series will address this gap and generate more comprehensive knowledge fields.

## Also in this Series

*'How Best Do We Survive?'*
*A Modern Political History*
*of the Tamil Muslims*
**Kenneth McPherson**
978-0-415-58913-0

*Health, Culture and Religion:*
*Critical Perspectives*
Editors: **Assa Doron and**
**Alex Broom**
978-81-89643-16-4

*Gujarat Beyond Gandhi:*
*Identity, Conflict and Society*
Editors: **Nalin Mehta and**
**Mona G. Mehta**
978-81-89643-17-1

*India's Foreign Relations,*
*1947–2007*
**Jayanta Kumar Ray**
978-0-415-59742-5

*Defining Andhra: Land, Water,*
*Language and Politics from 1850*
**Brian Stoddart**
978-0-415-67795-0

*Scoring off the Field: Football Culture in*
*Bengal, 1911–1980*
**Kausik Bandyopadhyay**
978-0-415-67800-1

*Religious Cultures in Early*
*Modern India: New Perspectives*
Editors: **Rosalind O'Hanlon and**
David Washbrook
978-81-89643-18-8

*Escaping the World: Women Renouncers*
*among Jains*
**Manisha Sethi**
978-0-415-50081-4

*South Asian Transnationalisms: Cultural*
*Exchange in the Twentieth Century*
**Babli Sinha**
978-81-89643-20-1

*Minority Nationalisms in South Asia*
Editor: **Tanweer Fazal**
978-81-89643-33-1

*Television at Large in South Asia*
Editors: **Aswin Punathambekar**
and Shanti Kumar
978-81-89643-35-5

# Indian Sisters

## A History of Nursing and the State, 1907–2007

Madelaine Healey

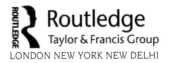
Routledge
Taylor & Francis Group
LONDON NEW YORK NEW DELHI

First published 2013 in India
by Routledge
912 Tolstoy House, 15–17 Tolstoy Marg, Connaught Place, New Delhi 110 001

Simultaneously published in the UK
by Routledge
2 Park Square, Milton Park, Abingdon, Oxfordshire OX14 4RN

First issued in paperback 2015

*Routledge is an imprint of the Taylor & Francis Group, an informa business*

© 2013 Madelaine Healey

*Typeset by*

Glyph Graphics Private Limited
23, Khosla Complex
Near Samrat Apartments
Vasundhara Enclave
Delhi 110 096

British Library Cataloguing-in-Publication Data
A catalogue record of this book is available from the British Library

ISBN 13: 978-1-138-66391-6 (pbk)
ISBN 13: 978-0-415-71040-4 (hbk)

# Contents

# List of Tables

# List of Figures

# List of Abbreviations

| | |
|---|---|
| AIDWA | All India Democratic Women's Association |
| AIGNF | All India Government Nurses' Federation |
| AIIMS | All India Institute of Medical Sciences |
| ANA | American Nurses Association |
| ANM | Auxiliary Nurse Midwife |
| ANMC | Australian Nursing and Midwifery Council |
| ANS | Auxiliary Nursing Service |
| ANSI | Association of Nursing Superintendents in India |
| BNE | Board of Nursing Education of the CMAI |
| CAHP | Coordinating Agency for Health Planning |
| CGFNS | Commission on Graduates of Foreign Nursing Schools |
| CHEB | Central Health Education Bureau |
| CIN | Central Institute of Nursing |
| CMAI | Christian Medical Association of India |
| CMC | Christian Medical College |
| CNF | Commonwealth Nurses Federation |
| CNL | Christian Nurses' League |
| COMPAS | Centre on Migration, Policy and Society, Oxford University |
| DGHS | Directorate General of Health Services |
| DGNU | Delhi Government Nurses' Union |
| EHA | Emmanuel Hospital Association |
| EU | European Union |
| GNM | General Nursing and Midwifery |
| ICN | International Council of Nurses |
| IELTS | International English Language Testing System |
| IHD | The International Health Division at the Rockefeller Foundation |
| ILO | International Labour Organization |
| IMNS | Indian Military Nursing Service |
| INC | Indian Nursing Council |

| | |
|---|---|
| INS | Indian Nursing Service |
| IRN | International registered nurse |
| JAC | Joint Action Committee |
| KEM | King Edward Memorial Hospital, Bombay |
| KGNA | Kerala Government Nurses Association |
| LMS | London Missionary Society |
| MCI | Medical Council of India |
| NARA | National Archives and Records Administration |
| NCIW | National Council of Women in India |
| NGO | Non-government organisation |
| NHS | National Health Service, UK |
| NICE | Nurses for International Cooperatives Exchange |
| *NJI* | *Nursing Journal of India* |
| NMC | Nursing and Midwifery Council, UK |
| NRI | Non-Resident Indian |
| PGIMER | Post-Graduate Institute of Medical Education and Research, Chandigarh |
| PTS | Preliminary Training School |
| QAs | Nurses belonging to the Queen Alexandra's Imperial Military Nursing Service |
| QAIMNS | Queen Alexandra's Imperial Military Nursing Service |
| RCN | Royal College of Nursing, UK |
| RCS | Royal Commonwealth Society |
| SANA | South African Nursing Association |
| SNA | Student Nurses' Association |
| TNAI | Trained Nurses' Association of India |
| TUC | Trade Unions Congress, UK |
| UN | United Nations |
| UNCTAD | United Nations Conference on Trade and Development |
| UNICEF | United Nations' Children's Fund |
| USAID | United States Agency for International Development |
| VAD | Voluntary Aid Detachment |
| WHO | World Health Organization |
| YWCA | Young Women's Christian Association |

# Acknowledgements

I would first like to thank Robin Jeffrey, my PhD supervisor. His enthusiasm, knowledge and generosity are surely without parallel in the world of PhD supervision. I am also indebted to Nalin Mehta for gently encouraging me to get my act together in finishing the book. The hospitality of P. Vijaya Kumar, Khyrunnisa A., their son Amar, and the extended family was also essential to the task of researching this book. They are wonderful friends who helped me so much with my research, while also bringing to life Kerala's history, cuisine, geography, and fashion.

At La Trobe, I benefited greatly from the advice of Priscilla Robinson at the School of Public Health. In the Politics Department, Judith Brett kindly and instructively commented on several early drafts. Sanjay Seth, Michael O'Keefe, Larry Marshall, Assa Doron, Leighton Vivian, Alanna Vivian, Anita Ray, Tom Weber, Sue Chaplin, and Dave Miller were all exceptionally supportive. Elisabeth Passmore, Maxine Loynd, Dave Miller, Cynthia Mackenzie, and Nitika Mansingh were my copy-editors and the best of friends.

In Delhi, Sreelekha Rajagopal Nair was a most informative colleague and a great friend. I owe much of my successful research in Delhi and in Kerala to her suggestions and contacts, and I have learned much from her about Malayali nurses and women.

I would also like to thank G. K. Khurana, who very generously shared with me the institutional files of the Delhi Government Nurses' Union and the All India Government Nurses Union, spoke with me at length about nursing politics and commented enthusiastically and knowledgeably on my work.

Evelyn Khannan and Nanthini Subbiah at the TNAI were also extremely generous and interesting in sharing their thoughts on Indian nursing, and kindly allowed me to set up shop in a corner of their Green Park headquarters in order to look at their extensive collection of journals.

The Centre for Women in Developing Societies in New Delhi allowed me to present some of my work, and the faculty there gave very useful guidance. I am also grateful to the Centre for Development Studies in Thiruvananthapuram, where I was able to use the library as well as speak with S. Irudaya Rajan and J. Devika. The Kerala Council for Historical Research also allowed me access to their collection and P. J. Cherian provided valuable suggestions and contacts.

I would like to thank all the nursing school and college principals in Kerala who spoke with me so openly and extensively. I am particularly indebted to the insight of A. Nirmal Jose at the Lisie Hospital College of Nursing in Kochi. C. Chandrakanthi was also exceptionally hospitable and informative. It was a great privilege to interview and to lunch with Aleyamma Kuruvilla and her close friend, Annamma Koshy, in Thiruvalla. At the Christian Medical College in Vellore, I am grateful to Shirley David for organising my visit and to the staff in charge of the college's exceptionally well-maintained archival collection.

In the UK, Shakuntala Bhansali, Daisy Lowe and Eileen Platts talked to me most interestingly of their experiences in India. Jennifer Doohan at the Royal College of Nursing assisted with my research on Indian nurse migrants. I also benefited particularly from the facilities and the assistance of the librarians at the British Library, the Cambridge University Library, the Wellcome Institute's Library for the History and Understanding of Medicine, the Imperial War Museum, and the UK National Archives.

In the US, Patricia d'Antonio at the Barbara Bates Center for the Study of the History of Nursing at University of Pennsylvania's School of Nursing was highly encouraging, and I found the seminar she arranged for me at the Center most helpful. Shortly before she died, Ruth Harnar gave me a lengthy telephonic interview from her home in Ohio, which was most enlightening and for which I am very grateful. Mary Ann Quinn at the Rockefeller Foundation Archives at Sleepy Hollow was very helpful in arranging my visit and focusing my research there. The librarians at Columbia University's Burke Library of the Union Theological Seminary in New York were also especially helpful in locating relevant missionary archives. I would also like to thank the librarians at the National Archives in College Park, Maryland, for their assistance in retrieving United States Agency for International Development (USAID) archives.

I received a generous grant from La Trobe University to conduct my research in India, and an Australian Postgraduate Award scholarship.

My parents were both very supportive. My mother helped with plentiful information on Australian nursing, and it is only due to my father that I am not in far worse debt than is the case. His generosity is truly wonderful. Finally, I would like to thank my husband, James Hewitt, whose technical nous, music and unflagging optimism have seen me through the final stretch of this project.

# Introduction

◾

*We the nurses of India, known as 'sisters' by the society, are not treated
equally with other professionals. Being women — a weaker section
of the society — we have never been given justice by the Ministry of
Health and Family Welfare. We face a lot of problems during our
service hours, but hardly any concern is shown for this community.*[1]

This book is a history of the development of the nursing profession
in India over the past 100 years. It charts the uneven, problematic
relationship of professional nursing organisations with governments
throughout the period. The complex nature of this task is, I hope,
indicated by the title of this book. 'Sister' is a term still very much
in use in India, as a title given to a nurse in-charge and as an expression of respect. Throughout this period, however, the nursing sisters
of India have struggled to achieve the authority and autonomy that
the title implies. 'Sister' also, of course, evokes the image of the
religious sister, who has in important ways influenced the cultural
heritage and the practical development of Indian nursing. Politicians
delivering speeches to nurses, promising improvements in conditions and salary that have rarely been delivered, have also always
addressed nurses as their 'noble sisters'. This repeated use seems to
have drained the term of its meaning, making the notion of nurses
as the nation's sisters a hollow joke. The relation of sister has also
been frequently deployed by international nursing organisations,
suggesting a cross-cultural continuity of care and a commonality of
purpose. This 'sisterhood' explains some of the weaknesses and some
of the strengths of Indian nursing, the culture, heritage and structure of which has been profoundly determined by Western women.
The notion of 'sisterhood' is also, evidently, at the heart of feminist

---

[1] All India Government Nurses' Federation (henceforth AIGNF), 'Representation to
Honourable Prime Minister, Government of India, in respect of Nursing Profession',
Fourth National Convention, 26–27 September 2000, New Delhi, p. 1.

organisation. Indian nursing leaders, however, have until quite recently only reluctantly identified themselves as feminist, and their evolving relationship with Indian women's movements has been complex and ambivalent. The different ways in which nurses can and cannot be captured by the term 'sister', therefore, suggest some of the questions at the heart of this book.

The book takes the 100 years between 1907 and 2007 as the period for study, responding to the self-perception of the Western nurses who first brought modern nursing to India. Many of these women viewed themselves as pioneers, building an institution for India that would provide rewarding, worthy careers for the women they could fit into the mould of the dutiful, service-oriented, frock-wearing Anglo-American nurse. Looking back from the early 21st century, it now seems apposite to consider the success of their project and the extent to which the institution they built has been remodelled by the nurses of India and by the post-colonial health establishment.

## Indian Nursing Organisations and the State

The story I have chosen to tell is of the relationship between the nursing leadership and the state. The threads of this narrative run through the entire period, with the post-colonial state replicating and perpetuating the colonial state's lack of engagement with nurses; and professional nursing organisations remaining largely weak and unrooted in the lives of nurses. On the one hand, the patriarchal state has proved consistently unwilling to recognise or focus on the development of the role of nursing in modern health systems. On the other hand, nursing inherited a professionalising culture of elitist leadership, which focused chiefly on education rather than conditions and which was insufficiently responsive to the actual experiences of nurses. It is my suggestion that the history of the state and of the leadership can explain, just as much as the oft-cited factors of culture and caste, the longstanding troubles of the nursing profession.

In telling this story I have attempted where possible to place the voices and views of nurses themselves in the foreground, something the state has repeatedly failed to do. Interviews with nurses and nurse leaders (carried out in Kerala, Delhi, Australia, and the UK) are used to tell the compelling and controversial story of the modern phenomenon of nurse emigration, to sometimes give shocking details of hospital conditions and to express the frustration of working within a system seemingly deaf to nurses' concerns. Archival materials such as the *Nursing Journal of India* (*NJI*), mission records and the papers of international organisations working in India have been used to give a strong sense of the struggles nurses faced in building up their profession.

The troubles of nurses in India are commonly ascribed to aspects of culture, seemingly accepted as immutable; the strength of the caste system, which stigmatises work with bodily fluids, strong limitations on female mobility in many parts of India, and disapproval of work that requires women to work intimately with male strangers. Ruth Harnar, a long-term American nurse leader in India, who worked for the World Health Organization (WHO) and a number of Indian hospitals, for example, wrote that

> the status of nursing as an occupation in India has suffered from the stigma attached to it by a society which could not approve of women working outside the home with tasks considered unworthy of all but the lowest caste people.[2]

As Chapter 1 explains, culture has certainly been an important part of this story. The introduction of the relatively youthful institution of modern nursing into colonial India involved a dramatic collision of concepts of gender at a historical moment when local gender practices were being vigorously defended and, to some extent, reified and hardened. Several historians of the late-colonial period have noted, as Srimati Basu writes, the 'centrality of the woman question as the marker of cultural authenticity or modernity, and a prime site of colonial domination and resistance'.[3] This meant that the challenge nursing posed — in asking 'respectable', high-caste women to care

---

[2] R. M. Harnar, 'Social Forces and Factors Influencing Nursing Education in India', *Nursing Journal of India* (*NJI*), vol. 67, no. 3, 1976, p. 54.

[3] Srimati Basu, 'Review Essay: Janaki Nair, Women and Law in Colonial India: A Social History', *Gender and History*, vol. 11, no. 1, 1999, p. 175. See also Tanika Sarkar, *Hindu Wife, Hindu Nation: Community, Religion and Cultural Nationalism*, Delhi: Permanent Black, 2001, p. 5; Antoinette Burton, *Burdens of History: British Feminists, Indian Women, and Imperial Culture, 1865–1915*, Chapel Hill: University of North Carolina Press, 1994, p. 31; Partha Chatterjee, *The Nation and its Fragments: Colonial and Postcolonial Histories*, Princeton: Princeton University Press, 1993, p. 119.

for strangers, and for men, and to expose themselves to polluting bodily substances, against all norms of higher caste communities — was unlikely to succeed. The reality was that nursing in the colonial period was an attractive career predominantly to Christian converts from communities considered untouchable under the caste system, and particularly to destitute orphans and widows from these communities. Social prejudices against these groups reinforced the public perception of nursing as 'dirty', low-status work (although for some of these women, at least, nursing represented an effective and even an enjoyable survival strategy).

The encounter between Indian society and nursing was also shaped by the nature of nursing as a recently evolved dimension of Western industrial modernity. Nursing has a long history of association with religious sisterhoods, which has heavily determined its symbolic culture. Its slow emergence from the middle of the 19th century as a career that could respectably be pursued by middle-class women was enabled by a heavily Christianised discourse of obedience and service. In India, where for a long time nurses were predominantly Christian, these aspects of nursing became firmly entrenched and to a large extent shaped the encounter between nursing and Indian society.

The persistently low social status of nursing, however, cannot be reduced to a story of caste, religion or gender. After all, the stern moral disapproval of nursing work is part of the professional history in almost every national context.[4] In both Western and non-Western societies, the early history of hospitals as a recourse for the desperately poor, combined with social restrictions on female work and mobility, invariably resulted in the stigmatisation of nursing. Extreme negative perceptions of nursing have persisted to a rare degree in

---

[4] See, for example, Barbara Melosh, *'The Physician's Hand': Work Culture and Conflict in American Nursing*, Philadelphia: Temple University Press, 1982, pp. 42–43; Charles E. Rosenberg, *The Care of Strangers: The Rise of America's Hospital System*, Baltimore and London: The Johns Hopkins University Press, 1987, p. 214; Judith Moore, *A Zeal for Responsibility: The Struggle for Professional Nursing in Victorian England, 1868–1883*, Athens: University of Georgia Press, 1988; Aya Takahashi, *The Development of the Japanese Nursing Profession: Adopting and Adapting Western Influences*, London and New York: Routledge and Curzon, 2004, p. 27; Catherine Ceniza Choy, *Empire of Care: Nursing and Migration in Filipino American History*, London: Duke University Press, p. 25.

India, however, and I suggest that this must be viewed, at least partly, as the result of an under-achieved relationship between a patriarchal state unusually unwilling to accept the need for quality nursing, and a weak mode of professional organisation determined by its colonial roots that was unable to adequately represent nurses.

The colonial nursing leadership was weakened by its failure to mobilise either Indian or Western nurses and by its adherence to a professionalising agenda that had relatively little real application in the Indian context (see Chapter 2). At the same time, the colonial state willingly and consistently tolerated an extremely underdeveloped nursing system and engaged only minimally with the concerns of nurses until the late 1930s. On their own terms, however, colonial nursing organisations cannot be judged to have been entirely unsuccessful. Although the organisational and representative structures they created were weak, their professionalising ideology determined the future of nursing in India. This was because the dying years of colonial rule brought nursing into the spotlight to an unprecedented degree. The war highlighted the shocking absence of nurses to care for the wounded soldiers pouring into Indian hospitals, focusing policymakers' attention on the need to develop nursing, and forcing them to consult with the leadership. In general, there was also a rush to reform the colonial health system that was to be independent India's legacy.[5] In this context, leaders' professionalising agenda, which was perceived as modern, progressive and desirable, found a strong theoretical place in the health-planning discourse. A professionalised nursing service was to remain the goal, if not the reality, throughout the ensuing decades.

The internationalist, professional orientation of Indian nursing was reinforced by the post-Independence arrival of nursing advisors in India, working for government and non-government development agencies. Rockefeller, WHO and the United States Agency for International Development (USAID)[6] nurses devoted much of their time and resources to the establishment of university degrees in

---

[5] For an account of this, see David Arnold, 'Crisis and Contradiction in India's Public Health', in Dorothy Porter (ed.), *The History of Public Health and the Modern State*, Amsterdam, Atlanta: Rodopi, 1994, p. 349.

[6] The international aid arm of the US government underwent a number of organisational and name changes during the period under discussion, but for consistency's sake, I have referred to it as USAID throughout the book.

nursing, to the development of advanced public health nursing and to the sponsorship of Indian nurses for training in the West. Chapter 3 examines the ways in which these post-Independence projects shaped the Indian nursing leadership. It is suggested that although the practical successes of international agency projects were limited, they contributed to the further institutionalisation of an outwardly focused, internationalist, professionalising nursing culture, through the preparation of an elite thoroughly schooled in such ideas. This had some positive effects — the relatively fast preparation of a local leadership, the promotion of quality education for nurses, an excellent theoretical understanding of the importance of public health nursing — but at the same time, such projects did not foster the growth of a responsive leadership focused on local issues and the concerns of working nurses.

Chapter 4 explores the activities and the ethos of a post-colonial leadership which was profoundly influenced by both colonial as well as international agency nurses. The Indian Nursing Council (INC), the Trained Nurses' Association of India (TNAI) and the Christian Nurses' League (CNL) of the Christian Medical Association of India (CMAI) have all developed according to the professionalising agenda promoted by Western leaders and advisors. Organisational activity centres above all on education, with the solution to poor conditions and the low status of nursing consistently viewed to be the creation of more educated, more highly skilled nurses. This has been accompanied by a theoretical, under-researched commitment to an enlarged public health role and a strong focus on nursing internationalism. Meanwhile, activism over working conditions has largely continued along the lines set out by colonial leaders: the genteel lobbying of those in power through the dispatching of petitions and memoranda. Unsurprisingly, nurse organisations have been neither powerful nor popular. Nevertheless, nursing leaders have had some significant achievements. They have institutionalised and defended the professionalist ethos, and have ensured a theoretical agreement (if not practical action) at all levels of government, that nurses require a good-quality education, rather than an exploitative training. In general, however, they have wielded little power. High-level positions for nurses in government have been disregarded and left vacant. While those in government have periodically endorsed leaders' plans and initiatives, they have rarely implemented them.

Since the early post-colonial years a rising groundswell of dissatis-faction with nursing leaders has been evident. Ward nurses have rejected a leadership distant from their own concerns about danger-ous workplaces, sexual harassment, poor accommodation, low salaries, and stagnant careers. This can partly be understood as a result of the youth and immaturity of the profession in India, which did not see the emergence of a strong Indian leadership until the early 1960s. At the same time, the recent development of stronger, nurse-led and nurse-managed trade unions has suggested, at least to some degree, the rejection of a leadership style profoundly shaped by nursing's colonial, Western inheritance. It seems that hope for the future lies substantially in the evolution of this kind of solid, issue-based leadership grounded in the concerns of nurses working in hospital wards, rather than with a degree-educated elite focused on professionalism.

The limitations of the nursing leadership have been compounded by, and in part determined by, a disengaged post-colonial state. The early years after Independence saw, at least in some quarters, a high level of respect for the importance of nursing in the context of a general atmosphere of optimism about the potential of the new state to build a more equitable, accessible and better quality health system. The commitment to better nursing and professional development remained abstract rather than actual, however, and by the mid-1960s, even this abstract commitment disappeared. A long series of committees, from the 1940s to the present day, produced reports lamenting the neglect of nursing and echoing nursing leaders' protests, but few resulted in substantial action. Chapter 5 analyses the post-colonial state's approach to nursing, examining the planning process of modern India to reveal an astonishing degree of blindness to nurses and nursing. Over time, this political neglect of nursing has become self-reinforcing. With nurses never seriously encouraged to work in public health, the planners and politicians of contemporary India now effectively accept that they are not needed in the nation's primary healthcare system. As hospitals have never employed enough nurses, it is generally accepted as the status quo that they should func-tion with only the most minimal nursing staff. With such small value ascribed to nursing skill, there is very little concern that emigration may further reduce the quality of nurses' education.

Struggling at home with poor conditions, unstimulating careers and low social status, the nurses of India, and especially of the south-western state of Kerala, have historically been an internally and internationally mobile group. Chapter 6 examines the phenomenon of nurse migration, particularly its increase since the late 1990s. It suggests that, although migration has brought dramatically improved social status to nursing, the willingness of the state to allow the rapid emigration of large numbers of nurses, while paying little policy attention to the consequences of this, illustrates the general disdain for nurses and their work identified throughout this book.

## India in Nursing History: The Global Context

This account of India's nurses is shaped by the sub-discipline of nursing history, which has become increasingly popular since the 1980s, enriched by the often unexplored written archives left by nurses, and the enormous potential offered by oral history work. Scholars of nursing history recognise that the study of nursing represents a unique opportunity to understand the social status of women. Eva Gamarnikow comments on nursing that it 'represents the patriarchal nature of the sexual division of labour in relatively pristine form'.[7] Indeed, E. D. Baer writes that for many years, feminist historians in the US ignored nursing because it painfully embodied the undervaluing of women in society, reflecting the 'deeply negative status of women'.[8] The devaluation of the uniquely feminised work of nursing, its subordination to the medical profession and its permeation by notions of service, vocationalism and obedience reflect the suspicion historically attached, in every national context, to women performing caring work in the public sphere. The story of nursing everywhere is that of subordination of nurses' interests and often, nurses' understandings of patient interests, to the (often economic) imperatives identified by male hospital administrators.

---

[7] Eva Gamarnikow, 'Sexual Division of Labour: The Case of Nursing', in Annette Kuhn and AnnMarie Wolpe (eds), *Feminism and Materialism: Women and Modes of Production*, London and Boston: Routledge and Kegan Paul, 1978, p. 121.

[8] E. D. Baer, quoted in Linda C. Andrist, 'The History of the Relationship between Feminism and Nursing', in Linda C. Andrist, Patrice K. Nicholas and Karen A. Wolf (eds), *A History of Nursing Ideas*, Sudbury, MA: Jones and Bartlett, 2006, p. 6.

At the same time, nursing history also offers the potential to explore very early stories of women's creativity, responsibility, leadership, and courage.

Within this field, according to Cynthia Connolly, authors have often chosen to strongly focus on social history, while neglecting the political histories that are key to positive action.[9] This book, therefore, aims to provide a political history of nursing that will highlight the reasons for the underdeveloped relationship between the profession and the state. I have drawn particularly on nursing academics' extensive work on professionalisation as the definitive concern of the modern nursing leadership since the beginning of the 20th century.[10] In her account of nursing in the US, for example, Barbara Melosh acknowledges the achievements of the exponents of professionalism in promoting an ideology of commitment and of entitlement to authority. By and large, however, she views professionalism as a divisive and ineffective strategy, with a history of marginalising the concerns of nurses working in the traditional apprentice system of hospital education.[11]

---

[9] Cynthia Connolly, 'Beyond Social History: New Approaches to Understanding the State of and the State in Nursing History', *Nursing History Review*, vol. 12, 2004, pp. 5–24.

[10] An important account of the work of the leadership in the UK has been provided by Brian Abel-Smith in *A History of the Nursing Profession*, London: Heinemann, 1960. He argues that leaders' focus on professionalism and drive for high standards has meant that healthcare outcomes suffered. Robert Dingwall, Anne Marie Rafferty and Charles Webster in *An Introduction to the Social History of Nursing*, London: Routledge, 1988, give an excellent account of the history of the defeat of professionalising leaders by the economics of health care as practised by British hospital administrators. Celia Davies in *Gender and the Professional Predicament in Nursing*, Buckingham and Philadelphia: Open University Press, 1995, p. 61, deconstructs the concept of the profession, arguing that it is deeply masculinised and rests on a vision of the world that tries to eliminate the feminine and deny the place of nurturing, caring qualities. Her suggestion that 'nursing's long-term project may therefore be not to become a profession in the present sense of this term, but to challenge the gendered basis of the concept' has much strength. For an overview of the contemporary professionalising position, see Rozella M. Schlotfeldt, 'Structuring Nursing Knowledge: A Priority for Creating Nursing's Future', in Linda C. Andrist, Patrice K. Nicholas and Karen A. Wolf (eds), *A History of Nursing Ideas*, Sudbury, MA: Jones and Bartlett, 2006, pp. 287–91.

[11] Melosh, *'The Physician's Hand'*, p. 16.

In writing on the relationship between profession and state, I have been particularly influenced by the work of Catherine Ceniza Choy and Shula Marks, who are also concerned with a 'long view' of the nursing profession in former colonies, and with the long-term ramifications of colonial projects in nursing. Ceniza Choy, in her study of nursing migration from Philippines, proposes the concept of the 'empire of care', in which global structures of power now determine the distribution of nurses between wealthy and poor countries. For Ceniza Choy, the large migration flows that developed from the 1960s cannot be understood independently of the early 20th-century history of US colonialism, which involved the development of a Filipino profession closely modelled on its US counterpart. Filipino nursing was oriented outward, shaped by an 'individual and collective desire for a unique form of social, cultural and economic success obtainable only outside the national borders of the Philippines'.[12] Marks' analysis of South African nursing traces the evolution of nursing representation under colonial rule and the tensions of race and class with which organisations struggled. This historical analysis is linked to the modern South African profession and the internal divisions caused by apartheid and the development of a leadership elite removed from the concerns of their constituency.[13] According to Marks, South African nurses' historical legacy includes 'the authoritarian and hierarchical structure of the profession' and leaders' adherence to a set of 'inappropriate standards', which promotes an increasingly professionalised nursing service, while ignoring the fact that 'there are simply insufficient educated women to fill the qualified nursing role'.[14] This is strikingly similar to the case of India, which inherited a similar colonial tradition of genteel, professionalising leadership.

The history of colonial nursing is, of course, shaped by the increasingly rich work in the field of the history of colonial health. This sphere of scholarship has strongly emphasised the role of Western medicine in 'promoting the security and legitimacy of colonial rule', while also questioning the extent to which it was able to or intended

---

[12] Ceniza Choy, *Empire of Care*, pp. 6–7.

[13] Shula Marks, *Divided Sisterhood: Race, Class and Gender in the South African Nursing Profession*, London: Macmillan, 1994.

[14] Marks, *Divided Sisterhood*, pp. 200, 207.

to access the rural majority of the Indian population.[15] In recent years, a strong focus on gender and women's part in the health projects of Indian colonialism has emerged, forming a significant dimension of the also relatively new body of historical work on the role of Indian and Western women under British imperialism.[16] This body of literature has emphasised the emergence of India as a site of professional advancement and career development for British and North American women doctors, facilitated by missionaries' promotion of the idea that Indian women (whose different social locations

---

[15] David Arnold, *Colonizing the Body: State Medicine and Epidemic Disease in Nineteenth Century India*, Berkeley: University of California Press, 1993, p. 139. For accounts of colonial medicine and its role in regulating and disciplining colonial subjects see also Shula Marks, 'What is Colonial about Colonial Medicine? And What has Happened to Imperialism and Health?', *Social History of Medicine*, vol. 10, no. 2, 1997, pp. 205–19; W. Anderson, 'Excremental Colonialism: Public Health and the Poetics of Pollution', *Critical Inquiry*, vol. 21, 1995, pp. 640–69; Megan Vaughan, *Curing Their Ills: Colonial Power and African Illness*, Cambridge: Polity Press, 1991; Radhika Ramasubban, 'Imperial Health in British India, 1857–1900', in Roy McLeod and Milton Lewis (eds), *Disease, Medicine and Empire: Perspectives on Western Medicine and the Experience of European Expansion*, London: Routledge, 1988, pp. 38–60; Radhika Ramasubban, *Public Health and Medical Research in India: Their Origins and Development Under the Impact of British Colonial Policy*, Stockholm: SAREC, 1982; Mark Harrison, *Public Health in British India: Anglo-Indian Preventive Medicine, 1859–1914*, Cambridge: Cambridge University Press, 1993; Sanjoy Bhattacharya, Mark Harrison and Michael Worboys, *Fractured States: Smallpox, Public Health and Vaccination Policy in British India, 1800–1947*, Hyderabad: Orient Longman, 2005; Deepak Kumar (ed.), *Disease and Medicine in India: A Historical Overview*, New Delhi: Tulika, 2001; Mridula Ramanna, *Western Medicine and Public Health in Colonial Bombay, 1845–1895*, London: Sangam Books, 2002.

[16] For work on gender and imperialism in India, see, for example, Avril Powell and Siobhan Lambert-Hurley (eds), *Rhetoric and Reality: Gender and the Colonial Experience in South Asia*, New Delhi: Oxford University Press, 2006; Jane Haggis, 'White Women and Colonialism: Towards a Non-recuperative History', in Clare Midgley (ed.), *Gender and Imperialism*, Manchester and New York: Manchester University Press, 1998, pp. 45–78; Lata Mani, *Contentious Traditions: The Debate on Sati in Colonial India*, Berkeley: University of California Press, 1998; Bharati Ray (ed.), *From the Seams of History: Essays on Indian Women*, Delhi: Oxford University Press, 1995; Burton, *Burdens of History*; Barbara Ramusack, 'Cultural Missionaries, Maternal Imperialists, Feminist Allies: British Women Activists in India, 1865–1945', *Women's Studies International Forum*, vol. 13, no. 4, 1990, pp. 309–21; and Kumkum Sangari and Sudesh Vaid (eds), *Recasting Women, Essays in Colonial History*, New Delhi: Kali for Women, 1989.

and experiences were often reduced to the figure of the high-caste, upper-class inhabitant of the *zenana*[17]) required women doctors.[18] It has examined the ways in which women doctors participated in the ideological and cultural work of imperialism, through their involvement in schemes such as the Dufferin Fund, the private philanthropic body launched by the Vicereine Lady Dufferin in 1883 to promote the training of Indian women doctors and nurses and improved hospital care for women and children.[19] As Barbara Ramusack and Dagmar Engels have recorded, Indian and Western women also forged a role for themselves in maternal and child welfare public health projects, directed to the reshaping of Indian motherhood along Western lines, and even in the early promotion of contraception.[20]

This literature has also focused on the different kinds of relationships that emerged between Indian and Western medical women. Geraldine Forbes, for example, has emphasised the limitations imposed by the often elitist and exclusionary practices of Western women doctors, as well as highlighting the less visible but often highly successful work pursued by early Indian doctors.[21] This literature has also explored the role of the *dai*, the village midwife, focusing on the constant problems experienced in the various schemes launched from the late 19th century to retrain her in the techniques of Western

---

[17] The term *zenana* refers to the section of the house in which women were secluded in some, usually higher caste and class, communities. The inhabitants of the *zenana* were a particular focus of many women missionaries.

[18] See, for example, Geraldine Forbes, *Women in Colonial India: Essays on Politics, Medicine and Historiography*, New Delhi: Chronicle Books, 2005; Maneesha Lal, '"The Ignorance of Women is the House of Illness": Gender, Nationalism and Health Reform in Colonial North India', in M. Sutphen and B. Andrews (eds), *Medicine and Colonial Identity*, London: Routledge, 2003, pp. 14–40.

[19] Maneesha Lal, 'The Politics of Gender and Medicine in Colonial India: The Countess of Dufferin's Fund, 1885–1888', *Bulletin of the History of Medicine*, vol. 68, no. 1, 1994, pp. 29–66; Sean Lang, 'Saving India through its Women', *History Today*, vol. 55, no. 9, September 2005, p. 46.

[20] Dagmar Engels, 'The Politics of Childbirth: British and Bengali Women in Contest, 1890–1930', in P. Robb (ed.), *Society and Ideology: Essays in South Asian History Presented to Professor Kenneth Ballhatchet*, Delhi: Oxford University Press, 1993, pp. 222–46; Barbara Ramusack, 'Embattled Advocates: The Debate over Birth Control in India, 1920–40', *Journal of Women's History*, vol. 1, no. 2, 1989, pp. 34–64.

[21] Geraldine Forbes, 'Medical Careers and Health Care for Indian Women: Patterns of Control', *Women's History Review*, vol. 3, no. 4, 1994, pp. 515–30; Geraldine Forbes, *Women in Modern India*, Cambridge: Cambridge University Press, 1998;

midwifery, as well as her representation as the embodiment of superstition and barbarity, and a crucial opponent in the battle to replace indigenous health practices with allopathic medicine.[22]

In general, however, the neglect of nursing in academic work on the role of women in the colonial medical system has been outstanding. This may be as a result of, first, the relatively fewer sources relating to nursing as compared to medicine and midwifery, second, the lesser focus on nurses and nursing in the colonial public sphere, and last, the comparatively less empowered position of nurses as compared to women doctors or women activists, who were usually privileged in class terms. It is perhaps also the case that perceptions of nurses as conservative, intensely bound to the missions, deeply identified with Christianity, and unlikely to challenge the orthodoxies of imperial rule has made them less popular subjects for feminist historians.

There are, however, important exceptions to this rule. Margaret Jones' research on nursing in Ceylon has emphasised the domination of leadership structures by British nurses during the late-colonial period. She suggests that this dominance retarded the acceptance of nursing as an attractive career option for Ceylonese women.[23] The major exception to the neglect of colonial nursing in India has been Rosemary Fitzgerald's pioneering historical work on nursing and the crucial role played by missionaries in its establishment.[24] Fitzgerald's

---

Geraldine Forbes, 'Negotiating Modernities: The Public and Private Worlds of Dr Haimabati Sen', in Avril Powell and Siobhan Lambert-Hurley (eds), *Rhetoric and Reality: Gender and the Colonial Experience in South Asia*, New Delhi: Oxford University Press, 2006, pp. 223–46.

[22] Sean Lang, 'Drop the Demon *Dai*: Maternal Mortality and the State in Colonial Madras, 1840–1875', *Social History of Medicine*, vol. 18, 2005, pp. 357–78; Geraldine Forbes, 'Managing Midwifery in India', in Dagmar Engels and Shula Marks (eds), *Contesting Colonial Hegemony: State and Society in Africa and India*, London: British Academic Press, 1994, pp. 152–72.

[23] Margaret Jones, 'Heroines of Lonely Outposts or Tools of the Empire? British Nurses in Britain's Model Colony: Ceylon, 1878–1948', *Nursing Inquiry*, vol. 11, no. 3, 2004, pp. 148–60.

[24] Rosemary Fitzgerald, '"Making and Moulding the Nursing of the Indian Empire": Re-casting Nurses in Colonial India', in Avril Powell and Siobhan Lambert-Hurley (eds), *Rhetoric and Reality: Gender and the Colonial Experience in South Asia*, New Delhi: Oxford University Press, 2006; Rosemary Fitzgerald, 'Rescue and Redemption:

work is particularly useful in highlighting the arrival in India from the early 20th century of nurses who perceived themselves as emissaries of a professionalised version of nursing, with a role to play in the cultural mission of imperialism. My work traces the results of this trend up to 1947, and emphasises the extent to which the internationalist, professionalist nursing ethos highlighted in Fitzgerald's work continued to define nursing organisation.

This book elucidates the influential role of international organisations in directing the development of nursing, and thus forms a contribution to the small but growing literature on the effects in India and other developing countries of the post-World War II internationalisation of medicine. According to Randall Packard, international health bodies such as the WHO and other United Nations (UN) organisations prevented former colonies from making a decisive break with the ideology and practice of colonial medicine.[25] In the case of nursing, the vague, theoretical and radically underachieved plans held by colonial leaders for professionalising nursing were strengthened by these international agencies, whose focus on nursing was strong in the 1950s and 1960s.

The literature on health and the post-colonial state has also been crucial in situating the story of nurses' neglect after Independence.[26] Sunil Amrith's work on the post-colonial history of medicine, for example, has emphasised the utopian possibilities expressed by the post-Independence nationalist government, and the nature of this

---

The Rise of Female Medical Missions in Colonial India during the late Nineteenth and early Twentieth Century', in Anne Marie Rafferty, Jane Robinson and Ruth Elkan (eds), *Nursing History and the Politics of Welfare*, London: Routledge, 1997, pp. 64–79; Rosemary Fitzgerald, 'A "Peculiar and Exceptional Measure": The Call for Women Medical Missionaries for India in the later Nineteenth Century', in Robert A. Bickers and Rosemary Seton (eds), *Missionary Encounters: Sources and Issues*, Richmond: Curzon Press, 1996, pp. 174–96.

[25] Randall Packard, 'Postcolonial Medicine', in R. Cooter and J. Pickstone (eds), *Medicine in the Twentieth Century*, Amsterdam: Rodopi, 2000, p. 98.

[26] For an indispensable account of the post-colonial health system, see Roger Jeffery, *The Politics of Health in India*, Berkeley: University of California Press, 1988. Amiya Kumar Bagchi and Krishna Soman's edited collection on Indian public health debates is also useful: Amiya Kumar Bagchi and Krishna Soman, *Maladies, Preventives and Curatives: Debates in Public Health in India*, New Delhi: Tulika, 2005.

commitment to a disease-free world, as 'both short-lived and inherently limited'.[27] According to Amrith, 'the patient, unglamorous task of building up local health services' was later sacrificed at the altar of the large and expensive 'vertical' programmes launched to eradicate particular diseases such as malaria and smallpox.[28] David Arnold's analysis of post-Independence public health emphasises that the transfer of the governance of health from British to Indian elites was 'unaccompanied by any radical overhaul of existing institutions or even a major shift in attitudes and personnel'.[29] The hitherto largely untold history of the politics of nursing forms an important contribution to this story of the evolution of a post-colonial health system. Nursing suffered from wholesale delegation to the states, and also witnessed the sidelining of what was initially a fervently proclaimed commitment to the building of a strong nursing service, in favour of an all-consuming commitment to vertical programmes, family planning programmes and later, the attempted reorientation of health services to rural needs.

The literature on Indian nursing after Independence is minimal, and the politics of nursing and any account of leadership are almost completely neglected. Though there is a small body of useful sociological work, including studies of nurses' status and career motivations.[30] Meera Abraham's monograph on south Indian nursing provides valuable information on the work of mission hospitals

[27] Sunil Amrith, 'Political Culture of Health in India: A Historical Perspective', *Economic and Political Weekly*, 13 January 2007, p. 114. See also Sunil Amrith, *Decolonizing International Health*, Basingstoke: Palgrave Macmillan, 2006; Sunil Amrith, 'Development and Disease: The United Nations and Public Health, c. 1945–1955', in Martin Daunton and Frank Trentmann (eds), *Worlds of Political Economy: Power and Knowledge, Eighteenth Century to the Present*, Basingstoke and New York: Palgrave Macmillan, 2004, pp. 217–40; Sunil Amrith, 'The United Nations and Public Health in Asia, c. 1940–1960', PhD dissertation, Christ's College, Cambridge University, 2004.

[28] Amrith, 'Political Culture of Health in India', p. 119.

[29] Arnold, 'Crisis and Contradiction', p. 351.

[30] See T. K. Oommen, *Doctors and Nurses: A Study in Occupational Role Structures*, Delhi: Macmillan, 1978; Shantha N. Mohan, *Status of Nurses in India*, New Delhi: Uppal Pub. House, 1985; Ranjana Raghavachari, *Conflicts and Adjustments: Indian Nurses in an Urban Milieu*, Delhi: Academic Foundation, 1990.

before and after Independence.[31] The survey conducted jointly by the
Coordinating Agency for Health Planning (CAHP) and the TNAI,
published in 1974, offers a rare and important source of hard data
on the profession.[32] Some attention has also been paid to nursing as a
dimension of the unique developmental successes of the south Indian
state of Kerala, where women have been much more highly educated
than elsewhere in India and encouraged to pursue paid employment.[33]
Most of the existing work, however, does not substantially examine
the role of the leadership or the political treatment of nurses.[34] There
is as yet no detailed account of the growth and development of the
profession post-Independence.

My analysis of the post-colonial fortunes of nurses also adds to
the literature on women and the Indian state, documenting the extent
to which a large, relatively well-educated group of working women
has been rendered voiceless by governments that have at all levels
proved persistently anti-woman. Shirin Rai's account of the state
proved particularly useful. She writes:

> I use the term 'the state' not as signifying a unity of structure and
> power. The state is used here as a shorthand term to describe a network
> of power relations existing in cooperation and also in tension. I do
> not regard these relations as based on a reductionist explanation of
> socio-economic systems but rather situate these power relations within

---

[31] Meera Abraham, *Religion, Caste and Gender: Missionaries and Nursing History in South India*, Bangalore: B. I. Publications, 1996.

[32] Coordinating Agency for Health Planning (CAHP), 'Report of a Nursing Survey in India Carried out under the Auspices of the Coordinating Agency for Health Planning and the Trained Nurses' Association of India', New Delhi, 1974.

[33] There is a brief but useful section on this in Robin Jeffrey, *Politics, Women and Well-Being: How Kerala Became 'a Model'*, London: Macmillan, 1992, pp. 193–95; see also Robin Jeffrey, 'Legacies of Matriliny: The Place of Women and the "Kerala Model"', *Pacific Affairs*, vol. 77, no. 4, 2004–5, p. 655; Gita Aravamudan, 'Nurses and Nuns of Kerala', in Devaki Jain (ed.), *Indian Women*, Delhi: Publications Division, Ministry of Information and Broadcasting, Government of India, 1975, pp. 251–59.

[34] Jeffery's account of the post-colonial politics of health contains a useful section on nurses: see Jeffery, *The Politics of Health in India*, p. 242.

a grid which is composed of economic, political, legal and cultural forms all interacting on, with and against each other.[35]

This usefully captures the potential of the state to simultaneously support the development of an empowered nursing profession, through its series of sympathetic committees, while displaying a consistent incapacity and unwillingness to implement its own findings. This is confirmed in the analysis of Rajeswari Sunder Rajan, who comments on the 'benign and progressive intent' of the state, expressed in its frequent and much-proclaimed commitment to international norms of gender equality, which is countermanded by its 'dismal failures' in achieving substantial improvements to women's status.[36]

This literature on the Indian state has been well complemented by international analyses of the politics of nursing. The elimination of nursing from the national health discourse in India provides stark evidence for the cross-national resonance of this body of scholarship. The suggestion by feminist scholars of nursing, such as Celia Davies, Karen A. Wolf and Chris Hart, that the gendered nature of nursing work can render it invisible to those in 'masculinised' positions of power and authority are particularly relevant.[37]

The historically high mobility of nurses has led to the creation of an important literature around the topic of nurse migration. Recent escalation in the global movement of nurses has meant increasing attention to this topic. The last chapter in this book addresses the question of the domestic effects of migration and is very much informed by this literature. In the Indian context, Sheba George and Marie Percot have conducted important anthropological and

---

[35] Shirin M. Rai, 'Women and the State in the Third World: Some Issues for Debate', in Shirin M. Rai and Geraldine Lievesley (eds), *Women and the State: International Perspectives*, London: Taylor and Francis, 1996, p. 5.

[36] Rajeswari Sunder Rajan, *The Scandal of the State: Women, Law, and Citizenship in Postcolonial India*, Durham: Duke University Press, 2003, p. x.

[37] See Davies, *Gender and the Professional Predicament*; Celia Davies, 'Introduction', in Celia Davies (ed.), *Rewriting Nursing History*, London: Croom Helm, 1980; Celia Davies, 'The Sociology of Professions and the Professions of Gender', *Sociology*, vol. 30, 1996, pp. 661–78; Karen A. Wolf, 'The Slow March to Professional Practice', in Linda C. Andrist, Patrice K. Nicholas and Karen A. Wolf (eds), *A History of Nursing*

sociological work on Keralite nurses' migration to the West and the Gulf States, and the resulting changes to nurses' individual levels of autonomy and family structures.[38] More broadly, other scholars have drawn attention to the increasing 'feminisation of migration', the rise of woman-led migration and the particular benefits and dangers of this new aspect of globalisation.[39] In my analysis, however, I have taken a more political and more national focus, examining the domestic ramifications of nurse emigration and the significance of state policy on the issue.

## Nursing Archives

In establishing this story, I have sought to accentuate the accounts of nurses themselves, while also tracing the history of nursing policy through the official correspondence and planning documents of the colonial and the post-colonial states in India. Despite frequent

*Ideas*, Sudbury, MA: Jones and Bartlett, 2006, pp. 305–18; Chris Hart, *Nurses and Politics: The Impact of Power and Practice*, New York: Palgrave Macmillan, 2004.

[38] Marie Percot, 'Indian Nurses in the Gulf: Two Generations of Female Migration', *South Asia Research*, vol. 26, no. 1, 2006, pp. 41–62; Marie Percot, 'Indian Nurses in the Gulf: From Job Opportunity to Life Strategy', in Anuja Agarwal (ed.), *Migrant Women and Work*, New Delhi: Sage Publications, 2006, pp. 155–76; Sheba George, *When Women Come First: Gender and Class in Transnational Migration*, Berkeley: University of California Press, 2005.

[39] See, for example, Nana Oishi, *Women in Motion: Globalization, State Policies and Labor Migration in Asia*, Stanford: Stanford University Press, 2005; Leela Gulati, 'Asian Women Workers in International Labour Migration: An Overview', in Anuja Agarwal (ed.), *Migrant Women and Work*, New Delhi: Sage Publications, 2006, pp. 46–72; B. Ehrenreich and A. R. Hochschild, *Global Women: Nannies, Maids and Sex Workers in the New Economy*, London: Granta Books, 2003; Susie Jolly, Emma Bell and Lata Narayanswamy, *Gender and Migration in Asia: Overview and Annotated Bibliography*, BRIDGE, Institute of Development Studies, 2003, at http://www.bridge.ids.ac.uk/reports_gend_sect.htm (accessed 26 March 2006); Anupama Roy and Sadhna Arya, 'When Poor Women Migrate: Unravelling Issues and Concerns', in Anupama Roy and Sadhna Arya (eds), *Poverty, Gender and Migration*, London: Sage Publications, 2006, pp. 19–48; Ken Young, 'Globalization and the Changing Management of Migrating Service Workers in the Asia-Pacific', in Kevin Hewison and Ken Young (eds), *Transnational Migration and Work in Asia*, Abingdon and New York: Routledge, 2006, pp. 15–36.

warnings that there is little material available on Indian nursing, I found a rich and extensive archive, which would reward further investigation. A crucial source has been the *NJI*, the monthly journal published by the TNAI since 1910. This journal is a somewhat unique resource of women's history, in that it is an almost uninterrupted record of close to a century of women's organisational work and professional identity. The TNAI headquarters at Green Park in New Delhi hold a continuous run of the journal in their library, to which they provided generous access. I have also used the Oriental and India Office Collections at the British Library in London, the archives of the Imperial War Museum in London, the archives and collection of the Wellcome Institute Library for the History and Understanding of Medicine in London, the British National Archives in Kew, the Church Missionary Society Archives at the University of Birmingham, the Royal Commonwealth Society Library collection held at Cambridge University Library, the Rockefeller Foundation archives in New York, the archives at Columbia University's Burke Library of the Union Theological Seminary, the USAID archives in Washington, DC, records at the Nehru Memorial Library in Delhi, and the archives of the Christian Medical College (CMC) in Vellore.

I interviewed nurses and nursing leaders in the UK and in India. Indian nurses in Britain gave accounts of their education in India and their passage to the West; nursing leaders in India described the benefits and challenges of the phenomenon of migration that increasingly defines the profession, and testified to the poor conditions under which most nurses continue to work. Retired leaders described their relationships with Western advisors and teachers and their commitment to the creation of a strong profession in India. Leaders in the new nurse-led unions expressed a whole new ethos, which combined much of the symbolic language of service, nobility and duty with a new and radical language of rights that was clearly informed by the growth of the feminist movement since the late 1970s.

In general, Indian nurses have few local heroines and the stories of nurses are little known. In an attempt to subvert this, and also to suggest the immense variety of individual stories that underlie my narrative of a century of professional development, I have included brief profiles of individual nurses at the start of each chapter. Some are eminent leaders, others are relatively anonymous. It is my hope that the life story of each will enliven the succeeding chapter, by suggesting some of the ways in which individuals might experience, reflect or contest the themes identified in it.

## Choices and Limits

In addressing such a lengthy time period and such a large subject, there have inevitably been choices of focus to be made. My analysis is of trained or registered hospital nurses, and in referring to 'nurses' I mean only those who have received either a three-year diploma in general nursing and midwifery or a four-year BSc (nursing) degree. This means that the history of Auxiliary Nurse Midwives (ANMs, later in some cases referred to as multipurpose health workers [female] or female health workers), the 18-month trained health carers who have worked in the public health system and in hospitals, has not been a main focus. Similarly, the histories of the health visitor and the two-year trained public health worker (trained from the first decade of the 20th century), who preceded the ANM, have not been included. I have, however, written on public health nursing, because nurses' exclusion from the public health system and the radical underdevelopment of this branch of nursing has been a consistent concern of the nursing leadership. My analysis of Indian nursing organisation also attempts to suggest that a closer alliance between nurses and the other grades of female health worker will be crucial to more effective professional activism, improvements in conditions for both, and the evolution of a sustainable, meaningful role for nurses in public health.

I have chosen to write the history of the profession at a national level, but am conscious that this has meant the sacrifice of rich local detail. There are many stories still to be told about the development of nursing in particular regions and states — the role and experience of south Indian nurses in north India, the choice to run a state nursing service in West Bengal, the prominent role of male nurses in Rajasthan and Punjab, the exclusion of Keralite students from the schools of Andhra Pradesh, and the different social attitudes towards nursing that characterise the north-eastern states.

Throughout this book, I have chosen to refer to Indian nursing as a profession, despite frequent suggestions that this was an inaccurate use of the term, and that 'nursing service' or the rather unattractive 'semi-profession' would be more accurate. Michael Burrage, Konrad Jarausch and Hannes Siegrist cite the German scholar Jurgen Kocka's definition of the profession as the most accurate, in that it incorporates not only the characteristics of professions, but also the demands and claims that they make:

> Profession means a largely non manual, full time occupation whose practice presupposes specialized, systematic and scholarly training ... Access depends upon passing certain examinations which entitle to titles and diploma, thereby sanctioning its role in the division of labour ... [Professions] tend to demand a monopoly of services as well as freedom from control by others such as laymen, the state, etc. .... Based upon competence, professional ethics and the special importance of their work for society and common weal, the professions claim specific material rewards and higher social prestige.[40]

It is clear that by any analysis, the nurses of India do not qualify all of these criteria. At the same time, they very strongly satisfy the element of the *claim* to 'higher social prestige'. Leaders themselves have not generally been blind to the fact that they do not fulfil the oft-identified criteria of autonomy and occupational monopoly usually suggested in definitions of the concept of the profession. Kamal Joglekar, for example, in her textbook for nursing students, writes that 'in general, Nursing in India has made sufficient progress to meet the criteria for a profession to some extent. Perhaps the future nurses will be able to help the profession to attain its status as profession fully.'[41] At the same time, the concept of nursing as a profession has been at the heart of nursing's identity, taking a central place in TNAI's work since the drawing up of its constitution in the first decade of the 20th century. Joglekar, despite her recognition of the

[40] Jurgen Kocka, quoted in Michael Burrage, Konrad Jarausch and Hannes Siegrist, 'An Actor-based Framework for the Study of the Professions', in Michael Burrage and Rolf Torstendahl (eds), *Professions in Theory and History: Rethinking the Study of the Professions*, London: Sage Publications, 1990, p. 205.

[41] Kamal S. Joglekar, *Hospital Ward Management, Professional Adjustments and Trends in Nursing*, Bombay: Vora Medical Publications, 1990, p. 84.

definitional problems of nursing as a profession, proceeds to advise students, 'during the course of your study and practice, evaluate your work regularly and make sure that you are a professional nurse and you are practising a profession'.[42] It is obvious that the concept of nursing as a profession has been a source of self-esteem and a key aspect of nurses' identity and I have therefore not felt it appropriate to refuse the use of a term so frequently employed by those on whom my research has focused. The search for professional status, moreover, is at the heart of all that follows. Respect, status, a decent education, and authority over the field of practice are the goals which, for better or worse, have animated leaders from the time of the first professional meeting in Lucknow in 1907.

---

[42] Joglekar, *Hospital Ward Management*, p. 86.

# A Nurse Abroad
## Shakuntala Bhansali

SHAKUNTALA BHANSALI (nee Dutt) was born in a high-caste Hindu family, but her mother died soon after giving birth to her, leaving her an orphan.[1] Her grandparents took her to the mission hospital in Bhowani, in the princely state of Bikaner (now in Rajasthan). Bhansali was adopted by an unmarried woman doctor at the mission, who she referred to as 'my missionary mother'. According to Bhansali, the practice of single lady missionaries adopting Indian girls was very common, and most ensured that their adopted daughters went on to become doctors, nurses or teachers. Her Indian grandparents contributed the money for her upbringing and would initially visit often. As she grew older, the visits grew shorter and shorter before stopping entirely. Bhansali felt that her adoptive mother had not told her the full story; this was confirmed when she found, after her mother died, that all records of her birth family had been destroyed. This was a source of considerable unhappiness, as she had nothing to tell her children and grandchildren about her own family.

Her adoptive mother was very proud of Bhansali and constantly encouraged her in her studies. She was an exceptional student and her mother hoped that she would take a medical degree. Bhansali, however, strongly felt that she wanted to be a nurse, because she had grown up in a mission hospital and had been around nurses all her life. She had always been impressed by the way they cared for patients and by the happy environment they

[1] This section is a record of my interview with Shakuntala Bhansali, London, 23 August 2005.

created. She took her nurse-training at the highly regarded Christian Medical College (CMC) Hospital in Ludhiana, Punjab, between 1952 and 1956. She was encouraged to study abroad and hence completed her midwifery training in Aberdeen and then took nursing jobs in Edinburgh and at Guy's Hospital in London. She trained as a health visitor in London and as a midwifery tutor in Bristol. Bhansali paid for all the post-certificate training herself, by working hard and saving, so that she would not need to accept financial support from her missionary mother.

Bhansali vividly remembered her early student experience in Ludhiana. Her first three months were awful. She was 17 years old and had never left home before. On night duty, she struggled to stay awake and was often in trouble for dozing off. She had frequent fainting attacks, one in an operating theatre and one while watching an earlobe being stitched. The superintendent at Ludhiana wrote to her mother saying that she thought she would never make a nurse. Her mother suggested putting her on the children's ward for the first three months. This was done and Bhansali began to thrive.

The Ludhiana teachers, all Western women, were intent on training Indian nurses to the highest standards possible. When Bhansali arrived in Aberdeen to do her midwifery course, she found herself well-prepared by their efforts. All her missionary teachers were single women, who she felt had lived hard lives. She particularly remembered Christina Allen, from Dundee in Scotland, an excellent tutor with strictly enforced high standards. Bhansali still has several friends from her Ludhiana days. In her class of 20, 19 of the student nurses were Christians and one was a Sikh. She felt that the Punjabis were quite advanced compared to other states, in that they were beginning to accept the idea of modern nursing at that stage. Working at CMC Ludhiana, she was encouraged to join the TNAI and had enjoyed reading the *NJI*.

Bhansali had planned to return to India, but clashed with Margaretta Craig, the Canadian principal of the Delhi College of Nursing (by all contemporary accounts, a prickly personality). She refused Bhansali a job at the

College on the grounds that she could have attained her post-certificate qualifications there, rather than abroad. As it turned out, there were many opportunities in the UK, and Bhansali went on greatly to enjoy her lengthy career there. She joked about her pleasure in the discovery that there were machines instead of nurses in British hospitals to sluice bedpans. Bhansali felt thoroughly appreciated by her patients throughout her career and was glad that she had not become a doctor, because she had been able to get very close to her patients as a nurse. She was very proud of the independence she had attained through her nursing career.

Bhansali wished to emphasise to me the low status of nursing in India. When she had worked as a staff nurse at CMC Ludhiana in the 1950s, she had been paid ₹13 per month, whereas government teachers got ₹300–400. Teaching, she felt, would have been most women's first choice, because it would have provided better for their family. The low status of a nurse came from the fact that she had to do menial tasks, such as giving bedpans. She related returning to Bombay from Britain in 1977 and being asked by her husband to present herself to her in-laws as a teacher rather than a nurse. This was true as she was a midwifery tutor, but illustrated the low regard held for nursing in India. In the mission environment, however, she had been protected from this, as 'no one in that world thought about nursing in that way'. At the same time, she commented that even in the missions doctors treated nurses quite badly. She felt that most Indian doctors, women and men, considered themselves above nurses and treated them 'like skivvies'.

Patients at Ludhiana, in contrast, had always been intensely appreciative of the care they received. She recalled a time when she had privately nursed a baby with tetanus back to health, and in return the family had gifted her of an enormous basket of fruit. This was rather embarrassing as nurses were strictly forbidden to accept gifts, but on this instance it was allowed and shared by all at the hospital.

When I interviewed her in August 2005, Bhansali was rather down. She had recently lost her daughter (who had carried on the family tradition of medical work by becoming a doctor) in a tragic accident. Yet, she looked back on her career as a nurse as stimulating and intensely rewarding. She said that she had enjoyed 'every minute'.

◼

# 1

# The Institution of Modern Nursing in Indian Society

▣

When Western nurses came to India as emissaries of the profession, they brought with them an extensive cultural heritage. The role of a nurse in the West had been profoundly determined by its roots in the Christian religion and by the reworking of the professional role during the Victorian age. Nursing was associated with ideals of self-sacrifice, subservience and Christian duty, all to be practised by spotlessly clean, well-trained, white-frocked 'ministering angels'. This heritage meant that those seeking to develop nursing in India came up against, on the one hand, very different local ideas about gender and caring, and on the other, the reality of an impoverished and exploitative health system in which these ideals of modern nursing were almost impossible to realise. This chapter examines the institution of modern nursing and the ways in which it encountered Indian culture. It ranges in its analysis over the whole of the period under discussion, 1907–2007, and provides the theoretical foundations for subsequent chapters. It first describes the nature of the Western institution of modern nursing and then addresses the social and cultural environment that complicated attempts to recreate it in the Indian society.

## The Culture of Modern Nursing

This section seeks to understand the heritage of modern, three-year trained nursing, and the results of its partial and problematic translation into the Indian context. It surveys important elements of nursing culture — professionalism, internationalism and notions of service — and considers their impact and effects on Indian nursing.

As is outlined in further detail in Chapter 2, from the late 19th century better-trained and more skilled nurses began to arrive in India. These more competent nurses reflected the increasingly import-ant role that nursing was playing as a dimension of Western medical modernity. Between roughly 1870 and 1920, according to Charles Rosenberg, the hospital 'assumed its modern shape'.[1] From the late 19th century, medicine became increasingly technological in nature and the hospital was transformed from a refuge for the poor to a desirable site for treatment across the social classes. This brought about a new dependence on the nurse, who came to play an integral role in the more complex modes of treatment now required.[2] In Britain and America, the work of the nurse in war had also raised her social status since Florence Nightingale famously introduced women nurses into the Crimean War. Both the world wars cemented the key role of the nurse in modern warfare and, moreover, dramatically elevated the practical and symbolic importance of the profession.[3]

## Modern nursing and the Empire

The British Empire played a significant role as an arena in which this new importance and professional confidence could be played out. As the systematisation of nursing increased and its importance became more generally accepted, the profession sought to express

---

[1] Rosenberg, *The Care of Strangers*, p. 234.

[2] Melosh, 'The Physician's Hand', p. 184.

[3] For an account of the evolving role of the British Army nurse, see Anne Summers, *Angels and Citizens: British Women as Military Nurses 1854–1914*, London and New York: Routledge and Kegan Paul, 1988. For World War I in Britain, see Dingwall et al., *Social History of Nursing*, pp. 71–72. World War I, according to Kalisch and Kalisch, resulted in a 25 per cent increase in admissions to schools of nursing in America. Clara Noyes, the leader of the American Red Cross' wartime Bureau of Nursing, wrote to nurse leader and feminist Adelaide Nutting of the success of recruitment campaigns, which had created 'hysterical desire on the part of thousands, literally thousands, to get into nursing, or their hands upon it' (Phillip A. Kalisch and Beatrice J. Kalisch, *The Advance of American Nursing*, Boston: Little, Brown and Co., 2nd ed., 1986, pp. 329, 337). Julia Hallam's analysis shows that in Britain during World War II, the status of nursing was at an all-time high. Wartime films and recruitment literature from the period show 'high-minded moral seriousness and cultural esteem, emphasizing nursing as a distinguished and vital service to the nation and a prestigious position for women' (Julia Hallam, 'From Angels to Handmaidens: Changing Constructions of Nursing's Public Image in Post-war Britain', *Nursing Inquiry*, vol. 5, 1998, p. 35. For World War II in the US, see Melosh, *The Physician's Hand*, p. 67.

its newfound confidence more widely. Anne Summers writes that nurses in the late 19th century

> accepted the definition of the empire as the public arena in which they themselves should seek distinction. They not only supported every measure promoted to strengthen and protect the empire, but demanded equal rights with men to participate in these measures.[4]

In her work on the early development of nursing, Rosemary Fitzgerald describes the arrival in India, at the end of the 19th century and the early 20th century, of a number of 'professionalising' style of nurses, who were bent on defining a role for nurses in the project of Empire, and on making use of India as a field in which they could assert their new models of highly-trained and highly-skilled nursing.[5] There was, thus, a strong sense felt by some nurses of their role as the bearers of enlightened, progressive scientised models, both of care and of emancipated womanhood. Western nurses felt committed to the notion of reproducing in India their exciting new role in the modern institution of the hospital.

Western nurse leaders in India thus proclaimed themselves as strongly committed to notions of professionalism, replicating the activities of their colleagues in Britain and America by organising around the issues of nurse representation in the government and higher standards of nurse education. Modern nursing in the West was characterised by a set of recently evolved ideal standards: a three-year training programme in which nurses received classroom instruction and were viewed by hospital administrators as students, rather than just a cheap labour force; nursing schools that had some degree of independence from hospital administrators; and a registration system that would protect the graduates of this programme from less trained competition. Western nurse leaders were also increasingly animated by the desire to win better nurse representation in health departments and in the US, by educational experiments such as degree programmes for nurses.

In its ideal form, 'modern nursing' was certainly not universally practised in the West, where numerous sub-standard nursing schools continued to exist and untrained or less trained 'nurses' were still employed. Hospitals continued to prioritise their labour needs over

---

[4] Summers, *Angels and Citizens*, p. 200.
[5] Fitzgerald, 'Making and Moulding the Nursing'.

the educational requirements of their nursing students. Yet this idealised version of modern nursing was what animated India's nursing leaders from the beginning, and it determined their projects and endeavours throughout most of the 20th century.

## Nursing internationalism

Modern nursing was characterised by the growth and development of internationalism and the perception of nursing as a sisterhood that could transcend the boundaries of nationalities. This ethos was most prominently espoused by the International Council of Nurses (ICN), which was enthusiastically supported by the Western nurses who represented the TNAI at its conferences from 1912.[6] Whilst purporting to eliminate the relevance of nationality, the ICN's brand of internationalism presumed a strong cultural hierarchy. Renowned nurse reformer Lavinia Dock, explaining the role of the US, stated in 1911 that Americans went as a 'reinforcing army' to assist nurses of other nations in their 'campaign for a higher civilization'.[7] Nursing internationalism defined a role for nurses in the cultural project of imperialism, proposing that they could promote enlightened versions of care throughout the world. Basic tenets of nurse internationalism were: the principles of nursing the sick could be cross-cultural in their application; nursing transcended the national; nurses had an important role to play in 'civilising' the colonies; and the standardisation of education and establishment of nurse registration were the crucial goals to be achieved in each national context. This ideology proved complementary to the brand of paternalistic, benevolent internationalism increasingly espoused by the missions from the early 20th century, which were beginning to proclaim the end of 'overstressed, hard, exclusive, self-centred' nationalism, and the birth of 'world-patriotism' and an 'international mind'.[8]

---

[6] Anonymous, 'Calendar', *NJI*, vol. 49, no. 10, 1958, p. 343.

[7] Quoted in Anne Marie Rafferty and Geertje Boschma, 'The Essential Idea', in Barbara Brush, Joan E. Lynaugh, Geertje Boschma, Meryn Stuart, Anne Marie Rafferty, and Nancy J. Tomes (eds), *Nurses of All Nations: A History of the International Council of Nurses, 1899–1999*, Philadelphia: Lippincott, 1999, p. 42.

[8] Belle Jane Allen, *A Crusade of Compassion for the Healing of the Nations*, West Medford, MA: Central Committee of the United Study of Foreign Missions, 1919, p. 17.

Nurse internationalism allowed the elision and avoidance of uncomfortable issues of politics and the location of authority. The ICN, as Anne Marie Rafferty writes, promoted the notion that nurses' first loyalty was to 'some superordinate ideal of professionalism that went beyond nationalistic concerns'.[9] Indian nationalism rapidly gained support and influence from the first decades of the 20th century and was the cause of considerable anxiety in both missionary and government institutions. For nurse leaders, the notion of universal sisterhood of care became useful in this context. Abraham writes that Veera Pitman, superintendent of nursing at CMC Vellore, felt concerned about the extent of nationalist sentiment among her students during the 1920s and 1930s. Pitman wrote that in response she attempted to create an understanding 'that national feeling is only a step towards International feeling and that we may all strive together to bring India into God's Kingdom'.[10] Similarly, in the pages of the *NJI*, constant emphasis on the progress of 'the profession' as a transnational entity could eliminate the need to examine thorny issues of hierarchy, discrimination and domination closer to home.

Succeeding chapters explore the persistence of this internationalist ethos in Indian nursing. Colonial emphasis on internationalism was dramatically reinforced by the participation of Western nurses in the post-colonial international development programmes described in Chapter 3. In a context of widespread local prejudice against nursing and state neglect, the support proffered by international nursing and other development organisations had a strong appeal, and emerged as a source of legitimacy and of career development for nursing leaders, as is discussed in Chapter 4. Meanwhile, as Indian nurses graduated from programmes designed by British and American nurses, they were recruited to the hospitals of the Middle East and the West in increasing numbers. Chapter 6 shows that connections with Britain, Canada and the US were ubiquitous and served to reinforce the early philosophy of nursing internationalism. The idea of nursing as an international sisterhood proved an ideology with resonance and utility in India, and it persisted strongly.

---

[9] Rafferty and Boschma, 'The Essential Idea', pp. 46–47.
[10] Abraham, *Religion, Caste and Gender*, p. 96.

## *Modern nursing and the ideology of self-sacrifice*

Modern nursing bore a complex ideological legacy centred on moral purity and the nobility of service; a legacy which permeates Indian nursing. This ethos was initially very much a part of the work of the Protestant missionary nurses who monopolised the training of Indian women. The CNL states that its purpose is to 'promote Nursing as a Christian Vocation'.[11] Its forerunner, the Nurses' Auxiliary, in 1930 proclaimed its mission as promoting 'the highest efficiency in Christian nursing work in the relief of human suffering' and disseminating 'information concerning the need of nursing work and its place as an integral part of the Christian message to India'.[12] Although many mission leaders were also committed to high standards in professional development, this was framed by a commitment to a Christianised discourse of duty, service and self-effacement.

This ideology has a lengthy history in the nursing work of Christian religious orders, which played an extensive role in the development of Western nursing since organised religious nursing began in 17th-century France.[13] This religious emphasis on nursing as Christian service deriving from the work of religious women took particularly strong hold in India, because of the small but significant role played by nursing nuns there. Religious orders, Roman Catholic and Protestant, supplied nurses and nurse training in both Christian and government hospitals, especially in south India. A 1911 observer of nursing in India recorded that

> the most satisfactory results I have seen as regards nursing in Zenana Hospitals were those run by nuns, where the bulk of the work was done by these ladies, and a certain number of native girls were trained under them.[14]

It was often the case that hospitals or provincial authorities would invite particular religious orders to provide nursing services. In

---

[11] Abraham, *Religion, Caste and Gender*, p. 18.

[12] Ibid.

[13] For an account of the role of religious women in the development of nursing, see Sioban Nelson, *Say Little, Do Much: Nurses, Nuns and Hospitals in the Nineteenth Century*, Philadelphia: University of Pennsylvania Press, 2001.

[14] Anonymous, 'Women's Hospitals in India and their Nursing', *NJI*, vol. 96, no. 4, 2005 [April 1911], p. 77.

Bombay Presidency, the Protestant Sisters of the Community of All Saints were invited to supply nursing services to the JJ Group of Hospitals there. In 1916, Sister Eleanor Mary of the order received a Kaiser-i-Hind silver medal for her work in the development of nursing in Bombay.[15] In Poona, the sisters of St Mary the Virgin, Wantage, ran a nursing school. In Bangalore, the Roman Catholic order of St Joseph of Tarbes trained nurses.[16] In 1944, Weldon Dalrymple-Champney, a British doctor touring India as an expert advisor to the government's Bhore Committee on health planning, was impressed by the standard of nursing at the Cuttack Hospital in Orissa. In this hospital, French sisters of the Order of St Joseph provided clinical nursing and instruction. The sisters trained large numbers of Indian women, maintained impressively sanitary and orderly conditions and all their nurses looked after both men and women (in contrast to many parts of India in which Indian nurses nursed only women and children).[17]

The history of nursing in the south-western state of Kerala, which went on to supply the majority of nursing students post-Independence, is particularly closely tied to the work of European religious orders. The Maharaja of Travancore invited the Catholic Sisters of the Holy Cross from Switzerland to supply nursing services at the Trivandrum General Hospital as well as to run the school of nursing, and accordingly they arrived in 1906. According to Abraham, the Order had been unable to provide trained nurses, but sent nuns anyway because, as the Bishop of Quilon commented, 'a true sense of dedication counted much more than a diploma'.[18] J. Axel Hojer, a Swedish doctor working in Trivandrum in the early 1950s, reported that although the standard of nursing service was low among the nuns, they had 'made themselves beloved and respected for their devotion both in their care of the individual patient and in assisting the doctors'.[19]

---

[15] Milly Burke, Letter to the Editor, *NJI*, vol. 8, no. 1, January 1917, p. 21.

[16] Abraham, *Religion, Caste and Gender*, p. 83.

[17] Weldon Dalrymple-Champneys, 'India 1944', Wellcome Institute Library for the History and Understanding of Medicine, GC/139/H.2/1 File of Sir Weldon Dalrymple-Champney, Box 1, 79–80.

[18] Abraham, *Religion, Caste and Gender*, p. 84.

[19] J. Axel Hojer to Gerda Hojer, 14 January 1954, Rockefeller Foundation Archives, Sleepy Hollow, NY (henceforth RF), RG1.2, Series 464C, Box 53, Folder 493, 'India, Trivandrum School of Nursing, Equipment, 1953–1958'.

The role of nuns in nurse training continues to be significant in contemporary India. In 1978 the Kerala government still maintained a division for 'honorary nursing sisters and head sisters', which provided for the payment of an 'honorarium', or a much lower than average salary, to religious sisters who were nurses.[20] Numerous schools in Kerala and Karnataka are run by Catholic and Protestant orders, and there is a significant number of religious sisters among the nursing school principals and staff of India.

In many parts of India, a strong association developed between nurses and nuns. In writing an account of Kerala women for a 1975 government-sponsored publication on the women of India, Gita Aravamudan chose 'Nurses and Nuns' as her focus. Her account made the cultural proximity of the two very evident. In the early post-Independence decades, women joining religious sisterhoods were motivated similarly to those becoming nurses; the decision to join a convent was often also determined by the need for economic security.[21] In the late 1940s and early 1950s, it was even the case that the nurse similarly surrendered her chances of marriage, because the stigma against the profession was such that it was difficult for nurses to find husbands. Nuns and nurses have been similarly marked out by Western uniforms, similarly bound to an institutional life and similarly defined by notions of service. Hilda Lazarus (an Indian-Christian doctor who was the first Indian director of CMC, president of the CMAI and who retired in 1947 as the chief medical officer of the Women's Medical Service in India) commented that the recruitment of nurses had in fact been impeded by the strict discipline they faced, with a common perception that becoming a nurse was like joining 'the nunnery'.[22]

The legacy of this association of nurses with nuns was profound. Mrs Chandramathy, pioneer of nursing in Kerala and the first assistant director of nursing appointed there, felt that the strong association of nursing with Catholic nuns in the early days of its development left a problematic legacy for the state and encouraged the migration of Malayali nurses to other states. The nuns, with their strong emphasis

---

[20] Government of Kerala, 'Report of the Third Kerala Pay Commission', Trivandrum: Government of Kerala, 1978, p. 161.

[21] Aravamudan, 'Nurses and Nuns of Kerala', p. 259.

[22] Hilda Lazarus, *Our Nursing Services*, Aundh: Aundh Pub. Trust, for the All India Women's Conference, 1945, p. 11.

on service and self-sacrifice, had been willing to work in such poor conditions that they had reinforced the stigmatisation of nurses and created a tradition of low pay and exploitation.[23]

In general, the connection of Indian nursing with religious sisters linked the work of nursing still more firmly to the Christian community and strengthened the discourse of obedience, service and self-sacrifice that already infused nursing and the work of the Protestant missionary nurses.

## Nursing reform and Victorian womanhood

The service ethos promoted by the work of religious nursing sisters was complemented by the nursing reforms of the 19th century. Modern nursing was defined and circumscribed by the Victorian patriarchy under which it emerged; and in the US, by similarly restrictive ideas of the conditions under which it might be suitable for 'ladies' to work. From the mid to the late 19th century, middle-class reformers wrested the professional image (if not always the reality) of nursing away from working-class handywomen nurses. This refashioning of nursing into an occupation suitable for 'ladies' depended on a highly religious discourse of self-sacrifice and service that could legitimate women's work in the public sphere under Victorian patriarchy. 'Lady-nurses' could not be seen to work for money, but they could do it for suffering humanity. Carol Helmstadter writes of Britain that:

> In the 1840s and 1850s the religious revival, which stressed the philanthropic role for women, the widespread belief that nursing was an inherited part of ladies' natures, and the growing dissatisfaction of many ladies with their very constrained domestic role, merged with the need of the new scientific medicine for better educated nurses. This merger provided ladies with the possibility of finding a place for themselves in the public sphere.[24]

The remaking of nursing as a respectable profession by Nightingale and other reformers at this time, thus, involved a heavily Christianised

---

[23] Cited in Aravamudan, 'Nurses and Nuns of Kerala', p. 255.

[24] Carol Helmstadter, 'From the Private to the Public Sphere: The First Generation of Lady Nurses in England', *Nursing History Review*, vol. 9, 2001, p. 130.

discourse of vocationalism, service and obedience. As Chris Hart writes of British nurses' historical legacies — 'caring, nurturing, death, accepting hardship, suffering, subservience and subordination are all part of the myth'.[25]

The ethos of the 'noble profession', service, purity, and vocation took a powerful hold in India. Mission nurses promoted it vigorously in all their activities and it was at the heart of nurses' self-definition. The TNAI was wedded to ideas about vocationalism and its writings were often characterised by traditional ideas of nursing as inspired, selfless service. The organisational motto is 'Lighted to Lighten', invoking this idea of selfless service and also the 'lady with the lamp' culture of Nightingalism that characterises Indian nursing. British leaders in India enthusiastically promoted the notion of nurses as 'ladies', whose purity and honour must be guarded and defended. The organisation was heavily invested in conservative and traditional symbols — starched white frocks and winged caps were viewed as integral to the person of the nurse.

The service ethos, above all, took root in a powerful cultural attachment to the figure of Florence Nightingale, who in contemporary India remains the central professional role model. Early leaders vigorously promoted Nightingale as the exemplar of service, self-sacrifice and professionalism. It is possible to suggest several reasons for this strong attachment to Nightingale as a professional heroine. First, she had strong connections with India. Nightingale participated in the Royal Sanitary Commission on the Health of the Army in India, which presented its report in 1863, including detailed recommendations for improvements in military nursing. She also spent decades corresponding with viceroys and provincial governors, promoting health and sanitation and, later, supporting the Indianisation of the British administration.[26] More tellingly, as Anne Marie Rafferty and Geertje Boschma suggest, during the first half of the 20th century, the influential leaders of the ICN shaped Nightingale into a professional heroine who was 'above nationality, belonging to every age and country'.[27] As Rosenberg also points out, the exciting and dramatic work of Nightingale in Crimea, which

---

[25] Hart, *Nurses and Politics*, p. 85.

[26] For an account of Nightingale's work in India, see Jharna Gourlay, *Florence Nightingale and the Health of the Raj*, Aldershot: Ashgate, 2003.

[27] Rafferty and Boschma, 'The Essential Idea', p. 54.

nursing leaders mainly focused on, made a highly 'usable history'.[28] The TNAI, which increasingly had to present itself (however unconvincingly) as non-religious and non-partisan, could make the story of Nightingale's life embody notions of vocationalism, selfless service and pious obedience without the need to directly refer to any aspect of Christian religion. Aya Takahashi highlights a strikingly similar process in Japan, where a state trying to develop a modern nursing profession shaped Nightingale as a professional heroine. According to Takahashi, the state 'separated her career from Christianity and the English cultural background, and put some of her "great conduct", particularly that in the Crimea, into the context of Confucian moral ethics'.[29]

Most Indian nurses, of course, are likely to make their career choice at least partly on pragmatic and instrumental grounds, attracted by the reliable income and inexpensive training required. In terms of self-definition and the construction of a professional culture, however, the rhetoric of service and self-sacrifice is paramount. In the context of a society generally hostile to nurses and nursing and in which, until recently, the majority of recruits have been Christians, the notion of nursing as social service has been an important dimension of nurses' self-perception. This was reflected in T. K. Oommen's rather coldly expressed 1978 finding that nurses 'seem to develop an emotional-affectual bond with their occupation by assuming or even rationalizing that their life is dedicated to serve the sick and ailing'.[30] P. Arora, a nurse, wrote in the *NJI* in 1976 of nursing as requiring women who were 'religious minded, pious and missionary in work'.[31] A 1985 TNAI 'Career Guide for Nurses' asserted that the nursing profession '*lives* to serve *the needs* of all people' [original italics], that '[n]ursing is essentially a profession of courage, dedication, love for humanity and faith' and it is a profession of 'service and giving'.[32]

It is also unquestionable that the discourse of the noble profession has been deployed in the oppression of nurses, as has been the case

---

[28] Rosenberg, *The Care of Strangers*, p. 212.

[29] Takahashi, *The Development of Japanese Nursing*, p. 53.

[30] Oommen, *Doctors and Nurses*, p. 77.

[31] P. Arora, 'Perspectives on Indian Nursing', *NJI*, vol. 47, no. 9, 1976, pp. 223–24.

[32] Anonymous, 'A Career Guide for Nurses', in Narender Nagpal (ed.), *Nursing Perspectives: Indian Nursing Year Book: 1984–85*, Delhi: TNAI, 1985, p. SC 5.

in the history of nursing in most nations. Professional models based on service and subordination, in a context of radical gender inequality, have facilitated an extreme oppression of nurses by the medical profession. Moreover, the discourse of selflessness, service and subordination has been enthusiastically seized on by politicians. Invariably, communications with nurses from members of government and bureaucrats have included patronising instructions to nurses not to forget their duty of service and the 'nobility' of their profession.[33] So insistent has this repetition been, that the term 'noble profession' has come to seem emptied of whatever meaning it may once have had, so frequently and cynically has it been deployed by those in power to encourage nurses to continue working in dreadful conditions. Rajkumari Amrit Kaur, first health minister in independent India and an enthusiastic champion of nurses (particularly in comparison to those who followed), identified this danger in 1958:

> It is so easy to talk of nursing as a noble profession. It is indeed one of the greatest of all professions. But if we are to encourage girls filled with the right spirit to come into the profession, we must also see to it that working in the profession is not a drudgery but a real privilege and pleasure.[34]

This easy manipulation of the discourse of vocationalism and noble, selfless service has, unfortunately, continued apace since Rajkumari Amrit Kaur identified it back in 1958. In 1975, for example, then Member of Parliament Sheila Kaul addressed Lucknow nurses on the occasion of Florence Nightingale's birthday. She told them that 'it was their primary duty to serve their motherland' and exhorted them 'to follow the high ideals of the noble profession to which they have the honour and privilege to belong'. She finished with a brief mention of the fact that she was 'aware of the many problems which the nurses are facing'.[35] Whenever political attention has been directed to nurses, it has been considered necessary to remind them that 'noble' service is their destiny.

---

[33] Jeffery describes a similar tendency for politicians to deploy the notion of the noble profession against doctors, who are also encouraged to live up to high standards of self-effacing service. See Roger Jeffery, 'Allopathic Medicine in India a Case of Deprofessionalisation?', *Society, Science and Medicine*, vol. 11, 1977, p. 536.

[34] Rajkumari Amrit Kaur, in Anonymous, 'Greetings and Messages', *NJI*, vol. 49, no. 10, 1958, p. 319.

[35] Anonymous, 'Branch Affairs', *NJI*, vol. 66, no. 7, 1975, p. 181.

# Modern Nursing in Indian Society

Indian nursing was thus internally strongly defined by the culture of modern Western nursing, permeated by the ideals of internationalism, professionalism and service, in spite of the fact that the actual practice of nursing was a very different experience. Outside the profession, however, people understood nursing very differently. Attempts to promote the development of modern nursing in India were attended by a variety of social and cultural difficulties and by a continuing state and societal refusal of nursing leaders' status claims. Chapter 2 develops the argument that such social and cultural difficulties were too readily blamed for the slow progress of nursing. The rejection of nursing by polite Indian society was certainly, to some extent, determined by a very reasonable distaste for the often dreadful conditions in which nurses worked. Nonetheless, the social and cultural environment in which leaders attempted to develop nursing was clearly of profound importance. This section, therefore, discusses this socio-cultural environment and the challenges it posed.

## Local traditions of care

Pre-colonial India offered few cultural parallels for the caring role of the trained hospital nurse. It was somewhat different in ancient India, which had one of the oldest traditions of paid nursing, in which both women and men performed the role of a caring assistant that came relatively close to the modern figure of the nurse. Julia Leslie and Dominik Wujastyk write that the Sanskrit manual, the *Charaka Samhita* (estimated dates for which range between 600 BCE and 100 CE), records the role of the *upasthatr* or medical assistant. The four vital qualities of the assistant were: knowing how to wait on or attend on someone, dexterity, loyalty to the doctor, and cleanliness. Leslie and Wujastyk also describe the role of the nurse as specified in the *Sushruta Samhita* (dated between 600–350 BCE). In this text, the assistant is described as friendly, non-critical, able in the care of the sick, physically strong, obedient, and tireless. In this text it is made clear that male assistants nursed men and female assistants women. The *Sushruta Samhita* also describes midwives, who were to be mature, not easily upset, experienced at assisting during childbirth, and with short fingernails. An early military text, the *Arthasastra*, described a female military caring role, 'women in charge of food and drink and capable of filling men with enthusiasm, should be stationed in the rear'. Leslie and Wujastyk conclude from their analysis of these early texts that nursing was viewed as an important necessity, that men cared for men and women for women and 'there was a degree of autonomy in their attendance on the sick'.[36] This is a tradition described with some pride in the historical sections of Indian nursing textbooks, but it was not an aspect of ancient medical history that survived.

## Modern nursing and the dai

The most obvious existing indigenous equivalent to the modern nurse was the *dai*, the village midwife. Hindu *dai*s were usually members of castes considered untouchable, especially barber castes, and have been among the most oppressed, stigmatised and disempowered in society. Muslim *dai*s have also been among the poorest, lowest-status women. As has been widely documented, the *dai* was the frequent subject of lurid mission propaganda, which described her as unhygienic, ignorant and cruel. Notoriously, the American journalist Katherine Mayo's account of her six-week tour of India, *Mother India*, drew on sensationalist depictions of the obstetric practices of the *dai* as evidence for her argument that Indians were incapable of self-rule.[37] Although Mahatma Gandhi described her book as a 'drain-inspector's report', its rejection of the *dai* ultimately came to be shared by upper-class, upper-caste Indian society. As Geraldine Forbes documents, replacing *dai*s with trained midwives became the official goal of all of the national women's organisations by the 1930s.[38]

Underlying the rhetoric of the *dai* as ignorant, cruel and dangerous, there was also, however, a certain degree of fear among the Western medical establishment. The repeated failure of most *dai* retraining initiatives suggested the impossibility of bringing *dai*s into the allopathic fold, while the project of replacing them with trained midwives was obviously extremely limited, as the number of such midwives was very small and concentrated in urban areas. In the context of a very limited allopathic health system, the *dai*

---

[36] Julia Leslie and Dominik Wujastyk, 'The Doctor's Assistant: Nursing in Ancient Indian Medical Texts', in Pat Holden and Jenny Littlewood (eds), *Anthropology and Nursing*, London: Routledge, 1991, pp. 25–30.

[37] Katherine Mayo, *Mother India*, London: Butler and Tanner, 1927.

[38] Forbes, 'Managing Midwifery in India', p. 167.

provided a universal, affordable and culturally comprehensible form of midwifery that was trusted and used by women of all classes all over India. She thus represented a considerable threat to the cultural project of Western medicine. In describing the difficulty of replacing the *dai*, rather than her undesirable obstetric techniques, a much more nuanced picture of a more serious and worrying competitor emerged, rather than the filthy, disempowered 'cord-cutter' of mission propaganda.[39] Edris Griffin, who launched a *dai* retraining programme in Delhi that became the Lady Reading Health School, wrote that in modernising midwifery it was essential to make allies of the *dai*s, because 'they have much influence in the homes of the people. They act as Family Doctor and general adviser and are consulted about everything'.[40] Maqbool Ali, the assistant director for public health and maternal and child welfare in Andhra Pradesh, described the role of the *dai* at a 1958 session for health visitors. He viewed her as rather powerful:

> Her importance and multifarious contributions to the life of the village as a person to be consulted on matters of vital importance to the family and community, makes it necessary to gain her confidence and co-operation so that she may be taught and guided in methods of safe midwifery.[41]

---

[39] It is also clear that the role and duties of the *dai* and her status in the community differed to some degree in different parts of India. Patricia and Roger Jeffery and Andrew Lyon found the north Indian *dai*s, with whom they did extensive fieldwork, to be disempowered and of such low status that they suggested retraining programmes were unlikely to ever succeed (Patricia Jeffery, Roger Jeffery and Andrew Lyon, *Labour Pains and Labour Power: Women and Childbearing in India*, New Delhi: Manohar, 1989, p. 219). In other areas, descriptions of the *dai* are rather different. Abraham interviewed a third generation *dai* working for Brahmin families in Vellore district in Tamil Nadu who, as her mother and grandmother had done, remained with the mother and baby for 40 days following the delivery, assisting with washing and bathing each day (Abraham, *Religion, Caste and Gender*, p. 131). S. X. Charles, a senior obstetrician at CMC Vellore, in an article generally ambivalent about the worth of *dai* training, recorded that the advantages of a *dai* in Vellore district included her willingness to remain with the mother throughout the labour, her provision of supportive services such as cleaning the house and washing linen, her continuing regular visits with the mother after birth and her assistance with breastfeeding (S. X. Charles, 'Mode of Delivery by Untrained Dais in and around Vellore', *Journal of the Christian Medical Association of India*, vol. 46, no. 2, 1971, pp. 86–87).

[40] Edris Griffin, 'Health Visitors' League', *NJI*, vol. 13, no. 8, 1922, pp. 194–95.

[41] Maqbool Ali, 'The Role and Training of Dais (2)', *NJI*, vol. 50, no. 5, 1959, pp. 168–69.

For nurses, the *dai* was an obvious competitor, as she was far and away the dominant provider of obstetric services to the women of India. Nurses defined themselves against the *dai*s, but at the same time encountered some of the same stigma that they did. As Fitzgerald has suggested, while in the West professionalising projects took the working class apprentice nurse as their definitive 'other', in India the *dai* could serve this purpose. As Fitzgerald comments, 'the language employed to demolish the "old" nurse in the West was exactly the same as that used to condemn the Indian *dai* as careless, crude, unclean and criminally incompetent'.[42] Nurses thus joined in the general excoriation of the *dai* as the representation of ignorance, dirt and superstition, which, as Fitzgerald suggests, was held up in contrast to the idealised Western cleanliness and rationality. In a 1923 exhibition in Delhi sponsored by the Victoria Memorial Scholarship Fund, a nurse exhibit made this explicit by displaying a 'good' (retrained, clean and Westernised) *dai* and a 'bad' *dai* (dirty, with long, ragged fingernails).[43] Nurse leaders eagerly portrayed the profession as part of a scientific, modern, Westernised future, in opposition to the *dai*s, viewed as part of a dark, superstition-filled past.

By the 1920s and 1930s, the issue of health provision had become increasingly politicised and the neglect of public health and of maternal and child health was an important issue. Nurses eagerly sought a role in the new public health discourse as part of their general desire to define a significant role for nurses in national health plans (as is discussed in Chapter 2), and the *dai* played an important role in this quest. Although nurses' involvement in public health was almost non-existent, leaders still perceived the *dai* as an important future target in their professionalising project and as a way into a more substantial public health role for nurses. Some nurses did become involved in *dai* retraining projects; Griffin, for example, played a key role in the establishment of the Lady Reading Health School, and participated extensively in the school's work with local *dai*s. For most nurses, however, involvement with *dai*s was minimal and the battle to replace them mainly theoretical. Colonial nurse leaders optimistically perceived themselves as engaged in a long-term battle, not yet really underway, to replace the *dai* with trained midwives and public health nurses, which regrettably involved accommodating

---

[42] Fitzgerald, 'Making and Moulding the Nursing'.
[43] Edris Griffin, 'Health Visitors' Page', *NJI*, vol. 14, no. 2, 1923, p. 49.

*dais*' presence until a critical mass of better educated, higher caste replacements became available.

The increasing tendency of hospitals through this period to employ *dais* instead of nurses also provided what nursing leaders interpreted as a worrying indication of the contempt of the state for the skills of nurses. In a context of extreme shortage, hospital administrators drew on trained *dais* to provide nursing services. This was the start of a trend that has persisted through to the present; as later chapters show, the unqualified continue to be employed in large numbers throughout India, particularly in private hospitals. The employment of *dais* in hospitals during the colonial period presented nursing leaders with an early rejection of their claim to professional control over the employment of women in hospitals, making a mockery of their victories in achieving state registration acts and causing serious status anxieties. In 1941, the Punjab branch of the TNAI protested the employment of 'nurse-*dais*' and claimed that 'many of them are attempting work far above their knowledge and experience'.[44] An article written towards the end of World War II illustrated the status anxiety that the employment of *dais* caused. It urged all nurses to join the TNAI so that they would have strong common ground from which to protect themselves from state governments that might legislate their rights away, meaning that 'nurses who have enjoyed the privileges of being Army Sisters may be reduced to the rank of *ayahs* or *dais*'.[45]

The *dai* and the nurse led quite different lives, in general, but it is also important to recognise the commonalities in their experience of stigma, pollution and a society deeply concerned with the control of female sexuality. The powerful stigma attached to the role of the *dai*, to some degree, determined the stigmatisation of the new Western-style trained midwives in India. A 2005 report on the status of public health nursing records that

> the origin of the midwife and association with *dais* have not helped in the development of midwifery in India. Even to this day, the word midwife does not have prestige because in many Indian languages it is equivalent with the *dai*.[46]

---

[44] Anonymous, 'Précis of Honorary Provincial Secretaries' Reports', *NJI*, vol. 32, no. 4, 1941, p. 131.

[45] Anonymous, 'News and Notes', *NJI*, vol. 33, no. 8, 1942, p. 200.

[46] Academy for Nursing Studies, 'Situational Analysis of Public Health Nursing Personnel in India: Based on National Review and Consultation in Six States',

Trained nurses were not, it seems, so directly associated with the figure of the *dai*. Nurses and other commentators tended to relate the early low status of nursing more to the proximity of sweepers on the ward, the requirement of female mobility, the wearing of Western dress, and perceptions of moral laxity. Nonetheless, they suffered from the same caste and gender practices that determined the *dai*'s disempowered position. The *dai* was stigmatised due to her close contact with the processes and fluids of birth, which were considered intensely polluting. As Anu Gupta, Bharti Roy Choudhury and Indira Balachandran point out, pollution is 'an instrument of both gender and caste subordination' and 'a classic tool of the dominant, patriarchal hierarchy to weaken the power of women, a societal safety valve to distance men from women's sexuality'.[47] Although the school-educated, frock-wearing, hospital-bound trained nurse of the 1950s may have seemed a thousand miles from the village *dai*, both suffered intense social opprobrium due to their involvement with bodies, polluting bodily matter and the birth process.

## Women's work, patriarchy and the shadow of prostitution

Modern nursing also posed a significant challenge to local gender practices. The role of the nurse, as Western nurses presented it, conflicted with Indian understandings of the role of upper-caste, higher-class women. Recent scholarship has emphasised how crucial the maintenance of an idealised Hindu domestic with virtuous Indian women at its centre was to the nationalist critique of colonialism.[48] Antoinette Burton, for example, writes that idealised, reified Indian women emerged as 'guarantors of traditional values in nationalist discourse'.[49] Sudipta Kaviraj describes the way in which Indian society laid claim to social autonomy under political colonisation.[50]

---

conducted for Training Division, Ministry of Health and Family Welfare, Government of India, with support from UNFPA India (the UN Population Fund), Hyderabad, 2005, http://www.whoindia.org/LinkFiles/HSD_Resources_Situation_Analysis_of_Public_Health_Nursing_Personnel.pdf (accessed 3 January 2007).

[47] Anu Gupta, Bharti Roy Choudhury and Indira Balachandran, 'Women's Beliefs about Disease and Health', 1997, http://www.hsph.harvard.edu/grhf/SAsia/suchana/1299/rh402.html (accessed 30 January 2007).

[48] See, for example, Sarkar, *Hindu Wife, Hindu Nation*, p. 5; Chatterjee, *The Nation and its Fragments*, p. 119.

[49] Burton, *Burdens of History*, p. 31.

[50] Sudipta Kaviraj, 'Modernity and Politics in India', *Daedalus*, vol. 129, no. 1, 2000, p. 148.

A key dimension of this was the maintenance of a strong private patriarchy, defined by control over women's mobility and sexuality. As Meredith Borthwick writes, 'in Hindu society the position of women had always been a symbol of male honor, to be maintained by careful control over female sexuality'.[51]

In upper-caste and middle-class society, the care of the sick was seen as an important dimension of women's work in this controlled, feminised private sphere. The substance of the caring dimension of this role is a relatively little explored subject, but accounts of the lives of 19th- and early 20th-century Indian women refer to the importance of knowledge of home cures, remedies and care of the sick for wives and mothers. Borthwick writes that the shared responsibilities of the *bhadralok* or upper-middle class in 19th-century Bengal included the care of children and the sick. She details the considerable familiarity that middle-class Bengali women had with a number of systems of medicine — the Hindu *kabiraji* system, the Islamic *hakimi*, as well as allopathic and homeopathic medicine. Although commentators during the late 19th and early 20th century lamented the loss of much of this knowledge, women still had considerable familiarity with local herbal remedies. Bengali magazines published simple recipes for herbal medicines, and the average household in 1885 contained 'measuring glasses, scales and weights . . . a wooden syringe, and a thermometer, as well as a long list of basic drugs'.[52] Judith E. Walsh describes a 1900 advice manual for women, written by the female poet Nagendrabala Dasi, which contained a six-page section with advice on Ayurvedic medicines suitable for children's illnesses.[53] J. Devika's collection of the early writings of Malayali women contains some mention of the role of women in caring for the ill,

---

[51] Meredith Borthwick, *The Changing Role of Women in Bengal, 1849–1905*, Princeton: Princeton University Press, 1984, p. 6. A clear manifestation of this anxiety about female sexuality in the public domain of a hospital was the restriction on Indian nurses in many parts of India to only nurse women and children. In 1952, there were still 53 schools of nursing which did not teach the nursing of men (T. K. Adranvala, 'Nursing Profession in India', in Usha Sharma and B. M. Sharma (eds), *Encyclopaedia of Women and Education: Volume 3, Women and Professions*, New Delhi: Commonwealth, 2001 [circa 1957], p. 175. Sharma and Sharma do not give the date of this extracted piece but the contents indicate it was written between 1957–60).

[52] Borthwick, *The Changing Role of Women in Bengal*, pp. 216–20.

[53] Judith E. Walsh, *Domesticity in Colonial India: What Women Learned When Men Gave Them Advice*, Lanham: Rowman and Littlefield, 2004, p. 161.

including Manntaraveetil Lakshmy Amma's statement that know-ledge of home remedies was considered imperative for mothers.[54] The displacement of this key element of women's domestic work into the public environment of the hospital occasioned considerable discomfort and engendered moral suspicion of women willing to provide care to strangers.

The extent to which middle-class women might participate in any kind of work and in public activity was heavily circumscribed and, disappointingly for leaders, nursing did not emerge as one of the respectable routes by which the small minority of educated women might gain a career. This was in clear contrast to the medical profes-sion and even to teaching, where women did 'men's work', whereas nurses did (in public and for strangers) work that was firmly associ-ated with the private world of the family. Women doctors initially, as Arnold wrote, fought 'against the low-caste and polluting asso-ciations of the medical profession'. As was the case with nurses, the 'difficulty of attracting and keeping high-status, especially Brahmin, women as medical students was frequently remarked upon'. Although middle-class or elite women who took up professional employment as teachers, doctors or lawyers often 'gained respect, independence and personal satisfaction', most also faced disapproval, discrimination and harassment.[55] Gradually, however, medicine became an occupa-tion of considerable prestige for women.[56] As Forbes describes, even in the late 19th century, once women doctors made it through the difficulties of medical school, they 'graduated into a world that held them in high esteem and offered positions with high salaries'.[57] It was no surprise to anyone that, as Sarah Tooley wrote in her history of nursing in the Empire, the 'modern' Indian woman was 'more ambi-tious to use her new-found wings of learning to soar into the medical or some other profession rather than that of nursing'.[58] As doctors,

[54] Lakshmy Amma Manntaraveetil, 'An Account of My Life and My Home-Making', in J. Devika (ed.), *Her-Self: Gender and Early Writings of Malayalee Women*, Kolkata: Stree, 2005, pp. 10–21.

[55] Forbes, *Women in Modern India*, p. 186. See also Geraldine Forbes' account of pioneer women doctors in *Women in Colonial India*, pp. 85–90.

[56] Arnold, *Colonizing the Body*, pp. 266–67.

[57] Forbes, *Women in Modern India*, p. 166.

[58] Sarah Tooley, *The History of Nursing in the British Empire*, London: S. H. Bousfield & Co., 1906, p. 346.

women could access some of the power and prestige of a masculine profession, associated with intelligence, rationality and science. The extent of the moral suspicion attached to nursing as intimate caring work and the challenge it posed to private patriarchies was made evident in several ways. In many parts of India a 'B' grade of nurse arose for women trained only to nurse women and children.[59] Although this limited employment opportunities and kept Indian women out of positions of authority, as is discussed in the next chapter, it was by far the most popular training option for them. A persistent discourse also arose that associated nurses and prostitutes, partly based on the real susceptibility of some nurses to brothel owners but also on the nature of nursing work itself. Among missionaries, it was often commented that nursing students and nurses were susceptible to the agents of brothels. Lazarus commented about nurses in a pamphlet for the All India Women's Conference:

> Their task was arduous and irksome . . . The strain was great, and when temptation came in the guise of a kind invitation from a generous-hearted man, it was accepted . . . Repeated invitations came, she could not resist the temptation and she fell — a ruined woman, a greater outcaste in Society, the finger pointed at her. Was the profession such! How could any self-respecting parents countenance their daughters going in for nursing or midwifery![60]

Ethel Bleakley, a doctor from Manchester working at a mission hospital in Ratnapur, in her article about the first nurse from their hospital to qualify as a three-year trained and registered nurse, wrote that the early death of the nurse from beriberi in the mid-1940s could be viewed as a blessing. Her mother had been about to move her away from the mission to 'the city', which Bleakley presumed would result in succumbing to prostitution. She wrote that this move, 'would have had only one ending; and so, bitter though our grief was, we could and did give thanks to our Heavenly Father that "one of His little ones" had been taken away from the evil to come'.[61] In 1939, E. M. Tomkinson wrote in the *NJI*:

> When we have heard of nurse-probationers and nurses who have fallen into sin we have felt their disgrace to be our shame, and the dishonoring

---

[59] Adranvala, 'Nursing Profession in India', pp. 168–79.
[60] Lazarus, *Our Nursing Services*, p. 10.
[61] Ethel Bleakley, *Meet the Indian Nurse*, London: Zenith Press, 1949, p. 40.

of our Nursing Profession . . . Why has the Nursing profession in India been dragged so often into the mire of immorality?[62]

This association of nursing with prostitution has been longstanding and persistent. Jyotsna Chatterjee in 1985 described a nurses' union meeting at which she 'came face to face with the agony of women in the nursing profession who, though in a profession considered "noble", were looked upon as sex objects, easily available and cheap by society at large'.[63] In 1975, Aravamudan's study of Kerala nurses observed that 'in Indian society which still places a lot of emphasis on segregation of sexes nursing was looked down upon because girls had to look after men and often perform intimate chores for them'.[64] It is clear that the work of nurses, which required caring intimately for strangers, living outside the home and working night shifts, has been an ongoing threat to a patriarchal society that emphasised the confinement and restriction of women's sexuality — a threat that has led to a continuing, painful discourse associating nursing with prostitution.

With their work viewed as unprestigious, undemanding, dirty 'women's work', Indian nurses experienced particularly difficult relations with doctors. Celia Davies suggests that the self-perception of the 'masculine professions' as the autonomous, independent deliverers of essential expertise requires that 'women's work in organisations — some of it called nursing — has to be ignored, trivialised and devalued'.[65] Hart writes of the Victorian origins of nursing that nurses, taking on the role of the 'oppressed mother', were

> replicating the patriarchal Victorian society that shaped them, while aping that most important of Victorian institutions, the family. The doctor adopted the controlling, penetrative, dominating role of the father and it was the role, or 'duty' of the nurse to subordinate herself to, and support him, nurture and care for the patient and manage the anxiety of the patient as well as that of the doctor and her own.[66]

---

[62] E. M. Tomkinson, 'The Work of the "Association for Moral and Social Hygiene"', *NJI*, vol. 30, no. 2, 1939, p. 57.

[63] Jyotsna Chatterjee, 'Foreword', in Mohan, *Status of Nurses in India*.

[64] Aravamudan, 'Nurses and Nuns of Kerala', pp. 251–59.

[65] Davies, *Gender and the Professional Predicament*, p. 62.

[66] Hart, *Nurses and Politics*, p. 103.

In India, as elsewhere, the doctor–nurse relationship has been troubled, oppressive and restrictive. Yet, the medical establishment of India, as is described in succeeding chapters, has been particularly slow even to recognise the need for high-quality nursing and has since the colonial period actively attempted to limit nurses' authority. Efforts to realise the practice of 'modern nursing' — with nurses in charge of nurse education programmes, with clearly defined clinical responsibilities, with nursing superintendents administering hospital nursing — have continually stumbled against this seemingly unassailable power-relationship. B. G. Link and J. C. Phelan suggest that the process of stigmatisation is 'entirely dependent on social, economic and political power', because 'power . . . is essential to the social production of stigma'.[67] The continuing difficulty in raising nursing's status has to a large degree foundered in the face of its proximity to the dominant, controlling and heavily masculinised medical profession.

## Class and Caste in Nursing

Attempts to develop modern nursing also suffered from the feeling in polite Indian society that the work of nurses in hospitals was very close to that of servant castes considered untouchable. Leaders' hopes that nursing would be accepted as skilled, respectable work stumbled against the reality of Indian hospitals, in which nurses in general provided unskilled labour and worked alongside sweepers. This, of course, had also been a definitive aspect of the development of nursing in the West. Abel-Smith writes that the early history of modern nursing in Britain was defined by an ongoing preoccupation with distancing the public image of the nurse from that of the servant.[68] The recent history of nursing in Britain and America was strongly associated with the lower working classes. Rosenberg writes of the US:

> The line between nursing and domestic service could hardly be drawn in the mid-nineteenth century . . . Emptying bedpans, cleaning and

---

[67] B. G. Link and J. C. Phelan, 'Conceptualizing Stigma', *Annual Review of Sociology*, vol. 27, 2001.

[68] Abel-Smith, *A History of the Nursing Profession*, p. 242.

cooking, changing sheets and removing vomit and bloodstains were all tasks that guaranteed a humble status in this class-conscious society.[69]

The work of late 19th-century nurse reformers revolved around distancing nursing from these earthy beginnings (famously captured by Charles Dickens in the character of Sairey Gamp, the gin-sodden, snuff-taking drab of *Martin Chuzzlewit*). Nursing was claimed for the middle classes and portrayed as ideal work for religious 'ladies'. However, this was a battle that was only ever partially won. At the turn of the century, as Monica Baly points out, 'ladies and trained' dominated the leadership, but the majority continued to be working-class and often partially or questionably trained.[70]

In India, a similar process occurred. As in the West, hospital nursing developed into a survival strategy for the most disadvantaged. Until at least the 1930s, the majority of candidates for nursing were widows, orphans or destitute converts who had no other option. According to Lazarus,

> those in charge of orphans were anxious about their future and decided thus: if a girl were pretty she was sure to get married, if good at passing examinations she was made a teacher; and if she possessed neither of the former she was sent to be trained as a nurse or midwife.[71]

The association with widows was particularly problematic in a society where widowhood was intensely stigmatised and in which, as Uma Chakravarti describes, upper-caste widows were subject to marginalisation and extreme forms of social exclusion.[72] The monopolisation of the profession by such groups did little to raise its public image and reinforced the notion of it as polluting work, making it unlikely that either non-Christian or 'respectable' Christian families would allow their daughters to train as nurses. According to Lazarus, a central problem that faced nursing when India achieved

---

[69] Rosenberg, *The Care of Strangers*, p. 214.

[70] Monica Baly, *Florence Nightingale and the Nursing Legacy*, London: Croom Helm, 1986, p. 4.

[71] Lazarus, *Our Nursing Services*, p. 10.

[72] Uma Chakravarti, 'Gender, Caste and Labour: The Ideological and Material Structure of Widowhood', in Martha Alter Chen (ed.), *Widows in India: Social Neglect and Public Action*, London: Sage Publications, 1998, pp. 63–92.

independence was to dissociate nursing from its low-class, low-caste origins and to attempt to attract 'the beautiful and the cultured, the educated and the intelligent, the sympathetic and the understanding' into the ranks of nurses.[73]

In the Indian context, the stigmatisation of nursing as servant work took on added force under the caste system. Nurses were often linked disparagingly to the sweepers, who were employed along with them and played a vital role in the functioning of the wards. John Carman, a missionary doctor in India from 1928 until the 1950s, wrote of the nurses in his hospital at Ongole:

> They are eager to pass on the menial but essential tasks to the new probationers . . . to the patient's relatives, or to some scrub-woman. They don't want to be ridiculed, called by the various names which people apply to sweepers, no, not even if their grandparents did have to do that work before they became Christians. In that case, as a matter of fact, they are even more sensitive.

As nursing began to attract the more educated, 'respectable' candidates that leaders desired so deeply, the perception of nursing work as polluting and associated with untouchability became increasingly painful. Most detailed accounts of the education of Indian nursing students during this period discuss the difficulty of persuading Indian students to attend to the personal care of patients. Disputes were frequent between Western nurses, who believed that the nobility of nursing lay in a willingness to tend to every need of the human body, and their Indian students, who often felt that their experience of life within the hospital and society would be much easier if bedpans and baths could be delegated to sweepers and ward-boys. In the early 1950s, the Western director of the School of Nursing at Vrindaban wrote to the *NJI*, demanding to know, after decades of professional development in India, 'why cannot we dignify all tasks that are necessary in caring for the human body in illness?'[74] Despite all the educational emphasis on the desirability of nurses personally caring for patients, she had observed that in most hospital wards it was common practice for nurses, reluctant to undertake polluting work, to delegate the bathing and personal care of the patients and even the giving of enemas to the sweepers.

---

[73] Lazarus, *Our Nursing Services*, p. 25.
[74] Elda M. Barry, 'Letter to the Editor', *NJI*, vol. 44, no. 8, 1953, p. 203.

Issues of caste and pollution thus clearly formed part of the daily experience of the average Indian nursing student, who strove to distance herself from the polluting aspects of the work. It seems that the same anxieties about the proximity of nursing to servants' work, that had so strongly informed the growth of professional nursing in the West, found new manifestations in India, where under the rigid hierarchy of the caste system this proximity had even graver consequences. Milton Singer writes that pollution involves 'not simply a categorical contrast between "untouchables" and "clean" castes; it is pervasively implicated in status hierarchies of people, jobs and products'.[75] It is clear that pollution emerged as a crucial aspect of the subordination of nurses and the perpetuation of their inferior status relative to the medical profession.

Indian perceptions of nursing as unclean work pursued by marginalised, morally suspect, low-caste women were heavily internalised by the white nurse leadership, who were constantly anxious about the standard of recruit they were able to attract. Central to the reform of nursing in the West had been the acceptance of nursing work as a respectable endeavour for 'ladies', and the leadership in India was continually discouraged by the failure of polite Indian society similarly to accept nurses' claims to respectability. Diana Hartley, a British nurse who played an important role in promoting and developing the work of the TNAI, felt that 'the status of the nurse has always been a vexed question . . . nurses in other countries had to fight to gain and maintain their position; things were even more difficult in India'.[76] In 1947, nurse leaders from the Nurses' Auxiliary of the CMAI wrote of 'the fact that nursing is not publicly accepted as a profession but looked upon as a lower menial service', the urgent need to obtain students from 'higher cultural and social backgrounds', and the lamentable failure of the public to understand the 'fine history of service which has been attached to this profession since the days of Florence Nightingale'.[77] Nurses at the American

---

[75] Milton Singer, 'Introduction: The Modernization of Occupational Cultures in South Asia', in Milton Singer (ed.), *Entrepreneurship and Modernization of Occupational Cultures in South Asia*, Durham, NC: Duke University, 1973, p. 3.

[76] Diana Hartley, 'The First General Secretary Looks Back', *NJI*, vol. 69, no. 10, 1958, p. 337.

[77] Committee from the Christian Medical Association of India, Burma and Ceylon and the Nurses' Auxiliary (CMAI Committee), 'A Survey of Nursing and Nursing Education in Mission Hospitals and Schools of Nursing in India', Mysore: Wesley Press and Publishing House, 1947, pp. 6, 9.

Baptist Mission Hospital in Nellore during the 1930s reported being 'compelled to take girls of a lower grade' because in wider society 'nursing was not considered a profession'. This, they said, was discouraging for both teachers and the students themselves, who 'had to endure many taunting remarks about "taking nurses' training"'.[78] A committee of mission nurses constituted in 1947 to plan for the post-Independence future of the profession commented that 'for many, many years Mission nursing sisters have struggled toward the goal of procuring more desirable and better nursing candidates' from 'the higher cultural and social backgrounds'.[79] This quest for better students was not only about improving the educational base of probationers, but also about attracting higher caste women who would dignify the profession in the eyes of local elites.

This relentless focus on overcoming caste-based beliefs about pollution and attracting a 'better class' of candidate disguises a history in which it is quite likely that many of the low-status women blamed for the stigmatisation of nursing found it a useful, rewarding and even a status-enhancing occupation. As Padma Anagol emphasises, missionaries 'did not encounter a docile set of Indian Christians who could be manipulated at will'.[80] Although the perspective of nurse converts is generally not a focus of accounts of missionary work, the occasional glimpse can be found of women finding personal fulfilment through their training as nurses. Bleakley's book on the lives of Indian nurses working at her Bengali mission hospital during the 1930s and 1940s gives valuable detail of this kind. She records, for example, the work of Shoila, a Muslim widow who converted and took nurse training. Shoila arranged to hold a weekly clinic in her home village, which meant that local children became free of the seasonal sore eyes and skin diseases that had long afflicted them.[81]

---

[78] Annie S. Magilton, Helen M. Benjamin, Lena A. Benjamin and Lena M. English, 'American Baptist Mission Hospital for Women and Children', 1930, by courtesy of the Burke Library of Union Theological Seminary in the City of New York, Rh. India A — American Baptist Mission, Hospital for Women and Children and School of Nursing, Reports, p. 9.

[79] CMAI Committee, 'A Survey of Nursing', p. 6.

[80] Padma Anagol, 'Indian Christian Women and Indigenous Feminism, c.1850–c.1920', in Clare Midgely (ed.), *Gender and Imperialism*, Manchester: Manchester University Press, 1998, p. 94.

[81] Bleakley, *Meet the Indian Nurse*, p. 33.

Shubala, a Christian from Calcutta who had made a socially well-regarded marriage but was deserted by her husband for a wealthier woman, was brought to the mission by penurious relatives keen to ensure her safety.[82] She proved a highly capable nurse and was put in charge of a new maternity hospital opened by the mission. It was estimated that this hospital treated between 15,000 and 20,000 outpatients annually. Although Bleakley's book also reflects the maladjustments, stresses and relentless propaganda that formed part of the experience of conversion, the health training imparted to these women also made them figures of some power in the eyes of their own communities. For these women, nursing was in some cases a route to personal influence and also to social mobility, as their children were able to attend Christian schools and forge good careers. In 1951, Catherine E. White, the Superintendent of Nursing at St Columba's Hospital in Hazaribagh, wrote to protest the relentless promotion by the leadership of the search for the better educated:

> We must not forget the very real contribution to the health and happiness of the ordinary villager that is made by the 'B' grade or 'Assistant' nurse . . . I wonder how many 'A' Grade nurses, or those who have attained degree standards, would be content to live in a village and run, with very little or no assistance, a small dispensary, helping poor women in difficult childbirth, treating sores and bad eyes and dispensing malaria drugs in places where doctors only rarely come, and with very little supervision, and at the same time, bring up their own children, cook for their husbands and mind their own houses . . . justice demands that we acknowledge the real debt of gratitude we owe to these pioneers who have faced so many problems and difficulties in the early days with self-sacrifice and devotion.[83]

As has so often been the case throughout its history, nursing probably proved a successful life-strategy for numerous women in difficult circumstances, who provided useful and essential nursing services. As is also the case in the West, histories of the uses made of nursing by the non-elite have not usually found a place in the official record. Instead, those recording the advance of modern nursing have focused

---

[82] Bleakley, *Meet the Indian Nurse*, pp. 60–63.
[83] Catherine E. White, 'Letter to the Editor', *NJI*, vol. 42, no. 4, 1951, p. 100.

on the negative effects of these women's early work and on the positive results of their replacement by more 'respectable' women.

## Anglo-Indians and Malayalis: India's First Modern Nurses

Given the widespread stigmatisation of nursing, the mainstream of Hindu and Muslim Indian society was in general unlikely to provide a reliable recruitment base for the modern nursing service envisaged by Western leaders. It was women from atypical or minority communities who, for various reasons, overcame cultural dissonance to form the nucleus of the hoped-for profession. The Anglo-Indian or Eurasian community, with its Western-style gender practices, emerged as the colonial basis for the recruitment of a nursing cadre for government hospitals. It is not clear when this process of 'occupational capture' began, but O. P. Jaggi cites a Madras General Hospital record from 1895 that 'the better class of Eurasians seems to be awakening to the fact that the Hospital nursing is a suitable employment for their unmarried daughters'.[84] This was ascribed to the recent arrival of particularly skilled and impressive English nurses, and it is probably the case that Anglo-Indian girls were increasingly drawn to nursing as the numbers of British nurses grew and local educational opportunities expanded. Frank Anthony, a political leader and historian of the community, claimed that at Independence 80 per cent of civilian and military nurses were Anglo-Indian women.[85] Among the Indian Military Nursing Service (IMNS) and Auxiliary Nursing Service (ANS) nurses during the war, 70 per cent were Anglo-Indian.[86] To some extent, as the political climate in the last decades of colonial rule demanded the Indianisation of institutions, this became problematic. In 1945, Janet Corwin, nursing advisor at the Rockefeller Foundation, made a five-month tour of Indian hospitals. She found plentiful evidence of discrimination in favour of Anglo-Indians and wrote that government authorities still 'in certain places . . . tended to

---

[84] O. P. Jaggi, *Western Medicine in India: Medical Education and Research*, Lucknow: Atma Ram, 1979, p. 132.

[85] Frank Anthony, *Britain's Betrayal in India: The Story of the Anglo-Indian Community*, Bombay: Allied Publishers, 1969, pp. x–xi.

[86] Ibid., p. 141.

discourage those other than Anglo-Indians and domiciled Europeans from becoming nurses'.[87] Lazarus resented the easy policy of dependence on the Christian Anglo-Indian community to provide nursing services, which inhibited the development of more active initiatives to encourage Indian women to become nurses.[88]

In contrast, the Anglo-Indian community itself took pride in providing a local source of nurses, pointing to the early lack of alternatives and the enormous role played by Anglo-Indian women in running the civil and military hospitals of India. As Alison Blunt documents, the Anglo-Indian nurse was also deployed as a representation of the perceived superiority of the gender practices of her community. Blunt cites a 1937 article in *The Anglo-Indian Review*, which proudly claimed that the community's dominance of nursing was a result of 'their special aptitude for the kind of work the profession involves'. According to the author, 'women of other Indian communities have hitherto turned up their noses at the profession, partly because of religion and sentimental objections and partly due to their past traditions and social customs'.[89] Another article published in the same journal in 1939 optimistically claimed:

> The Lady of the Lamp raised the lamp in the Crimea. The Anglo-Indian woman has raised it in India permitting its lustre to fall on every caste and creed. She has eradicated the prejudicial opprobrium and held the lamp high until today the Indian woman sees the beacon to a high and noble profession.[90]

Some Anglo-Indians deployed their liberated women against what they viewed as the tradition-bound, oppressed Indian woman as a symbol of their own community's greater progressiveness and sophistication. Anglo-Indian women, however, were also often regarded by both the Indian and European communities as 'loose', and subjected

---

[87] Janet D. Corwin, 'Semiannual Report: Nursing: Feb 11–June 30 1945', RF, RG 5.3 (IHD) Series 464 C, Box 204, Folder 2493, by courtesy of the Rockefeller Foundation Archives, New York, p. 2.

[88] Forbes, *Women in Modern India*, p. 164.

[89] Cited in Alison Blunt, *Domicile and Diaspora: Anglo-Indian Women and the Spatial Politics of Home*, Melbourne: Blackwell, 2005, p. 61.

[90] Cited in ibid.

to what Dolores Chew describes as the stereotype of the 'Anglo-Indian whore'.[91] The strong association of Anglo-Indian women with nursing unfortunately heightened the persistent moral suspicion attached to the profession. Importantly, Anglo-Indian women, like nurses, almost universally wore Western dress. Blunt comments that, 'as well as marking Anglo-Indians as different from other Indians, Western dress is sometimes thought to represent Western licentiousness'.[92] In analyses of the fortunes of the profession in India, it was often obliquely stated that Anglo-Indians' longstanding association with nursing was rather unfortunate, and tended to deter Indian girls from good families from taking nurse training. Lazarus felt that it was most important to encourage educated Indian women to take nursing rather than continuing to rely on Anglo-Indians, 'the majority of whom take up nursing not as a vocation but as an easy means of livelihood'.[93]

Anglo-Indian women, with their different gender practices and strong identification with the British, provided an essential source of willing and reasonably well-educated candidates for the nurse training programmes of Indian government hospitals. They were not perceived as the long-term solution to providing a nursing workforce, due in part to a ubiquitous prejudice against women of mixed race and partly to their limited numbers and the large-scale post-Independence emigration of the community. At the same time, as the first local modern nurses, they shaped the profession in important ways. They reinforced the image of nursing as a Westernised, Christian pursuit and increased its association with the colonisers' practices of gender. The perception of Anglo-Indian women as 'loose' to some degree determined the similar stereotyping of nurses.

---

[91] Dolores Chew, 'The Search for Kathleen McNally and Other Chimerical Women: Colonial and Post-Colonial Gender Representations of Eurasians', in Brinda Bose (ed.), *Translating Desire: The Politics and Gender of Culture in India*, New Delhi: Katha, 2002, p. 3. Anglo-Indians often self-consciously pursued a lifestyle close to that of the British, and, according to W. T. Roy, represented a sub-culture with 'a tradition of fairly free mixing of the sexes'. It was common for Anglo-Indian women to pursue paid employment and they also dominated the ranks of air hostesses and clerical assistants (W. T. Roy, 'Hostages to Fortune [A Socio-political Study of the Anglo-Indian Remnant in India]', *Plural Societies*, no. 2, 1974, p. 60).

[92] Blunt, *Domicile and Diaspora*, p. 187.

[93] Lazarus, *Our Nursing Services*, p. 11.

## Malayali nurses: The face of nursing in modern India

A reliable supply of willing and able candidates for modern nurse training was ultimately found in the south-western state of Kerala. The willingness of Malayali women to become nurses has, perhaps more than anything, guaranteed the better position of nursing in India as compared to Pakistan and Bangladesh; unlike its neighbours, India was able to draw on a sizeable group of high-school educated women to form the basis of a modern, professional cadre of nurses.[94] At the same time, the strained and low-status position of the nurse within Kerala society has also been an important dimension of the generally low status of the profession in India.

Prior to Independence, the area that is now Kerala was made up of the two princely states of Travancore and Cochin and the Malabar district of the Madras Presidency. All of these areas were populated by ethnic Malayalis, speakers of the Malayalam language. Malayalis, too, had a distinctly non-mainstream and unique history of gender practices. A significant proportion of old Kerala society, including the Hindu Nair community and some Muslim groups, practised matriliny. Although the Kerala matrilineal system still involved considerable constraints on women, with household authority mainly vested in the *karanavan* or the male head of the matrilineal family unit, it is generally acknowledged to have brought with it a comparatively higher level of freedom and status for women than was the case in other parts of India. The extensive pre-colonial education system, for example, was open to girls. The different position of women in Kerala, combined with a high social respect for education and a ruling class keen to promote Western schooling, all contributed to Malayalis' remarkable and unique enthusiasm for sending their

---

[94] In Pakistan, working conditions for nurses are generally reported to be appalling, with extreme shortages (the nurse to population ratio is 1: 3,000) and endemic, unpoliced sexual harassment. Social prejudices against nurses remain virulent, and most of them are still unable to marry; Yusufzai describes the public perception of nurses as 'a group of disposable female sex objects' (Ashfaq Yusufzai, 'Pakistan: Nurses Get Little Training or Respect', 4 June 2006, The Center for Nursing Advocacy, http://www.nursingadvocacy.org/news/2006/jun04_pakistan.html [accessed 9 September 2006]). See also Marilyn B. Lee and Ismat Saeed, 'Oppression and Horizontal Violence: The Case of Nurses in Pakistan', *Nursing Forum*, vol. 36, no. 1, 2001.

daughters to school.[95] According to Robin Jeffrey, in 1921, 34 per cent of Nair women and 31 per cent of Syrian Christian women were literate. By 1941, in Travancore and Cochin one-third of all women were literate.[96] With a large base of educated women, many of whom were not from particularly well-off families, and a tradition of relatively pronounced female autonomy, Malayali women became increasingly willing to enter employment. Jeffrey writes that as early as 1941, 15 per cent of teachers in Travancore and 30 per cent in Cochin were women.[97]

Another important feature of Kerala history was the creation of a migrant tradition. World War II brought mass hunger to Travancore and Cochin, motivating thousands of Malayalis to travel all over India in search of work. Jeffrey writes that as a result, 'to move, to travel, to go off to seek one's fortune — these became part of a newly forming body of Malayali myths and dreams'. To some extent, this determined the willingness of Kerala women to travel to other states for the higher quality and less restrictive nurse education that was on offer elsewhere. A strong local Christian tradition was also important. Kerala contained a sizeable minority of indigenous Christians, members of the Syrian Christian religion, which claimed its roots in the evangelistic work of the apostle Thomas. In addition to this was a significant and longstanding missionary presence, meaning a network of mission schools and a community of low-caste converts. This meant not so much that Kerala Christian women did not share the pollution-based stigmatisation of nursing (most accounts of nursing there in fact heavily emphasise this), but that they were able to enter nursing schools without the well-grounded fears that Hindu or Muslim women and their families had of missionary evangelism or of conversion.

---

[95] For analysis of matriliny and the early education of women in Kerala see Jeffrey, 'Legacies of Matriliny', pp. 647–64; Jeffrey, *Politics, Women and Well-Being*; Robin Jeffrey, 'Culture and Governments: How Women Made Kerala Literate', *Pacific Affairs*, vol. 60, no. 3, 1987, pp. 447–72; Kunjulekshmi Saradamoni, *Matriliny Transformed: Family, Law and Ideology in Twentieth Century Travancore*, New Delhi: Sage Publications, 1999; G. Arunima, *There Comes Papa: Colonialism and the Transformation of Matriliny in Kerala, Malabar, c. 1850–1940*, New Delhi: Orient Longman, 2003.

[96] Jeffrey, 'Culture and Governments', pp. 463–65.

[97] Jeffrey, *Politics, Women and Well-Being*, p. 69.

This did not, however, mean that Travancore and Cochin were the sites of nursing's earliest development in India. Higher quality and more successful programmes for training Indian nurses were being run at an earlier stage in Bombay and Madras Presidencies. T. H. Somervell, a missionary doctor at the Neyyoor Hospital (run by the London Missionary Society's South Travancore Medical Mission), wrote that when he arrived in 1923 numbers of any kind of female nurses in Travancore hospitals, let alone trained ones, were very low. In 1933, Mary Beard, an associate director for nursing with the Rockefeller Foundation's International Health Division (IHD), who was touring India to survey nursing facilities, stated that the health unit run by the Foundation at Neyyattinkara had been unable to find any nurses willing to work there, and had instead had to employ four sub-assistant surgeons to perform nursing duties.[98]

Although the Travancore government undertook some progressive steps in health, such as its support for the health unit at Neyyattinkara and promotion of the training of women doctors, there was less emphasis on nursing. Haragovindan's article on women employed in the Travancore government's medical department shows that there was much greater emphasis on training women as doctors.[99] In 1933, Beard reported a discussion with F. E. Grose, the principal of the Maharaja's College for Women in Trivandrum.[100] They observed that well-educated, independent Travancore women were to be found working as doctors from Rangoon to Nagpur to Poona to Vellore, and had wondered how they might be similarly motivated to take to nursing, given that the need for nurses was very great. Until after Independence, the main facility for training nurses was the school of nursing at the general hospital in Trivandrum, at which often unqualified Swiss nuns gave Indian women the most basic training. Anna Noll, surveying India for the Rockefeller Foundation in February 1948, wrote that after having toured the hospitals of most

---

[98] 'Travancore: Memorandum on Public Health Nursing by Miss Mary Beard on her Visit to the State — February 14–18, 1933', RF, RG 5.2, Series 464, Box 49, Folder 304A.

[99] Narayani Harigovindan, 'Employment of Women in the Medical Department of the Government of Travancore', Proceedings Volume, XIX Annual Session, South Indian History Congress, 1999.

[100] 'Travancore: Memorandum on Public Health Nursing by Miss Mary Beard on her Visit to the State — February 14–18, 1933', RF, RG5.2, Series 464, Box 49, Folder 304A.

of south India, the general hospital at Trivandrum was 'the worst hospital I have seen so far', with a staff of about 12 fully trained nurses for 340 beds and 600 patients.[101] In 1949 it was reported that although things were slightly better in Cochin, nurses in Travancore were subject to 'unbelievably low salary scales' in comparison to the rest of India.[102]

The lack of high quality training at home meant that the pioneers of nursing in Kerala went elsewhere for their training (as indeed many continued to do even when better facilities were available). Women from Travancore and Cochin began to come forward in small numbers for training at CMC Vellore from around the mid-1920s. CMC Vellore was then already regarded as the pre-eminent Indian nursing school, with the strongest emphasis on the development of nursing and the highest level of nurse autonomy, and it has retained this reputation to the present day. From early in its history, many of its students were Malayali women. Abraham writes that students from Travancore began to join CMC from about 1924 (when college records documented Syrian Christian women's distaste for work with bandages and pus basins). From 1932, CMC instituted the requirement that candidates have secondary school leaving certificates, after which there was an influx of mostly Syrian Christian Malayali women.[103] A recruitment tour of the high schools of Travancore by Veera Pitman of CMC Vellore in 1932 was so successful that, according to Abraham, the nursing superintendent's report for that year recorded alarm, stating 'our Nursing School should be first and foremost for the Tamil student nurse, if we are to be a hospital that can make the village patient feel at home'.[104]

Several of these early nurses who came forward between the 1930s and the 1950s were idealistically motivated, defying their families to adopt nursing as a career and emerging as successful, forceful, career-driven post-Independence leaders. By the 1950s and 1960s, however, more utilitarian Kerala women were coming forward in large numbers, having witnessed the potential of nursing to provide

---

[101] Anna M. Noll, 'Diary, 1947–1948', RF, RG 12.1, Diaries, Anna M. Noll, volume 1 of 2.

[102] Anna M. Noll, 'Annual Report on Nursing in India, Pakistan and Ceylon 1949', RF, RG 5.3, Series 464C, Box 204, folder 2497, p. 4.

[103] Abraham, *Religion, Caste and Gender*, p. 91.

[104] Ibid., p. 94.

secure employment and a cost-free training during which a stipend was provided. Eileen Platts, a missionary nurse from 1953–88 at CMC Ludhiana in Punjab, told me that Malayali women began to arrive there for nursing training from the late 1950s. As had happened at Vellore, the initial trickle of students sent home positive reports, and was followed by a large cohort, to the extent that leaders at Ludhiana also became concerned at the dominance of non-Punjabi women.[105] The state of Andhra Pradesh until recently maintained a ban on candidates from outside the state joining nursing. A correspondent writing to the *NJI* in 1990 felt that without the ban, 'there would have been 50 percent Keralites, as we had prior to the formation of A.P'.[106]

Nursing's deep roots in Kerala have shaped the public image of the profession in important ways. Although Malayali women took up nursing careers in large numbers, this did not mean that nursing there was free of stigma. In fact, some of the strongest anti-nurse prejudice was, and is, to be found in Kerala society. The economic attractions of nursing as the source of a livelihood and a means of saving for the punitively high Syrian Christian dowry meant that thousands of Kerala women joined nursing despite this stigma. Such a decision, however, often involved considerable sacrifice. Sheba George, in her account of Malayali nurses in the US, records the common Kerala figure of the eldest daughter who took nursing in the knowledge that this would close off her own opportunities for marriage, in order to provide for the welfare of the family, which often included dowries for younger sisters.[107] In general, George characterises Kerala women's decisions to take nursing as a survival strategy, involving a willingness to undertake 'dirty' work in order to achieve social mobility for the family. Kurien comments on the rarity of second-generation nurses, suggesting that this survival strategy entails ensuring higher status career paths for one's children.[108] Lucrative opportunities for emigration and the introduction of more technology into nursing

---

[105] Author interview, London, 27 August 2005.

[106] T. Stephens, 'Point–Counter-Point: Socio-Economic Background of Nurses in a Hospital Organization', *NJI*, vol. 81, no. 7, 1990, p. 224.

[107] George, *When Women Come First*, pp. 47–48.

[108] Prema Kurien, *Kaleidoscopic Ethnicity: International Migration and the Reconstruction of Community Identities in India*, New Brunswick, NJ: Rutgers University Press, 2002, p. 156.

work have lifted the status of nursing, but it is generally agreed that in Kerala, nurses continue to experience low status.

The historically low social status of nursing in Kerala is strongly informed by class-based prejudice. Nursing has chiefly attracted lower middle class and working class Malayali women, often from poor rural families. Kurien wrote that the older nurses in the predominantly Christian village she studied who had taken training during the 1950s were predominantly from lower middle class agricultural families, who sent them to mission nursing schools to save for dowries. During her fieldwork in the 1990s, it was still only women from the poorer families who took nursing training.[109] Oommen wrote in 1978 that a large proportion of Kerala nurses came from poorer families, and strongly felt that their lower economic status contributed to their low social status.[110] The lower class origins of Kerala nurses has seemingly informed the wider perception in India that nursing is a 'low-class' occupation, in which, as Proshanta K. Nandi and Charles P. Loomis write, 'the requirements for respectable status of the professional person are seldom met'.[111]

One of the distinctive features of Malayali nurses has been their high level of mobility. Both at home and in other parts of India, the unusual mobility of Kerala nurses has contributed to the stereotype of the nurse-prostitute, with intense suspicion attached to women living independent lives away from home and family. George's account of Malayali nurses in the US confirmed that the unusually free movement of Kerala nurses, at home and abroad, created a strong social stigma, feeding the image within the Malayali community of the 'dirty nurse'.[112] Sreelekha Nair's research with contemporary Malayali nurses in Delhi shows that this continues to be a strain. Nurses reported negative comments from men at home in Kerala who insinuated that their travel abroad involved prostitution, such as 'who knows how they make so much money in the Gulf? . . . These Arabs have a lot of money', and 'she is a nurse from the Gulf — that

---

[109] Kurien, *Kaleidoscopic Ethnicity*, pp. 152, 156.
[110] Oommen, *Doctors and Nurses*, p. 59.
[111] Proshanta K. Nandi and Charles P. Loomis, 'Professionalization of Nursing in India: Deterring and Facilitating Aspects of Culture', *Journal of Asian and African Studies*, vol. 9, nos 1–2, 1977, pp. 43–59.
[112] George, *When Women Come First*, pp. 46–47.

is how they say it — contemptuously'.[113] Nair recorded that many of her interviewees felt that 'increased mobility also costs them their respectability'.[114] High mobility may have also contributed to the general disempowerment of nurses, as a large proportion of India's nursing staff have been women far from home, speaking their second or third language and, in the case of north India, living in very different cultures and environments.

# Conclusions

The development of modern nursing in India was partial and practically an often unsuccessful project. Nonetheless, professionalising leaders made sure that the culture and ideology of modern nursing took a firm hold. The ideals of the professionalising project — a high standard of education for nurses, effective state registration, nursing's character as a global sisterhood — had a profound impact on Indian nursing, shaping its culture and modes of organisation. The ideology of self-sacrifice and the ethos of service that had facilitated the emergence of professional nursing and which had longer roots in the nursing work of religious sisters also became a key dimension of nursing culture in India.

The agents of modern nursing encountered a challenging local socio-cultural context, which restricted their promotion of nursing as a respectable occupation for educated women of good family. Attempts to entrench the narrative of nursing as a 'noble profession', requiring service and self-sacrifice, took a strong cultural hold within nursing, coming to permeate nurses' education and professional self-image, but had little resonance in wider society. Indian society rejected nursing, directly associating it with the work of untouchable sweeper and midwife castes, with prostitution and the perceived 'looseness' of Anglo-Indian women. Nursing emerged as a distinctly undesirable pursuit for young women. Heavily Christianised, it was most strongly associated with the widows, orphans and low-status converts who were the only recruits most missionaries could find. In a context where it was rare for women to pursue any kind of work

---

[113] Sreelekha Nair and Madelaine Healey, 'A Profession on the Margins: Status Issues in Indian Nursing', Occasional Paper, Centre for Women in Developing Societies, 2006, p. 23.

[114] Ibid.

outside the domestic sphere, it brought none of the prestige or financial rewards that allowed some 'respectable' high-caste Hindu and Christian women to pursue careers in medicine or teaching.

The members of the fledgling modern nursing service, therefore, emerged from communities that were in various ways less affected by these aspects of society and culture. Anglo-Indian women, who were Christian and maintained Western style gender practices, emerged as the backbone of the government nursing workforce. Later, the state of Kerala provided a large group of educated but poor women who were comparatively mobile and independent, who needed the security and, later, the potential social mobility that nursing careers could provide. These predominantly Christian women could more easily enrol in the nursing schools that, even when government run, were heavily associated with Christianity. Thus, in spite of the anti-nursing stigma (probably less in Kerala than elsewhere but nonetheless virulent), they became a sustainable recruitment base for the Indian profession.

The next chapter describes more specifically the interactions between Western nursing leaders and the colonial state in developing a nursing system for India. It highlights the commitment of leaders to replicating the professional and the modern in India, and their general unwillingness to adjust their models to promote Indian nurses or to address the needs of Indian hospitals. On the other hand, the colonial state accepted that the obstacles to Indian participation in nursing were too great to overcome and willingly relied on a skeleton nursing staff, substantially composed of Anglo-Indian and domiciled European women. The unsatisfying relationship between profession and state meant, ultimately, that the story told in this chapter, of an idealised but difficult to realise nursing modernity encountering a hostile Indian society, continued to characterise the fortunes of nursing well into the post-Independence period.

# Upward Mobility
# Hemila

HEMILA was typical of the thousands of Indian widows, orphans and destitute wives who made up much of the staff in mission hospitals up until Independence and even beyond. These women were often illiterate and trained in basic nursing by Western nurses and doctors. Unusually, Hemila's mission employer, Dr Ethel Bleakley from Manchester, was fascinated by the life stories of Hemila and her fellow nurses, and recorded them in extensive detail.[1] Although Bleakley's book on Indian nurses was written as a piece of missionary propaganda, and was sentimental as well as viciously critical of local culture and Bengali women (who she felt were characterised by duplicity, unreliability and a predisposition to malicious gossip), it is nevertheless a goldmine of information on these nursing assistants, whose lives are otherwise very difficult to penetrate.

Hemila was a recent widow with six surviving children (others had fallen victim to cholera and malaria) when she walked several days to Ratnapur in West Bengal to find work at the local Protestant mission, bringing only the baby with her. Hemila was put to work in the mission's dispensary. Although she had no schooling, Bleakley recorded that she was intelligent and had an excellent memory. She was trained to assist in compounding, patient care, wound-dressing, and midwifery.

It is clear from Bleakley's account that Hemila became an effective and assertive cultural intermediary. Bleakley found local practices of purity and pollution ridiculous and records that if it was not for Hemila's advice, she would have disregarded many of them. Hemila, however,

---

[1] Bleakley, *Meet the Indian Nurse*, pp. 9–25.

ensured that when attending births, Bleakley left through a different door than she used to enter (as was the local practice) and explained to her the necessity of the vessels and utensils used in a delivery being destroyed. On the other hand, Hemila was also able, where Bleakley had failed, to dissuade the family of a patient from taking him out on the veranda to let his spirit escape and not return to trouble the family if he died. By preventing this patient from being moved at the most critical point of his illness, Bleakley felt that Hemila saved his life.

Later, Hemila brought her daughter, Sheshu, to Bleakley and asked that she be trained as a nurse. Bleakley objected, suggesting that the work was demeaning in Indian eyes, and it would be painful for Hemila to watch her being corrected by teachers on the wards. Sheshu, however, took her training and became one of the first two women from the mission to take the CMAI's examination, administered by the North India Board of Examiners. Sheshu did not work as a nurse for long, however, making a well-regarded marriage to the son of a Bengali pastor.

Hemila embodies the image of the nurse that the professional leadership tried so hard to overcome. She was ill-educated, socially outcast and extremely poor. We do not know how she felt about converting to Christianity, but it was clearly required of her. Yet, like so many nurses before and since, she was able to use her very basic training to secure a sustainable income and upward mobility for her family, while providing an important community service.

◼

# 2

# Lighting India's Lamp

## Nursing Leadership and
## the Colonial State, 1905–47

◘

*A further conviction possessed them, recruited as they were from other lands, that India's own Lamp must be lighted and trimmed and held high, if ever her Darkness and Disease are to be efficiently combated and dispelled.*[1]

The first half of the 20th century saw the rapid growth of nurse training programmes in mission and government hospitals, the implementation of registration acts, and the development of professional representation. All of this, however, was rather superficial. In practice, most nurses experienced an exploitative and exhausting apprenticeship training, and most of the caring work in hospitals was done by the untrained or the partially trained. Minimal progress was made in elevating nursing's status or attracting better educated candidates into the profession. This chapter, in exploring the reasons for this, identifies the two major fault lines that run through the 20th-century history of nursing — a disengaged state and an elitist, unrepresentative mode of leadership.

The chapter first offers some background to the early development of Indian nursing under colonial rule. It then explores the day-to-day experience of the working nurse in the first half of the 20th century, highlighting the strain of unsafe living quarters and the absence of effective education. The next section details the

---

[1] Ethel A. Watts, *The Handbook of the Trained Nurses' Association of India*, Madras: TNAI, 1931, p. 9.

response of the leadership to this situation, suggesting that it suffered from a lack of connection to its constituency, from the exclusion of Indian nurses, and from an excessive commitment to the ideals of nursing internationalism and professionalism. The final section looks at the orientation of the state towards nursing. It suggests that a pattern of detachment, followed by sporadic and unsustained interest, was formed, which would also characterise the approach of the post-colonial state. The crisis of care brought on by World War II, combined with the injection of new energy into health planning for a state on the cusp of independence, meant that leaders' plans for professional nursing ultimately found a strong theoretical place in the independent state's health system. The state's late engagement with nurses, however, was shallow, under-institutionalised and opportunistic, and did not provide a strong basis for the profession post-Independence.

## Nursing in Colonial India: An Overview

Western nurses of varying backgrounds and qualifications had been present in colonial India since the mid-19th century. White women, often the widows or wives of soldiers, took on basic nursing and midwifery work to cater for the British community. In 1859, the Royal Sanitary Commission on the Health of the Army in India was appointed. The Commission was famously driven by Florence Nightingale, who participated extensively in its research and reporting. Its report was issued in 1863, identifying an urgent need to provide proper nursing care for soldiers in India. As a result, the Indian Nursing Service (INS) was instituted, with a remit to provide care to British soldiers. The INS was officially launched with the arrival of 10 trained nurses in Bombay in 1888, under the leadership of the redoubtable Catharine Grace Loch, an assertive, upper class woman from a wealthy Manchester family who protested against army officers' perception that nurses should be 'ministering angels only without a definite responsibility or position of any sort or kind'.[2] In 1903 this INS was renamed the Queen Alexandra Military Nursing

---

[2] Catharine Grace Loch, *Catharine Grace Loch, Royal Red Cross, Senior Lady Superintendent, Queen Alexandra's Military Nursing Service for India: A Memoir (With an Introduction by Field-Marshal The Earl Roberts V.C., K.G., O.M.)*, London: Henry Frowde, 1905, p. 44.

Service for India. Later, it was replaced by nurses posted through the empire-wide service, the Queen Alexandra's Imperial Military Nursing Service (QAIMNS).[3] Indian nurses were not recruited for military service until World War I.[4] The Indian Military Nursing Service (IMNS), which employed domiciled European, Anglo-Indian and Indian three-year-trained nurses (who mainly cared for Indian soldiers), was not launched until 1927.[5]

Sporadic attempts at providing a trained, female nursing staff for government hospitals began from the mid-19th century. Margaret Balfour writes that the first mention of a hospital matron was in 1844 at the Madras Maternity Hospital, which, in 1854, was also the first to begin training midwives.[6] In 1858, the Allahabad General Hospital began employing women nurses.[7] In Calcutta, the Calcutta Hospital Nurses Institution trained probationers from 1859 for work in the Presidency General, Medical College and Eden Hospitals.[8] In 1864, the Sanitary Commission of Bengal recommended that female nurses should be hired in all large hospitals in India.[9] In 1870, the general hospital in Madras first appointed a permanent nursing staff, beginning the training of probationers in 1871.[10] By the late 19th century, as Rosemary Fitzgerald documents, better-trained, better-qualified 'new nurses' arrived in India from Britain, perceiving themselves, to some extent, as playing a role in the cultural mission of imperialism.[11] A number of these took work in government institutions, as well as in mission hospitals. In 1886, for example, Edith Atkinson started as the nursing superintendent at the Cama Hospital in Bombay, which by 1906 was running a three-year training programme for probationers.[12] Government hospital training schools gradually increased

---

[3] Watts, *Handbook of the Trained Nurses' Association*, p. 43.

[4] T. K. Adranvala, 'Nursing in India — 1908–1968', *NJI*, vol. 59, no. 11, 1968, pp. 369–71.

[5] Alice Wilkinson, *A Brief History of Nursing in India and Pakistan*, New Delhi: Trained Nurses' Association of India, 1958, p. 11.

[6] Margaret Balfour, 'Indian Nursing — Its Past and Future', *NJI*, vol. 14, no. 2, 1923, p. 29.

[7] Gourlay, *Florence Nightingale*, p. 66.

[8] Balfour, 'Indian Nursing', p. 29.

[9] Gourlay, *Florence Nightingale*, p. 66.

[10] Balfour, 'Indian Nursing', p. 30.

[11] Fitzgerald, 'Making and Moulding the Nursing'.

[12] Tooley, *The History of Nursing*, p. 346.

in number throughout the early 20th century, but in general schooled mainly domiciled European and Anglo-Indian trainees, playing little role in the training of Indian nurses.

Some private, charitable and philanthropic institutions also employed and trained nurses. Among these, the Dufferin Fund has attracted significant attention from historians. Lady Dufferin's National Association for Supplying Medical Aid by Women to the Women of India (the Dufferin Fund) was launched by the Vicereine Lady Dufferin at the direct request of Queen Victoria.[13] Soon after, the 'Dufferin hospitals' established by the fund began training Indian women as nurses — in Calcutta from 1885 and in Bombay from 1886.[14] Maneesha Lal has described the Dufferin Fund as a successful vehicle for the professional ambitions of English women doctors and an advertisement of the perceived superiority of British gender relations, but as ineffective in terms of improving women's health or providing medical training to Indian women.[15] Most reports of the standard of nursing and nursing training in the Dufferin hospitals attest to the fact that it was equally inadequate in preparing nurses. Indian candidates were not attracted to Dufferin hospitals because they were often discriminated against in admission processes, and the standard of training and living conditions for nurses and students were poor.

Several other private or philanthropic groups provided nursing care. In 1906, the Vicereine Lady Minto founded the Indian Nursing Association (incorporating the Up-Country Nursing Association, established in 1892). 'Minto Nurses', as they were known, provided private nursing care mainly to European families. In Bombay, several of the hospitals funded by Indian philanthropists trained nurses, including the Jamsetjee Jeejeebhoy group of hospitals (the JJ Group of Hospitals), which trained probationers from 1891. In 1921, the Matru Seva Sangh was established at Nagpur by two eminent women social workers, Kamalabai Hospet and Venutai Nene. It aimed to assist women, especially widows, to earn a living, and offered general nurse training, in association with the Dufferin hospitals.[16]

---

[13] For accounts of the Dufferin Fund, see Lal, 'The Politics of Gender and Medicine', pp. 29–66; Lang, 'Saving India'; Forbes, *Women in Modern India*.

[14] Balfour, 'Indian Nursing', p. 30.

[15] Lal, 'The Politics of Gender and Medicine', pp. 29–66.

[16] Joglekar, *Hospital Ward Management*, p. 142.

Meera Abraham reports that Ramabai Ranade's Seva Sadan also helped train Brahmin widows as nurses. In the 1930s, Muthulakshmi Reddy, in her Avvai Home in Madras, provided training in nursing and midwifery to some destitute women.[17] Local initiatives, therefore, strongly focused on the potential of nursing to provide an income for socially marginalised women in Indian society.

The training of Indian women as nurses was monopolised by Anglo-American Protestant missions, which by 1947 were running 75 schools of nursing in India.[18] While the colonial administration largely neglected women's health, according to Fitzgerald, 'missions developed energetic and often innovative approaches to this subject', and this included a strong focus on the need to provide a local corps of nurses.[19] St Stephen's Hospital in New Delhi (which still runs a highly regarded nursing school) began training Indian women as nurses from around 1867, with a systematic training course launched by a European nurse-deaconess, Deaconess Foltz, in 1874.[20] St Catherine's Hospital in Amritsar began training Indian nurses in 1872, as did the American hospital in Sialkot in 1887.[21] It was not until the late 19th and early 20th centuries, however, that nurses played a really significant role in the work of medical missions in India. From the beginnings of the 20th century, nursing had emerged as a key component of medical missionary work, and more professional and better trained nurses (products of the only recently reformed and standardised education systems of the West) were attracted to work in the empire, as was discussed in Chapter 1. Fitzgerald states that missions began to demand fully trained nurses who 'would not falter in their demonstration of the superior nursing skills of the West'.[22] Nurse education became an increasingly strong focus, so that in 1946, 80 per cent of Indian nurses had been trained under missionary programmes.[23]

Under the stewardship of mission nurses and, to some extent, their colleagues in government hospitals, nursing in India grew more

---

[17] Abraham, *Nursing History in South India*, p. 80.
[18] Ibid., p. 101.
[19] Fitzgerald, 'Rescue and Redemption', p. 65.
[20] Wilkinson, *A Brief History of Nursing*, p. 38.
[21] Balfour, 'Indian Nursing', p. 30.
[22] Fitzgerald, 'Rescue and Redemption', p. 75.
[23] Ibid., p. 76.

standardised and in theory more sophisticated (although in practice the majority of mission nurses continued to be trained under ad hoc, unrecognised programmes devised by the hospitals in which they worked). British and American nurses formed organisations focused on professional development and as a result, nurse registration acts were legislated by provincial governments from the late 1920s (beginning with Madras in 1926), regulated systems of examination were devised and there was some improvement in the standard of training offered.

Nonetheless, in 1947, nursing was stunningly underdeveloped. Of course, this was to some extent a consequence of wider under-development in public health and hospital care under colonial rule. During the 18th and early 19th centuries, there had been a general absence of state-provided health care for the Indian population, with allopathic medicine chiefly confined to European military and civil enclaves. Throughout the period of British rule, the vast bulk of the population, living in rural areas, had minimal access to allopathic medicine; village India relied on indigenous systems of medicine such as *ayurveda* and *unani*. From the late 19th century there was some expansion in health services, mainly focused on urban areas. David Arnold suggests that from this period onward there was an attempt to provide a public health and hospital system that catered to Indian as well as European needs, although Radhika Ramasubban has asserted the ongoing lack of state interest in Indian health needs.[24]

Whatever improvements occurred, they did not bring with them a strong focus on nursing. Even in this context of a generally inadequate health system, nursing was particularly neglected. As Fitzgerald writes, the colonial state's efforts in developing nursing were 'never more than lethargic, frugal, piecemeal and tentative'.[25] Central and state governments accepted a health system in which many hospitals functioned almost entirely without qualified nurses. Numerically, the profession remained tiny; in 1947, there were only 7,000 trained nurses working in India, a ratio of approximately one nurse to every 50,000 or 60,000 people.[26] Clearly, colonial Indian society had not

---

[24] See Ramasubban, 'Imperial Health in British India', and Ramasubban, *Public Health and Medical Research in India*.

[25] Fitzgerald, 'Making and Moulding the Nursing', p. 29.

[26] Wilkinson, *A Brief History of Nursing*, p. 96. It was suggested, however, by the eminent doctor and politician Sir Jivraj Mehta that although seven thousand nurses were on the register, double registration and marriages meant that the number of nurses

provided fruitful ground for the construction of an efficient cadre of nurses. The reasons for this are explored in the next section.

## 'Suffering More Than the Followers of Florence Nightingale Could Ever Have Done': The Lives of Nurses under British Rule

In the first two decades of the 20th century, it was widely accepted that few Indian women would be willing or able to become nurses. By the 1930s, however, the opinion began to be expressed that obstacles other than caste, religion and local gender practices were preventing them. Women who did become nurses lived and worked in dangerous, arduous conditions, and it was becoming clear that objections to nursing on the grounds of it being 'dirty', morally dangerous, low-status work in fact had considerable justification. It was worryingly clear that the low salaries paid to nurses, especially those trained in mission hospitals, left them vulnerable to brothel-keepers. Chapter 1 described the ways which the intimate nature of nursing work rendered it morally suspect and associated with prostitution, but this association was also to some extent grounded in reality. In 1939, the TNAI protested against the unethical practices increasingly common in private nursing homes, which actively recruited mission-trained nurses. Often, these 'hospitals' turned out to be brothels, and, the association recorded, they posed 'a source of grave moral danger to young and inexperienced nurses'.[27] A survey conducted by the Young Women's Christian Association (YWCA) in 1924 found evidence that nurses were not safe, inside or outside the hospitals in which they worked, and that 'conditions among nurses in large cities are appalling and require the earnest prayerful concern of every Christian nurse and doctor'.[28] According to the CMAI's survey of

---

actually working may have been closer to three thousand (Jivraj Narayan Mehta, 'Medical Services in India [The Sir George Birdwood Memorial Lecture]', *Journal of the Royal Society of Arts*, vol. 113, no. 5112, 1965, p. 1001).

[27] Anonymous, 'Minutes of the 28th Annual Conference of the Trained Nurses' Association of India (continued from the January issue)', *NJI*, vol. 30, no. 2, 1939, p. 50.

[28] CMAI Committee, 'A Survey of Nursing', p. 25.

nursing in 1947, these conditions persisted, and it remained the case that nurses who had graduated from the closely supervised life of a mission nursing student, struggled 'to live upright lives' when they moved alone to work in cities.[29]

Conditions in the wards in many hospitals were dangerous and unsanitary. A 1948 article in the Calcutta *Statesman* described small-pox wards with between four and six nurses to care for 300–400 patients. If family members did not collect the bodies of the deceased, they were liable to remain in the ward for days on end.[30] At the Campbell Hospital in Calcutta, it was widely recognised that 'the health of the students deteriorates noticeably during their training'.[31] Diana Hartley was a British nurse who was the Secretary of the TNAI and the editor of the *NJI* from 1935–44. She left behind a large collection of writings on her time in India and was one of the few colonial nurses who carefully documented both her work and personal impressions of the Indian health system. Hartley toured the hospitals of India extensively, and repeatedly protested against the conditions in which nurses were expected to live and work, describing the ill health, exhaustion and disillusionment of nurses again and again.[32]

The most basic need felt by most nurses was for clean, safe accommodation. In 1947, a survey conducted by the CMAI found that the recruitment difficulties experienced in mission hospitals could be ascribed to 'the ratio of work in the wards to lecture and laboratory hours, the lack of time for study and recreation . . . poor living quarters and low salary scales'.[33] Recording her initial impressions of Indian hospitals, in 1935 Hartley wrote that 'nurses' quarters are often more sordid than pigsties and quite unprotected'. The 'few better class Indian women' who were entering nursing were, she declared, 'suffering more than the followers of Florence Nightingale

---

[29] CMAI Committee, 'A Survey of Nursing', p. 25.

[30] Anonymous, 'Hospitals', *The Statesman*, Calcutta, 17 May 1948. Copy typed and included in Wellcome Institute Library for the History and Understanding of Medicine GC/139/H.2. File of Sir Weldon Dalrymple-Champney, Box 1.

[31] Anna M. Noll, Diary 1947–1948, RF, RG 12.1, Diaries, Anna M. Noll, volume 1 of 2, p. 39.

[32] See, for example, Diana Hartley, 'Tour from Nagpur to Delhi', circa 1935, Cambridge University Library: Royal Commonwealth Society Library (henceforth RCS), Indian nursing collection of Diana Hartley, RCMS 77/1/2, pp. 4–8.

[33] CMAI Committee, 'A Survey of Nursing', pp. 7–8.

could ever have done'.[34] Hartley felt that the first recourse of any economising hospital was to cut back on nursing staff, and the prevailing contempt for nursing services resulted in a universal reluctance to spend the often minimal sums needed to fund better buildings for nurses. She was particularly incensed when a major Delhi hospital which had pleaded a lack of funds to expand its 'overflowing' nurse quarters, proceeded to erect a 'completely unnecessary though spectacular clock tower'.[35]

Hartley's opinion was that conditions for nurses were very bad in the majority of government hospitals, and even worse in the private philanthropic hospitals set up by the Dufferin Fund (which had been established with a remit to focus on medical and nursing education for Indian women).[36] The Dufferin hospital at Benares was typical, according to Hartley. Living quarters consisted of 'a line of unprotected rather tumbledown, badly ventilated godowns'.[37] At the Dufferin hospital in Allahabad, the back windows of the nursing quarters faced onto a bazaar, and passersby were wont to 'throw things at the nurses through the bars'.[38] In the United Provinces (UPs), nurses working in Dufferin hospitals welcomed the 1947 handover of their hospitals to the government, because, although conditions continued to be worse than those in government hospitals, they at least received a significant pay-rise.[39]

Mission hospitals in general provided better living conditions for Indian nurses and students. At the same time, with their small and unreliable funding bases, they paid notoriously low salaries and relied heavily on the labour of Indian probationers. The 'training' that the students received was often exploitative, unrewarding and unrecognised by any authority. In 1914, Florence Gifford of the London Missionary Society (LMS) hospital in Murshidabad district,

---

[34] Diana Hartley, 'First Impressions of India', 1935, RCS, Indian nursing collection of Diana Hartley, RCMS 77/1/1a.

[35] Diana Hartley, 'Nursing in India', undated, RCS, Indian nursing collection of Diana Hartley, RCMS 77/2/2.

[36] For accounts of the Dufferin Fund, see Lal, 'The Politics of Gender and Medicine', pp. 29–66; Lang, 'Saving India Through its Women'; Forbes, *Women in Modern India*.

[37] Hartley, 'Tour from Nagpur to Delhi', p. 3.

[38] Ibid., p. 6.

[39] S. E. Farr, 'Improvements in the Provincial Nursing Service 1945–1946 of the United Provinces', *NJI*, vol. 38, no. 2, 1947, p. 57.

Bengal, wrote to the *NJI* to point out the neglect and mistreatment of Indian nursing students in mission nursing schools and the dire consequences this had for the care of patients. Gifford felt that Indian probationers were often cynically recruited as a means of cheaply staffing the wards. The average hospital, in her experience, had 60 beds, 10 probationers and one trained nurse, with the obvious consequence that the 'students' learnt very little. This led to a severe wastage problem; although the LMS had been training Indian women for years, none of the three hospitals with which Gifford was familiar had a single trained Indian nurse on staff. Students, receiving an exhausting and unstimulating 'training', tended not to stay in the profession. This problem continued up until the end of the colonial period; a 1947 survey of nursing by the CMAI commented that 'practically the whole nursing care' in mission hospitals was supplied by probationers.[40] Missions, moreover, barely paid their nurses a living wage. In 1947, the advertisements in the *NJI* for vacant positions indicated that a staff nurse in a mission hospital could expect to be paid around ₹40 per month, which was less than half of the salary paid by even the least generous government hospitals.[41] The CMAI's survey of nursing in 1947 found that only 40 per cent of nurses (from the 72 mission hospitals surveyed) were paid over ₹30 per month. It was concluded that the other 60 per cent did not receive a salary sufficient to maintain 'any suitable standard of living'.[42]

Hartley accepted the argument that 'caste and *purdah* systems' prevented the entry of educated Indian women into nursing in the first couple of decades of the 20th century, when, she wrote, 'it is wrong to say they would not, they simply and obviously could not become nurses'. She felt, however, that as the numbers of educated women grew, this position was no longer tenable. According to her, the 'lack of insight and parsimoniousness of the Government and other authorities has been the real cause of the present shortage of nurses'.[43] Alice Wilkinson, who was the nursing superintendent at St Stephens Hospital in Delhi from 1916–38 and then the president of the TNAI for much of the 1940s, similarly felt that the failure of Indian women to join nursing could be explained by the fact that

---

[40] CMAI Committee, 'A Survey of Nursing', p. 2.
[41] Anonymous, 'Wanted Advertisements', *NJI*, vol. 38, no. 2, 1947, inside front and back covers.
[42] CMAI Committee, 'A Survey of Nursing', p. 30.
[43] Hartley, 'Nursing in India'.

state-run hospitals had 'failed to supply a sufficient number of qualified nurses to teach and train' and that 'in many hospitals the accommodation provided is disgraceful'.[44] Major-General J. B. Hance, the
Director General of the Indian Medical Services, expressed the same
feeling with even greater vehemence:

> I will merely express my conviction based on a not inconsiderable
> experience that the alleged failure of the nursing profession to appeal
> to the right type of women in India is due far more to the attitude
> of the authorities responsible for the maintenance of hospitals, and
> to the conditions in which, too often, probationers are trained and
> nurses are expected to work, than to the alleged reluctance of educated
> Indian women to undertake the care of the sick. As long as trained
> nurses are regarded, paid and housed as menials it is not reasonable
> to expect that large numbers of Indian ladies will come forward to
> dedicate themselves to this work.[45]

Indian nurses during this period, therefore, often worked in dangerous and unsanitary conditions, receiving exceptionally low salaries.
This had come to be recognised by many observers as an obstacle
to professional development that was at least as relevant as local
understandings of caste and gender, and it was a hindrance that could
clearly be overcome more straightforwardly. The following sections
examine the response of leadership and the state to the development
of the nursing profession, suggesting that both displayed fundamental inadequacies, and were insufficiently shaped by the basic needs
identified here.

# Nursing Leadership
# in Colonial India, 1905–47

Although the average Indian nursing school was literally and
metaphorically thousands of miles from the experiments in nursing
happening in Toronto, New York and London, the work of leaders

[44] Alice Wilkinson, 'President's Address', in TNAI, 'Annual Report of the Trained
Nurses' Association of India, 1942–43, including the 32nd Annual General Meeting,
January 13th and 14th, 1944', RCS, Indian Nursing Collection of Diana Hartley,
RCMS 77/4/2, pp. 9–10.

[45] 'Major-General Hance's Speech', in TNAI, 'Annual Report of the TNAI 1942–43',
RCS, Indian nursing collection of Diana Hartley, RCMS 77/4/2, p. 8.

in India was shaped by them in important ways. As Fitzgerald has written, nurses working in India from the start of the 20th century increasingly viewed themselves as the emissaries of the reformed models of nursing that had developed in the West.[46] The earliest expression of this was when British nurses began the task of establishing professional infrastructure, shaping organisations similar in structure and purpose to those in Britain and the US. In 1905 in Lucknow a group of trained nurses from government and mission hospitals created the Association of Nursing Superintendents in India (ANSI), and then the TNAI at the annual conference in Bombay in 1908. The ANSI began as an association of superintendents from Punjab and United Provinces, but by 1906–7 had attracted members from all over India. It took the Matrons' Council of Great Britain and Ireland as its model, and hoped to engage the 'united efforts of every trained nurse in the country'.[47] Until 1910, ANSI and TNAI shared the same officers. In 1912 they combined for the purpose of representation at the International Council of Nurses (ICN), and in 1922 they were officially merged as the TNAI.[48] Conferences were held annually from 1907, except during World War I. The TNAI proposed a professional journal in 1908, launched it at the annual conference in Agra in 1909, and published the first issue of the *NJI* in 1910. The objectives of both the TNAI and the ANSI centred on lifting standards and elevating the social status of the profession. The ANSI hoped that it would be able to: 'Elevate nursing education by obtaining a better class of candidates, by raising the standard of training, and striving to bring about a more uniform system of education, examination and certification for trained nurses, both Indian and European'.[49]

Similarly, the TNAI aimed to 'uphold in every way the dignity and honour of the nursing profession, to promote a sense of *esprit de corps* among all nurses, to enable members to take counsel together on matters affecting their profession'.[50] Both organisations were

---

[46] Fitzgerald, 'Rescue and Redemption', p. 75.

[47] Association of Nursing Superintendents in India (ANSI), *Report of the Association of Nursing Superintendents of India 1907*, Cawnpore: ANSI, 1907, pp. 9–10.

[48] Anonymous, 'Calendar', *NJI*, vol. 49, no. 10, 1958, p. 343; Anonymous, 'The Trained Nurses' Association of India: An Introduction', *Indian Nursing Year Book 1996–97*, New Delhi: TNAI, 1998, p. 9.

[49] M. Barr, 'Editorial', *NJI*, vol. 8, no. 8, 1917, p. 164.

[50] Ibid.

characterised by a sense of excitement at the nursing reforms that were happening in Britain and the US and by an anxiety that colonial nurses should not miss out on the advances and professional developments occurring at home. In 1908, J. W. Thorpe of St Catherine's Hospital, Kanpur, the secretary of ANSI, proposed that the time for establishing a professional journal had come:

> I feel very strongly that we ought to take a still greater interest in our association. To read the Reports of the American Association of Superintendents how small their beginning was and how much they have accomplished is always an inspiration to me.
>
> We could do just the same, if we tried equally hard, perhaps not in such a short time, as the west moves much faster than the east, but the east does move. It is moving now in the direction of nursing reform and we ought to be ready to rise to the occasion, and order our own affairs.
>
> It might not be out of place for me to here throw out the suggestion that a Nursing Journal for India, managed by Nurses, would do a good deal toward this.[51]

The CMAI (which was originally the Medical Missionary Association of India) also had a nursing association, the Nurses' Auxiliary (which became the CNL in 1964). The Nurses' Auxiliary shared the aims, orientation and much of the membership and leadership of the TNAI. It was formed in 1930, with a governing committee of 15 British, three Canadian, nine American, one New Zealand, and a couple of Swedish and Norwegian nurses.[52] Meera Abraham records that in 1930 the Nurses' Auxiliary declared as its aim 'the highest efficiency in Christian nursing work in the relief of human suffering' and the dissemination of 'information concerning the need of nursing work and its place as an integral part of the Christian message to India'.[53] The Nurses' Auxiliary shared the TNAI's emphasis on professionalism, but had a more sustained and practical involvement in the lives of nurses. It conducted examinations and awarded diplomas for missionary hospital nursing trainees (it continues to be the only non-governmental authority to certify nurses). The Nurses' Auxiliary benefited from a stronger missionary emphasis on the development

---

[51] ANSI, *Report of ANSI 1907*, pp. 12–13.
[52] Abraham, *Nursing History in South India*, p. 99.
[53] Ibid., p. 18.

of nursing, which included some recognition of the need for nurse authority. Just as the Christian mission hospitals have played a vital role throughout the 20th century and in contemporary India, going some way to fill the enormous gap in health provision left by the state, so have the mission nurse organisations profoundly contributed to the shape of nursing education in India.

State registration boards and nursing councils were also instituted from the first decade of the 20th century. It is difficult, however, to regard these as 'nursing organisations', since (as has continued to be the case even to the present day in some states) they were dominated by doctors, often with a small minority of nurse membership. The Bombay Presidency Nursing Association was probably the first of its kind, appointed in 1909, but was consistently dominated by the medical profession. In 1916, it appointed 17 official examiners, of whom two were nurses.[54] In 1923 the United Provinces government had not a single nurse on its board of examiners, motivating a letter of protest from the TNAI.[55] Abraham records that the first Madras Nurses and Midwives Council, appointed in 1928, had five members, of whom three were doctors.[56]

Until the 1930s, nursing organisation in India was very weak; plans for the professionalisation of Indian nursing were clearly mainly rhetorical and leaders seemed to feel little faith in their own ambitions. Prior to World War I, at least, substantive achievements mostly lay in providing genteel social interaction and news of professional developments at home for lonely British and American nurses working in India. Dora Revell, who came to south India to nurse in 1912 (she remained until the 1940s), wrote that she and her colleagues 'looked forward eagerly' to receiving the *NJI* as 'there was no way of meeting other nurses or medically interested people' in the remote area in which she worked. The annual TNAI picnic, held each May in a holiday resort in the Nilgiris, was keenly anticipated.[57]

---

[54] Anonymous, 'Bombay Presidency Nursing Association: Half-Yearly Examination for Nurses and Midwives, August and September, 1916', *NJI*, vol. 7, no. 9, 1916, p. 194.

[55] M. Thacker, 'Annual Conference', *NJI*, vol. 14, no. 1, 1923, p. 10.

[56] Abraham, *Nursing History in South India*, p. 99.

[57] Dora M. Revell, in Anonymous, 'Greetings and Messages', *NJI*, vol. 49, no. 10, 1958, p. 325.

The 1930s brought a reorientation and vivification of nurse organisation, which meant that nurses increasingly desired and sought a more serious role in public health and in the development of health and medicine in India. Hartley referred to 1931 as 'the year of true awakening', after which leaders viewed their role more seriously and membership began to expand rapidly. This reorientation was the result of factors both internal and external to nursing. Internally, nurse organisations had suffered after World War I, during which many nurses returned home to Britain and large numbers who might have come to India as missionaries enlisted in the army instead.[58] This led to an at least partial redefinition of the TNAI as an organisation that would depend, for its finances as well as its *raison d'être*, on the substantial participation of Indian, not just Western nurses. In 1931, the membership of the TNAI stood at 600, a healthy figure compared to the immediate post-war years, but nonetheless it was recognised as insufficient to exert much political influence.[59] In 1935, Hartley arrived in India to take up a position as TNAI secretary and editor of the *NJI*. Her papers do not record the conditions of her employment or her personal reasons for embarking on work in India, but it seems that she was the first TNAI office-holder to be employed exclusively by the organisation, without also working as a nurse. She worked enthusiastically documenting conditions and researching metropolitan nursing developments and promoted a more substantial and practical engagement with Indian conditions. Her work gave the TNAI a more convincing voice. In addition, the founding of the Nurses' Auxiliary meant the emergence of a new forum solidly focused on the education of Indian women as nurses, and more removed from the 'colonial ladies' club' character that still to some degree infused the TNAI. The ICN was also growing stronger and better organised. India's nurse leaders, heavily invested in their affiliation to it, were increasingly aware of the expectation of the ICN that the cause of professional nursing should be promoted by Western nurses in colonised states. There were thus a variety of forces inside the profession that determined the emergence of a more locally focused and more serious mode of nurse organisation from the early 1930s.

---

[58] M. Thacker, 'Editorial', *NJI*, vol. 13, no. 4, 1922, p. 74.
[59] Watts, *Handbook of the Trained Nurses' Association*, p. 9.

Outside the politics of the nursing world, health had in general become the site of intense political contention, which inevitably affected the work of nursing leaders. The poor state of India's health system emerged as a key concern for Indian nationalists; as David Arnold writes, public health and 'its neglect under the British became part of the unfolding critique of colonial rule'.[60] Hartley's hospital tours throughout India during the late 1930s recorded the pervasive presence of nationalist politics in government hospitals and the strong nationalist orientation of many doctors.[61] This political climate and the accompanying opposition to evangelism curtailed and reshaped the work of missionaries. Margaret Balfour and Ruth Young, both eminent British doctors, in 1929 described this change as the reorientation of missionary medicine from 'a means to an end' into 'a service to be performed for its own sake'.[62] A general emphasis on high quality professional medicine rather than on evangelism had begun to develop, besides an awareness of the compelling need to 'Indianise' mission hospitals and locate a sustainable place for them in the national health system.

Nursing organisations were also shaped by a colonial public sphere that became more open to women's participation. The 1920s and 1930s saw the emergence of a variety of increasingly vocal and effective Indian women's organisations; in general a greater ethos of associationalism was evident among both Indian and Western women.[63] In a context where women's groups were increasingly well-organised and articulate on issues of women's health and maternal and child welfare, there was pressure on nursing organisations to develop similarly. From the early 1930s, therefore, nursing organisations responded to political and professional developments and attempted to define themselves as important contributors to Indian health debates.

---

[60] David Arnold, 'Public Health and Public Power: Medicine and Hegemony in Colonial India', in Dagmar Engels and Shula Marks (eds), *Contesting Colonial Hegemony: State and Society in Africa and India*, London: British Academic Press, 1994, p. 151.

[61] Hartley, 'Tour from Nagpur to Delhi', p. 13.

[62] Margaret I. Balfour and Ruth Young, *The Work of Medical Women in India*, London: Oxford University Press, 1929, p. 88.

[63] Ramusack, 'Embattled Advocates', p. 35.

## An international identity for Indian nursing

The TNAI enthusiastically supported the ICN, representing India at its conferences from 1912.[64] In the Indian context, where nurses were few and had minimal local power and influence, alignment with nursing internationalism was seen as crucial to successful advocacy for nurses and the ICN provided a valuable source of ideas and leverage for nurse leaders in India.[65] At the 1909 Conference in Agra, C. R. Mill, a prominent ANSI and TNAI leader, even declared that the TNAI would be a small-scale version of the ICN.[66] In 1914, Annie Goodrich, president of the ICN, was made an honorary member of the TNAI.[67] According to Ethel Watts, a British nurse leader who was editor of the *NJI* from 1929 and remained in India until 1953, membership of the ICN was an important source of legitimacy in the TNAI's more sustained efforts from the 1930s to portray itself as a source of expertise worthy of state consultation.[68] The ICN could be used as a source of arguments against the tendency of Indian-led state governments from the late 1930s to advocate lower standards in nurse training in order to facilitate the employment of more Indian women more economically. In 1944, Wilkinson, then president of the TNAI, emphasised the dangers of not meeting the professional standards of the ICN:

It is of the utmost importance for every nation when legislating for the nursing profession to do so in accordance with the International Council of Nurses — for this great and important Council comprises expert nursing representatives from every national nursing association throughout the world. It would be a sad and shameful day for India, if she refused to work up to the splendid standards for training set up by this International Council, or if she keeps the present level so low, that she will forfeit her right to belong to it.[69]

---

[64] Anonymous, 'Calendar', *NJI*, vol. 49, no. 10, 1958, p. 343.

[65] Rafferty and Boschma, 'The Essential Idea', p. 65.

[66] C. R. Mill, 'Some Advantages of Joining the "Trained Nurses' Association of India"', *NJI*, vol. 97, no. 2, 2006 [1910], p. 29.

[67] Annie Goodrich, 'Letter to the Editor — Miss Goodrich's Honorary Membership', *NJI*, vol. 5, no. 3, 1914, p. 98.

[68] Ethel A. Watts, 'The Years That Have Passed', *NJI*, vol. 49, no. 10, 1958, p. 333.

[69] Wilkinson, 'President's Address', p. 11.

While being deployed in arguments against a relaxation of standards which might have allowed the greater participation of Indian nurses, the ICN at the same time also pushed the TNAI into a more sustained focus on Indian nurses, as it generally viewed white nurses as bearing a heavy burden of responsibility to create a strong local profession. In 1930, Watts prepared an article for the ICN's journal that presented the TNAI as significantly more focused on and more advanced in the development of local nursing leadership than was the reality. She claimed that India had 'a supply of indigenous women, not only as probationers, but as leaders in this great profession', contradicting the more general and more honest tendency at this time to bemoan the almost complete absence of Indian leadership.[70] This instance of exaggeration for the purpose of international public relations suggests the positive pressure exerted by the ICN to show evidence of progress in encouraging local participation and leadership.

India's nurses also participated in a crucial practical experiment in nursing internationalism: the provision of British or American education to nurses from countries perceived as less advanced in nursing. During this period, Indian women were periodically sent to London to take the course in public health nursing at Bedford College, which was run by the League of Red Cross Societies and the Royal College of Nursing from 1912 until 1934, and then by the Florence Nightingale International Foundation. The Bedford College course was not widely viewed as effective. Anne Marie Rafferty records that international leaders described the course as 'ill-equipped to meet the needs of all nurses and poorly designed to translate findings across cultures'.[71] Despite these shortcomings, education abroad was enthusiastically promoted by leaders in India. From the late 1920s, the TNAI participated in the selection and preparation of Indian nurses for study abroad (the first to be sponsored by the TNAI for the Bedford course was a Mrs K. Phatak).[72] This was a project with strong official support; the Vicereine Lady Reading had begun a

---

[70] Ethel Watts, 'The Training of Nurses in India: Its Problems and Prospects', in Watts, *Handbook of the Trained Nurses' Association*, p. 55. Also published in *The International Nursing Review*, May 1930.

[71] Anne-Marie Rafferty, 'Internationalising Nursing Education during the Interwar Period', in Paul Weindling (ed.), *International Health Organisations and Movements, 1918–1939*, Cambridge: Cambridge University Press, 1995, pp. 275–76.

[72] Anonymous, 'Calendar', *NJI*, vol. 49, no. 10, 1958, p. 343.

scheme from the early 1920s to train Indian nurses in London as matrons and administrators.[73]

Nursing leaders saw education abroad as not merely a means for Indian candidates to receive advanced education, but as an opportunity for them to fully appreciate their status as members of an international sisterhood. Although only a minute number participated (leaders found it rather difficult to attract applicants for their scholarships), the promotion of international education was important, because it meant that some of the most senior post-Independence Indian nurse leaders were thoroughly schooled in the notion that nursing was an international, trans-cultural and transnational profession. Some of the graduates of these scholarships went on to occupy positions of considerable importance at home. In 1938, Edith Paull, an experienced Anglo-Indian nurse who had worked in Calcutta, Delhi and Allahabad, and M. Korah, an Indian graduate of the Christina Rainy School of Nursing and holder of a health visitor's certificate from the Madras Health School, were the first recipients of the Florence Nightingale Memorial Scholarship.[74] Paull went on to become president of the TNAI, the Director of Nurses at the GT Hospital in Bombay, and the staff officer for nursing at the Indian Red Cross in the late 1950s. Most importantly, Tehmina K. Adranvala, who later became nursing advisor to the Government of India, vice-president of the ICN and president of the TNAI, also participated in this programme. Adranvala — more than any other nurse, Western or Indian — oversaw the institutionalisation of nursing professionalism in India.

Shaping nursing into an international sisterhood was an integral part of Western leaders' work in India. This kind of activity, however, was based around a hoped-for future, in which the nursing practice of West would be replicated in India, and was far removed from the present. It had little relevance to the lives of nurses living and working in desperately difficult conditions.

## Representation and registration

Another aspect of nursing leaders' commitment to professionalism was a strong emphasis on nurse registration and representation

---

[73] Balfour, 'Indian Nursing', p. 35.

[74] Anonymous, 'Notices', *NJI*, vol. 29, no. 4, 1938, pp. 95–96.

in government. Nurse leaders in the West, particularly in Britain, were vigorously espousing these causes during this period. State-maintained registration was integral to the search for professional status; it meant protection from untrained competitors and higher status in the public eye. Western nursing leaders in India followed the progress of nursing activism at home and applied similar arguments in India. This was partly due to pragmatic self-interest. The disorganised, chaotic and neglected state of nursing in India gave the cause of registration a strong local resonance. In 1922, Mrs Chesney, then editor of the *NJI*, recorded that 'very many call themselves trained nurses who only possess a year's certificate for midwifery . . . demanding exorbitant fees, to the exploiting of the public and to the great detriment of Nursing as a profession'.[75] Sarah Tooley's 1906 history of nursing in the Empire described the problematic proliferation of women trained only in midwifery who were working as nurses in Indian hospitals and complained that semi-qualified or unqualified 'nurses' were able 'to claim the same fee as the highly trained English nurses from home'.[76] It is clear from Tooley's account that nurses trained in Britain were eager that their training be given appropriate

---

[75] Chesney, 'An Appeal to Trained Nurses', *NJI*, vol. 13, no. 1, 1922, p. 2. Anxieties about the threat from less trained competition were exacerbated in both world wars, when the government employed Voluntary Aid Detachment nurses (VADs), with 6–18 months training and often paid them higher salaries than fully qualified nurses working for the Indian government or army. In World War I, the VADs were paid ₹150 per month from their second month of employment, at a time when the average trained nurse in India did not expect to receive much more than ₹80 per month throughout her entire career (Lorna S. Mackenzie, 'Letter to the Editor', *NJI*, vol. 7, no. 10, 1916, pp. 206–7). Mrs Barr, the then editor of the *NJI*, reported that many trained nurses were refusing to teach important skills to the VADs, which she felt displayed a 'spirit of arrogance and selfishness and also we must own, an underlying sense of fear' (M. Barr, 'Editorial', *NJI*, vol. 7, no. 12, p. 243). The same issue arose again with more seriousness in World War II, when the ranks of trained Indian nurses had grown and the political sensitivity of paying them less than minimally trained British VADs had also increased. In both wars, these conflicts had a strong class dimension; many of the women who came to India as VADs represented a continuing tradition of upper-class women's voluntarism, and came from a quite different section of society than the often lower-middle class or working class nurses, who had to work for a living.

[76] Tooley, *The History of Nursing*, pp. 346–47. It seems that there was a similar willingness to disregard systems of qualification and training in the employment of women teachers. Borthwick, for example, writes that out of 3853 women, lower primary teachers in Bengal in 1904–5, only 207 had teacher training or university degrees or diplomas (Borthwick, *The Changing Role of Women in Bengal*, p. 315).

financial recognition and also that they should not be associated with the 'undesirable' and unqualified domiciled European and Anglo-Indian women who made up the ranks of their competitors.

The promotion of registration and of representation in government was not only motivated by self-interest, but also by the desire of leaders to put in place the structures of a Western-style profession. With the backing of registration, legislation and institutionalised representation in government, modern trained nursing would theoretically be defended from the initiatives sporadically produced by local politicians that proposed the lowering of training standards. The nursing leadership thus enthusiastically set about promoting the cause of nurse registration. An early meeting in 1908 involved the discussion of 'a register of all trained nurses in India', an ambitious proposal given that this was not achieved in England until 1919.[77] The TNAI's 1917 Constitution specified that the association should 'be the medium whereby nurses can make their voices heard in regard to legislation that affects the profession and safeguard nursing interests'.[78] The TNAI claimed the majority of the credit for the implementation of registration acts from the mid 1920s. In 1926, the first Registration Act was passed in Madras, Punjab followed in 1932, as did Bengal and Uttar Pradesh in 1933, Bihar, Orissa and Bombay in 1935, and Madhya Pradesh in 1936. State Nursing Services, with standardised pay and terms of service, were instituted in Madras in 1941, in Uttar Pradesh in 1944 and in Bengal in 1946. By 1944, proposals for an All India Nursing Council were being seriously entertained.[79] In theory these were important victories, but in practice hospitals were neither willing nor able to prioritise the employment of registered nurses. In reality, organisational lobbying for registration had little practical effect on the lives of Indian nurses. It did, however, ensure the reciprocity of qualifications earned in India and Britain, protecting the interests of nurses who envisaged returning home one day or, in the case of Anglo-Indian and Indian nurses, working abroad.

---

[77] ANSI, *Report of ANSI 1907*, p. 8.

[78] Watts, *Handbook of the Trained Nurses' Association*, p. 15.

[79] Diana Hartley, 'The General Secretary's Report', in TNAI, 'Annual Report of the TNAI 1942-43', RCS, Indian Nursing Collection of Diana Hartley, RCMS 77/4/2, 12.

Nurse leaders also protested against the medical profession's dominance of the organisation and administration of nursing. Doctors almost ubiquitously allowed minimal authority to nursing superintendents and school principals, and monopolised positions on nursing boards and councils. The TNAI contested this situation from relatively early on, dispatching letters to provincial governments from the early 1920s. In 1931, the TNAI passed a resolution that all registrars should be trained nurses.[80] As more attention was paid to the state of nursing, the TNAI formed a more ambitious set of goals. A 1938 article included among its aims respect for the ultimate authority of the nursing superintendent over her staff and the appointment of sister tutors in all schools of nursing (which often relied on doctors for lectures and tutorials).[81]

Gradually, the principle of greater nurse autonomy found official acceptance. By 1931, the South India Missionary Nurses' Examining Board even consisted of six nurses and two doctors.[82] The first nurse registrar, Miss Tyzack of the Medical College Hospital in Patna, Bihar, was appointed in 1938 (although the position was jointly held with a doctor).[83] Lillian Clarke, who had trained at the Presidency General Hospital in Calcutta, was chosen in 1938 as the Registrar of the Bengal Nurses' and Midwives' Council. Bengal TNAI members had helped to persuade the surgeon general that it was necessary that a nurse should occupy the position, and they hailed the appointment as 'recognition of the true status of nurses and nursing as a profession'.[84] Nursing superintendents were appointed in Madras in 1941, Bengal in 1944 and Uttar Pradesh in 1945.[85] Adranvala, writing in the late 1950s, attributed most of these advances to the work of the TNAI.[86] Although later chapters will reveal the extent to which the dominance of the medical profession continued, this was perhaps one of

---

[80] Watts, *Handbook of the Trained Nurses' Association*, p. 52.

[81] Diana Hartley, 'News and Notes', *NJI*, vol. 29, no. 3, 1938, p. 65.

[82] Watts, *Handbook of the Trained Nurses' Association*, p. 62.

[83] Diana Hartley, 'News and Notes', *NJI*, vol. 29, no. 6, 1938, p. 149.

[84] Diana Hartley, 'News and Notes', *NJI*, vol. 29, no. 3, 1938, p. 64.

[85] T. K. Adranvala, 'Nursing in India — 1908-1968', *NJI*, vol. 59, no. 11, 1968, p. 370.

[86] T. K. Adranvala, 'Nursing Profession in India', in Usha Sharma and B. M. Sharma (eds), *Encyclopaedia of Women and Education: Volume 3, Women and Professions*, New Delhi: Commonwealth, 2001, p. 175. Sharma and Sharma do not give the date of this extracted piece but the contents indicate it was written between 1957–60.

the more important aspects of Western nurses' work in India. They managed at the very least to enshrine in theory a very strong belief in nurses' right to self-governance, and to establish the beginnings of an institutional infrastructure to support this right.

## A nurse's role in community health

Despite the overwhelming concentration of nurses in hospitals, nursing leaders also tried to promote the role of a nurse in community health work. Leaders were aware of the role public health had played in the professional advancement of American nurses and were also exposed to the strong emphasis the ICN placed on it as a means of identifying the aims of organised nursing with the priorities of the state.[87] Moreover, within India, an increasing focus on the issue of maternal and child health was developing and it became clear from the 1920s that a role for nurses in community health would mean greater involvement in the politics of health. In 1918, Lady Chelmsford had extended her support to schemes for the training of health visitors and 'maternity supervisors'. With the support of government grants, a health school was opened in Delhi, which later became the Lady Reading Health School. This marked the beginning of an increased societal interest in maternal and child health, reflected in sporadic state support for small-scale programmes. By 1931, there were two other government-run training schools for health visitors — the Punjab Health School in Lahore and the Calcutta Health School. The Red Cross also ran three health schools, at Calcutta, Madras and Nagpur, and some of the missions trained skilled female health assistants for public health work.[88] The 1920s saw the beginnings of a variety of European women's organisations promoting infant and maternal welfare and the holding of 'baby weeks'. As Geraldine Forbes has documented, by the 1930s this interest was also reflected in the activities of middle-class Indian women's groups, which emphasised replacing the *dai* with Western-trained midwives.[89] There was thus an increasing awareness of maternal and child health, which, combined with international nursing leaders' heavy emphasis on

---

[87] For a discussion of public health and the ICN, see Rafferty and Boschma, 'The Essential Idea', p. 49.

[88] Watts, *Handbook of the Trained Nurses' Association*, pp. 123, 128.

[89] Forbes, 'Managing Midwifery in India', pp. 152–53.

public health, suggested that this might be a route to a more positive public image and stronger political influence for nurses.

In practice, though, nurse involvement in community health in India was minimal. Mission hospitals sometimes ran clinics, dispensaries and domiciliary midwifery programmes, but nurse participation in these was usually peripheral. The vast majority of nurses in both the mission and the government sector worked in hospitals rather than in community health programmes. Nonetheless, nursing leaders promoted community health rhetorically, at least, as an important branch of nursing. The registration acts passed at provincial level during this period generally contained sections for the registration of health visitors, midwives and *dais*, as well as for trained nurses. This was in accordance with a TNAI resolution passed in 1931, and ensured that in theory, public health workers would work under the authority of trained nurses.[90] Some attempt was also made to include principles of public and community health in the better nursing education programmes. In 1938, the examination for the Florence Nightingale Memorial Scholarship for further training in England required candidates to write a paper on a selection of public health topics, including the causes of maternal mortality in India, tuberculosis care, the diet of rural India, and the importance of school nurses.[91] In 1944, the TNAI was strongly espousing the inclusion of public health as a dimension of every nurse's basic training and regretting the continuing failure to establish training for rural, district, domiciliary, and school nursing.[92]

A small number of enterprising nurses did find work in community health work. The role of nurse leaders in the Lady Reading Health School, at least, was quite significant. Edris Griffin, as briefly discussed in Chapter 1, played a central role in its establishment, and documented some of the many concerns and difficulties it encountered through the 1920s in her column for health visitors in the *NJI*. Griffin attempted to create a wing of the TNAI for health visitors, launching a Health Visitor League in 1922 (which continued into the mid 1970s, when it was replaced by an association for ANMs). The main work of the League was to run lectures and events. The Bengal branch of the TNAI's Health Visitors League reported that

---

[90] Watts, *Handbook of the Trained Nurses' Association*, p. 52.

[91] Anonymous, 'Examination Questions Florence Nightingale Memorial Scholarship, 1938', *NJI*, vol. 29, no. 4, 1938, pp. 99–102.

[92] Wilkinson, 'President's Address', p. 9.

in 1942–43, they had held nine lectures. Among the speakers were Dr Sarala Ghose, who had spoken on 'Public Health Work in the City of London', Miss Bankart, who had discussed 'Gruel and Milk Kitchens for Famine Relief' and Mrs Aziz, who lectured on 'Social Service Work by Women in Russia'.[93] The Delhi branch of the Health Visitors' League held similar events, including a lecture by Dr Jean Orkney, a prominent medical advisor with the WHO and the Honorary Secretary and Treasurer of the Association of Medical Women in India, who spoke on 'social and economical problems in the homes'.[94]

The League, however, was not successful. In 1943, it had 113 members, out of 750 health visitors in India.[95] Even this small body of members was unenthusiastic. Griffin continuously criticised the health visitors of India for their refusal to report on their activities for the *NJI*. M. Korah, the first Indian nurse to head the League (she became the Superintendent of the Lady Reading Health School), reported in 1944 that the practice of writing invitations to rural health visitors was being discontinued due to their lack of interest in attending events. In general, relations between nurses and health visitors were insubstantial. Nonetheless, such initiatives to promote the idea of nurses as situated at the top of a hierarchy of female public health personnel reflected the keenness of the profession to reserve a place for itself in public health work, which, as became increasingly evident, would play an important part in future health planning for India. Again, however, this strong focus on a potential future role for nurses was unfortunately detached from the concerns of the majority of nurses, who had little to do with public health work.

### Improving nursing education

International nursing reformers at this time also focused very strongly on institutionalising good quality education for nurses, attempting to entrench the belief that the nurse deserved and would repay a proper education; and advocating an end to the practice of the

---

[93] P. J. Gazder, 'Report on Health Visitors' League, Bengal Branch, 1942–43', in TNAI, 'Annual Report of the TNAI 1942–43', RCS, Indian Nursing Collection of Diana Hartley, RCMS 77/4/2.

[94] M. Korah, 'Report of the Health Visitors' League, Delhi Branch', in TNAI, 'Annual Report of the TNAI 1942–43', RCS, Indian Nursing Collection of Diana Hartley, RCMS 77/4/2.

[95] Hartley, 'The General Secretary's Report', p. 11.

'apprenticeship' style of training, in which students provided long hours of inexpensive labour which kept hospitals' costs low.[96] A few substantive initiatives towards achieving the vision of a higher standard of education were made. From 1932, as Abraham records, CMC Vellore only admitted candidates with secondary school leaving certificates, which meant that their nursing course began to attract a steady stream of educated Malayali women.[97] From this point onwards, CMC was able to establish a reputation as the highest quality provider of nursing training in India, and one of the few institutions to focus at all on respect for the authority and autonomy of senior nurses. In the early 1930s, the Christina Rainy Hospital in Madras designed a programme that accepted only Indian women who had attained their matriculation standard. It reportedly taught a high standard of medical and surgical nursing (although only the care of women and children was covered). Nurses from this programme were the first mission-trained nurses to qualify for registration in Madras, representing the beginnings of a cadre of Indian women in the Presidency who were able to attain the same qualifications as Anglo-Indian and European graduates.[98]

The ultimate expression of professionalising ideology was the espousal of degree education for India. Leaders felt that university education for nurses would first serve the useful purpose of rapidly schooling an elite, which would provide some desperately needed Indian administrators and educators. The movement of nursing education into universities would also, it was hoped, do a great deal to improve the profession's image. Florence Taylor, Principal of the School of Nursing at CMC, felt that nursing degree programmes in India would form an 'acknowledgement to the general public of the dignity of the profession'.[99] It was difficult at this stage for most nursing schools to attract girls with more than an eighth standard education; many continued to accept girls with only primary schooling.[100] Yet, India was to become an international pioneer in degrees

---

[96] See, for example Janet D. Corwin, 'Semiannual Report: Nursing: Feb 11–June 30 1945', Rockefeller Foundation Archives, Sleepy Hollow, NY, RG 5.3 (IHD) Series 464 C, Box 204, Folder 2493.

[97] Abraham, *Nursing History in South India*, p. 91.

[98] Watts, *Handbook of the Trained Nurses' Association*, p. 63.

[99] Florence Taylor, cited in Abraham, *Nursing History in South India*, p. 105.

[100] A 1945 report on nursing in the British colonies pointed out that 'even in the United Kingdom it is not yet possible to insist even on the Junior School Certificate

for nurses. Clearly, university education had an urgency in colonial India that it did not have in the West. Education became, in the eyes of leaders, a potential 'quick-fix' to the solution of nursing's ongoing problem of dreadfully low social status. It was felt that if a higher standard of education could be instituted, leaders might be able to wrest the profession back from its dominance by former untouchables and low-status widows. It was predictable that the establishment of such programmes would be intensely difficult — by 1948 Noll was describing the Delhi degree programme as hindered by the 'almost total absence of qualified teaching staff and qualified nursing candidates, unsuitable hospital practice fields, and, most important, lack of understanding of the philosophy and purpose of nursing education on any level'[101] — but university education for nurses was still viewed as a vital strategy in the task of attracting higher caste and higher status candidates into nursing.

Leaders thus eagerly noted innovations and developments in nurse education in North America and Britain, considering their potential application in India. Preparation for degree education began at the TNAI from the mid-1930s, when Hartley wrote of collecting syllabi from the most progressive North American colleges in order to draft curricula for the hoped-for College of Nursing in Delhi.[102] In 1935, she visited Sir George Anderson, Commissioner of Education, to request the Government of India to consider making nurse education a responsibility of the Central Board of Education, as had been done in China, 'so bringing our training schools into line with women's colleges and universities, which would immediately raise the standard and status of nurses'.[103] Taylor worked from the mid-1940s with A. C. Mudaliar, a doctor and the vice-chancellor of University of Madras, in preparing a curriculum for a proposed degree course at CMC.[104] The pursuit of these plans in the general context of very low standards of education seems an extreme case

---

as a minimum standard of general education required prior to admission to a nurse training school' (*Report of the Committee on the Training of Nurses for the Colonies*, London: Colonial Office, 1945, p. 21).

[101] Anna M. Noll, 'Semi-Annual Report — Nursing (India and Ceylon), January 31 to June 30', 1948, RF, RG 5.3, Series 464C, Box 204, Folder 2496, p. 5.

[102] Hartley, 'The First General Secretary Looks Back', p. 337.

[103] Diana Hartley, 'Miss Hartley's Tours', 1935–38, RCS, Indian Nursing Collection of Diana Hartley, RCMS 77/1/4.

[104] Abraham, *Nursing History in South India*, p. 133.

of putting the cart before the horse. Again, although it could be suggested that the leadership valuably encouraged the view that nurses
deserved a good standard of education, the investment of research
and activism into such projects did little to address the more basic
concerns of the majority.

## A racial and professional elite

None of the nursing organisations were successful in creating enthusiasm among their members. This was in part due to lack of funds
and lack of time to spend on effective organisation. Importantly, it
was also because of the character of the nursing leadership as a racial
and a professional elite, distant from the lives and concerns of most
Indian and many Western nurses. Nursing leaders manifestly failed
to create effective, equal partnerships with their Indian colleagues.
Barbara Ramusack, in her analysis of five white women activists in
India, suggests that class barriers could prove a greater obstacle than
those of race.[105] Nurses were non-elite, lower middle-class women
with a somewhat tenuous position within colonial society and the
Indian women they worked with were from among the most economically and socially disadvantaged groups in local society. In contrast
with some of the wealthy, upper class white women described by
Ramusack, who were able to form alliances with high caste, educated
Indian women, nursing leaders rarely managed to consider themselves 'allies' with Indian colleagues. Indian women always remained
objects of plans for the professional development of nursing, and the
moment at which some might emerge as capable equals was often
envisaged but always postponed. The kinds of compromises and
negotiations which might have allowed the greater participation of
Indian nurses were consistently refused. This was to the great detriment of organisations, which remained, when independence arrived,
weak and un-rooted in the everyday lives of nurses.

Western nurse leaders emphasised the maintenance of what they
perceived to be adequate professional standards, and this functioned
as a means of excluding Indian women from authority and leadership.
In this respect nurses were similar to British women doctors, who
also excluded locally trained Indian colleagues. As Forbes writes,
the Indian Women's Medical Service also maintained a system of

---

[105] Ramusack, 'Cultural Missionaries', p. 320.

superior and inferior grades, which kept most Indian doctors out of positions of authority. 'Sisterhood' with Indian doctors was limited to the small minority with degrees earned in the West. British members were in general 'incapable of respecting the special skills and talents of Indian women doctors'.[106] The maintenance of a high standard of nurse education, as close as possible to that practised in the West, also kept Indian nurses out of positions of authority and the professional association. In general, any initiative to 'lower standards' of education, so that Indian women could more easily pass difficult English-language examinations, was resisted by the TNAI. In 1931, Watts wrote that the TNAI recognised two conditions that needed to be accounted for in organising Indian nursing: first, the upkeep of a 'standard of training and efficiency which will be recognised internationally'; second, 'the recognition of Indian conditions due to caste customs'. The leaders tended to consider the former as far more important than the latter, in part because it was a major concern for all Western nurses that those registered in India should easily be able to return to England or America and find work.

Indian nurses were most often excluded from the higher grades of training, pay and responsibility because of their reluctance to nurse male patients. Wherever Indian women were trained, it was viewed as necessary to establish a junior grade of nurses trained only in the care of female patients, which led to the establishment of a lower stratum of the profession occupied exclusively by Indian nurses. Missions, the majority of which maintained hospitals for women and children only, were frequently only able to teach the 'B' grade of nursing qualification, even if their Indian students had been willing to nurse men.[107] In the first decades of the well regarded school of nursing at St Stephen's in Delhi, for example, only 'B' nurses could be trained, until affiliation with the CMC Hospital at Ludhiana was gained, which meant that nurses could be posted there to gain the necessary experience in nursing men.[108] Similarly, the widespread

---

[106] Forbes, 'Medical Careers and Health Care', pp. 526–27.

[107] For example, out of the 40 hospitals affiliated to the North India United Board of Examiners for Mission and Other Hospitals, 35 were exclusively for women (Watts, *Handbook of the Trained Nurses' Association*, p. 77).

[108] 'St Stephen's Hospital Souvenir: Issued on the Occasion of the Foundation Stone Laying Ceremony of the New Building by Shri V. V. Giri, President of India, On Sunday the 13th February, 1972', New Delhi: St Stephen's Hospital, 1972.

requirement that government nurse examinations should be conducted in English often excluded Indian nurses from qualifying as fully trained nurses. Most provinces also legislated to create a junior register for those trained in the vernacular.[109] Madras Presidency was rare in that it had taken some deliberate steps to address these inequities. In the early 1930s, two registers were maintained, but unlike the usual vernacular qualification, inclusion on the vernacular trained register was, according to Watts, to be 'of equal value in India' (although not recognised internationally).[110] Even where Indian nurses held equal qualifications, however, they were often paid less than their white colleagues. In the princely state of Hyderabad, for example, a qualified Indian sister was paid half the salary of an English sister.[111]

The exclusion of Indian nurses from the structures of leadership could not entirely be justified on the grounds that there were no well-qualified or senior Indian nurses available. A small but significant number of Indian women had become nurses; by 1923, 1,262 Indian and 1,250 Anglo-Indian nurses had been trained, encompassing all educational sectors (an estimate considered conservative by Balfour[112]). Although the voices of Indian nurses were seldom heard in the *NJI*, there is evidence of capable individuals pursuing nursing careers outside the white-dominated universe of the leadership. In the city of Bombay, for example, nurses seemed to suffer less from the stigmatisation of the profession and the training and employment of Indian nurses was more acceptable and pursued more enthusiastically. A 1925 article published in the journal of the ICN suggested that, in Bombay, Parsi, Christian and Hindu women worked as private nurses within their communities and were well respected for the work.[113] Miss Jankibai Sabnis, a Bombay nurse, gave up marriage and family to pursue a career at the well-renowned Cama Hospital, where she worked from 1907–46. The author of her obituary

[109] Watts, *Handbook of the Trained Nurses' Association*, pp. 51–52.

[110] Ibid., p. 52.

[111] Ibid., p. 123.

[112] Balfour, 'Indian Nursing', pp. 28–35.

[113] M. Bonser, quoted in Meryn Stuart and Geertje Boschma, 'Seeking Stability in the Midst of Change', in B. L. Brush and J. E. Lynaugh (eds), *Nurses of All Nations*, Philadelphia: Lippincott, 1999, pp. 109–10.

wrote that 'as Lady Superintendent she did much to improve nursing conditions and her skill as a nurse was widely testified'.[114] Pirojbai S. D. Lakdawala was a ward sister at JJ Hospital from 1929–42, when she was appointed matron there.[115] In Calcutta in 1935, Hartley met Mrs Belwant Kaur, a nurse and Health Visitor who was in sole charge of a local infant welfare clinic.[116] In Delhi in 1930, the new Women's Medical College Hospital was said to be 'staffed almost entirely by well-educated Indian girls'. Their English superintendent, Miss Hogg, thus described them:

> The nurses appear happy and interested in their work, and it is very rare that they ever have to be corrected for unkindness of manner towards patients. They have a great sense of humour and are intolerant of any form of injustice. They can be led but cannot easily be coerced. I consider there is a good future for intelligent Indian women in the nursing profession; they have qualities on the whole which lend themselves to a successful career under efficient training.[117]

Almost no Indian women during this period, however, occupied leadership posts. Balfour felt that this was partly because many senior posts were in state hospitals which took both sexes, meaning that Indian women were either reluctant or unqualified to work in them. This, she suggested, was one of the reasons nursing found it so difficult to attract good Indian candidates. In comparison, the teaching and the medical profession both boasted many successful Indian women in their ranks. She felt that it was no surprise that Indian women did not come forward to train in a profession in which it was clear that they could not advance.[118]

The organisational structures of the TNAI reflected this institutionalised exclusion of Indian women. At the 1920 TNAI conference, there were no Indian or Anglo-Indian attendees.[119] It was not until the

---

[114] Anonymous, 'In Memoriam: Miss Jankibai Sabnis', *NJI*, vol. 42, no. 7, 1950, p. 203.

[115] Anonymous, 'Obituary', *NJI*, vol. 66, no. 2, 1975, p. 42.

[116] Hartley, 'Tour from Nagpur to Delhi', pp. 12–13.

[117] Watts, 'The Training of Nurses in India', p. 59.

[118] Balfour, 'Indian Nursing', pp. 31, 34.

[119] Wilhelmina Noordyk, 'Conferences of Other Days', *NJI*, vol. 49, no. 10, 1958, p. 339.

1939 conference at Mysore that Indian and European attendees of the TNAI's annual conference ate at the same table.[120] The TNAI did not appoint an Indian president, general secretary or *NJI* editor until 1948.[121] However, as the political climate transformed over the last quarter century or so of colonial rule, pressure for greater inclusiveness was felt. Other institutions dominated by the Anglo-Indian and domiciled European communities, such as the Indian Railways and the Telegraph Department had seen a dramatic shift.[122] The power-sharing system that began with the 1919 India Act meant that health became a provincial responsibility to be administered by Indian politicians, and the resultant widespread pressure to 'Indianise' institutions became a factor in nursing. Watts wrote in an article she prepared for the ICN's journal in 1930 of being 'challenged constantly for going slowly' in the promotion of nursing for Indians. Gradually, a shift in focus occurred so that larger-scale recruitment and more advanced training of better-educated Indian women was emphasised.[123] This new focus on Indian nurses was signified in the *Handbook of the Trained Nurses' Association* published by the TNAI in 1931. Watts declared in the Introduction to the volume that:

> The objective of the Training schools for nurses, be they Government or Missionary, is to provide for India, *from India*, a force of efficient, fully trained nurses sufficient to meet and satisfy the needs for nursing care for India's vast population, and to care for the future training of future generations of nurses [italics original].[124]

The Student Nurses' Association (SNA) was started in 1929 and became a means to channel Indian nurses into the TNAI, meaning that Indian membership of the TNAI began over the 1930s to balance numbers of foreign nurses.[125] In 1933, Ms B. J. Singh was

[120] Noordyk, 'Conferences of Other Days', p. 340.

[121] Anonymous, 'Calendar', *NJI*, vol. 49, no. 10, 1958, p. 344.

[122] McMenamin documents, for example, that between 1878 and 1928 in the Indian Telegraph Department the percentage of domiciled European or Anglo-Indian employees had fallen by 60 per cent, in part due to the 'eligibility of Indians to compete for these positions' (Dorothy McMenamin, 'Identifying Domiciled Europeans in Colonial India: Poor Whites or Privileged Community?', *New Zealand Journal of Asian Studies*, vol. 3, no. 1, 2001, p. 108.

[123] Watts, 'The Years That Have Passed', p. 333.

[124] Watts, *Handbook of the Trained Nurses' Association*, p. 3.

[125] Watts, 'The Years That Have Passed', p. 334.

one of two delegates sent to the ICN Congress in Rome — the first Indian to attend as a representative of the TNAI.[126] In 1944, Mrs Haining's offer to stand for re-election as Organising Secretary of the Health Visitors' League was rejected due to the nomination of two Indian candidates (of whom M. Korah from Delhi was successful).[127] In 1941, the TNAI became affiliated with the National Council of Women in India (NCIW), signalling an increased recognition that it must become an Indian organisation serving Indian women.[128]

It is questionable, however, whether leaders succeeded in remodelling the TNAI into an institution which could credibly be viewed as a representative organ for Indian nurses. It is telling that in 1944 Hartley reported one of the chief problems facing the TNAI as the reluctance of the members of the SNA (which by this stage had an Indian majority) to transfer their membership to the TNAI when they graduated. Another challenge, not adequately confronted, was the provision of promotional, professional and educational material in languages other than English.[129] At Independence the TNAI was in general remarkably devoid of high-level participation by Indians.[130] Janet Corwin, attending the TNAI conference in 1945, recorded that 'the Conference illustrated well the domination of nursing in India by a rather small group of non-Indian nurses. Although almost 50 percent of those attending were Indian, they were passive observers'.[131] Whilst presenting themselves as an organisation defined by the task of creating a strong local profession, the TNAI had remained closed to Indian participation on equal terms.

The Nurses' Auxiliary and the CMAI in general were more active in encouraging the involvement of Indian nurses in their activities. An important focus of the Nurses' Auxiliary was the inclusion of the vernacular trained nurse. In 1933, for example, the American Baptist Mission Hospital at Nellore recorded that the Auxiliary had begun

---

[126] Anonymous, 'Calendar', *NJI*, vol. 49, no. 10, 1958, p. 343.

[127] Anonymous, 'Summary of the Business conducted at the Second Annual General Meeting of the Health Visitor League, January 14th, 1944', in TNAI, 'Annual Report of the TNAI 1942–43', RCS, Indian Nursing Collection of Diana Hartley, RCMS 77/4/2, p. 24.

[128] Anonymous, 'Calendar', p. 344.

[129] Hartley, 'The General Secretary's Report', p. 11.

[130] CMAI Committee, 'A Survey of Nursing', p. 14.

[131] Corwin, 'Semiannual Report: Feb 11–June 30 1945'.

publishing a bimonthly Telugu language newspaper for vernacular trained nurses. In 1936 it had 64 subscribers, although reportedly it had been difficult to expand this subscription base to include 'the nurses who are in the villages in Government service'. In September 1936 a conference of Telugu-speaking nurses was organised, which was attended by 50 nurses from 16 local hospitals.[132] The leadership of mission hospitals and mission organisations, however, remained firmly in the hands of European nurses. The Nurses' Auxiliary of the CMAI, formed in 1930, took five years to admit its first Indian member.[133] The South India Board of the Nurses' Auxiliary maintained a rule from 1934 until 1948 that their examinations could only be taken by students who had trained in hospitals with European or American superintendents.[134] In this context, the spirit of associationalism among nurses in mission hospitals was weak; a 1947 CMAI survey found that 'there seems to be a lack of the sense of what could be done for or given to the profession' and that in general a corporate spirit was absent among Indian nurses.

Apart from Indian nurses, nursing leaders also struggled to attract the enthusiastic participation of Western nurses working in India. The educational work of mission nurses, at least, was often far removed from the professionalising concerns of the leadership. Whilst leaders wrote curricula, planned for university education and spoke constantly of attracting a 'better class of candidates', most of their colleagues throughout India were running courses of their own devising, training women with primary education or sometimes even less, and relying on widows or abandoned wives among convert communities to supply nursing labour.[135] The majority of mission

---

[132] Annie S. Magilton, Helen M. Benjamin, Lena M. English, and Lena A. Benjamin, 'American Baptist Mission Hospital for Women and Children and Nurses Training School', 1936, by courtesy of the Burke Library of Union Theological Seminary in the City of New York, Rh. India A — American Baptist Mission, Hospital for Women and Children and School of Nursing Reports.

[133] Abraham, *Nursing History in South India*, p. 99.

[134] Ibid.

[135] Throughout the British Empire, much nursing education work was of this ilk. A 1945 report on nursing in the colonies recorded that 'while the uneducated are poor material to turn into nurses, it has been proved again and again that, provided instruction is severely practical and teachers exercise great patience, they can be trained into surprisingly competent practical nurses' (*Report of the Committee on the Training of Nurses*, p. 21).

hospitals pursued basic, practical programmes, often taught in the vernacular through much of this period, only gradually raising the standard as better-educated women began to come forward from the mid 1930s. The nursing course at the LMS hospital in Neyyoor, run by a nurse called Ms Mills from 1926–46, was fairly typical. It involved training in the most basic principles of sick nursing, in which widows and male nurses with minimal education were taught with 'an immense amount of patience . . . entirely in the Tamil language'.[136] The work of the leadership, therefore, did not substantially reflect the nature of the nursing work or the difficulties encountered in the everyday lives of many of their white colleagues on the missions, let alone Indian nurses and students.

## The Colonial State and the Absence of Nursing

The other side of the equation in considering the underdevelopment of nursing was the state. This late colonial period saw a strange and unique blindness among both British and Indian politicians to the role of nursing and the absence of nurses in Indian hospitals. The centre took little interest in nursing affairs, and nor were provincial governments much interested in the ideas or the complaints of nursing leaders. Ultimately, the development of nursing was restricted by an over-strained colonial state that saw little imperative to act strongly to promote the need for a nursing profession.

The role of the state in contributing to nursing's low status is reinforced by comparisons of nursing's development in other non-Western countries. As had been the case with the early history of nursing in the West, in most non-Western countries the early development of nursing was accompanied by stigmatisation of work requiring women to care for male strangers. Takahashi refers to the 'unpleasant image of female hospital nursing' in late 19th- and early 20th-century Japan.[137] Catherine Ceniza Choy quotes Lavinia Dock's observation that 'the idea of women nursing was an entirely

---

[136] K. Rajasekharan Nair, *Evolution of Modern Medicine in Kerala*, Thiruvananthapuram: Published by Mrs T. Indira Nair, Medical College, Trivandrum, 2001, p. 66.

[137] Takahashi, *The Development of Japanese Nursing*, p. 27.

foreign one to the Filipino people. To them the work seemed menial and wholly beneath a person of any family or birth'.[138] In both cases, the participation of the state was vital in reshaping the status of nursing as a career. Japanese politicians, in the context of a modernising, militarising state, encouraged the work of the Japanese Red Cross in developing a strong nursing corps. This worked, where missionaries had failed, in promoting the emergence of nursing as a socially acceptable career for educated women.[139] In the Philippines, the development of nursing into a 'new and prestigious profession' depended on the promotion of nursing as a form of national service, which 'benefited Filipinos and the Philippine nation'.[140]

In India, however, nursing was regarded neither by the British servants of the colonial state nor by Indian politicians (whose roles in the government were increasing during the period) as an aspect of modernity worth pursuing and developing. In general, the state at central and provincial level accepted a situation in which the majority of hospitals functioned with either a minimal or no nursing staff at all. In 1938, an *NJI* editorial commented that 'nurses are still in common opinion a luxury to be provided when funds permit, not to be worried about otherwise'.[141] In areas of India without a strong mission presence, the number of nurses was woefully small. In Uttar Pradesh, the 1946 Bhore Report found that there were 257 nurses for a population of over 50 million.[142] In Orissa, there were only 38 nurses.[143] In 1944, Hartley recorded that in Uttar Pradesh the nurse to population ratio was one for 197,700 people; in England, which was considered to have a severe nurse shortage, there was one nurse for 375 people.[144] In 1944, Wilkinson wrote that of every 1,000 hospitals, 200 had no nurses at all.[145]

---

[138] Lavinia Dock, in Ceniza Choy, *Empire of Care*, p. 25.

[139] Takahashi, *The Development of Japanese Profession*, pp. 25–27.

[140] Ceniza Choy, *Empire of Care*, p. 31.

[141] Anonymous, 'From "The Statesman"', *NJI*, vol. 29, no. 5, 1938, p. 128.

[142] Government of India, 'Report of the Health Survey and Development Committee' (Bhore Report), New Delhi: Health Survey and Development Committee, 1946, p. 40.

[143] Bhore Report, p. 40.

[144] Diana Hartley, 'Facts and Figures', in TNAI, 'Annual Report of the TNAI 1942–43', RCS, Indian Nursing Collection of Diana Hartley, RCMS 77/4/2, p. 28.

[145] Wilkinson, 'President's Address', p. 9.

Given this extreme lack of nurses, the care of patients in Indian hospitals was in practice provided by relatives and by a range of semi-trained or untrained personnel, holding a series of titles, including ward boy, orderly, sweeper, compounder, and *ayah*. Many of these caregivers were men, holding varying levels of qualification, education or training.[146] In military hospitals, it was orderlies with a modicum of training and 'ward boys' who undertook practical nursing throughout this period. A 1945 memorandum produced by the Indian Army Nursing Service highlighted the continuing failure to make any substantive provision for the nursing of Indian soldiers. It stated that:

> Before the war the Nursing Service of the Indian Army had barely developed beyond the experimental stage. In 1939 the number of Garrison Hospital beds for Indian Troops was 6077 and a cadre of 55 Sisters was maintained to supervise the work of and instruct the male nursing orderlies. The sisters did not undertake the actual nursing of patients nor were their numbers adequate for such duties.[147]

Indian hospitals, both civil and military, were thus in many cases adapted to a mode of functioning that included only a minimal role for female trained nurses. The state was in many cases content with a system that functioned without them, relying instead on a haphazard group of semi-trained and untrained caregivers.

In general, the policies of the government expressed a willingness to rely on the domiciled European and Anglo-Indian communities for nurses. Arguments that Indian women would never take to nursing were willingly accepted, despite the growing numbers of better-educated women that some schools, such as that at CMC Vellore, were beginning to attract. Not only were few attempts being made to

---

[146] In Indian hospitals, male carers were frequently qualified as compounders, although the sphere of their operations was usually far wider than the preparation of drugs. It seems that untrained, partially trained and even three-year trained male nurses were sometimes given this more socially acceptable title rather than that of 'male nurse'. Formal training of male compounders was less in north India, but 'ward boys' and 'dressers' predominated. In north India in 1931, 'dressers' were allowed by the North India United Board of Examiners for Mission and Other Hospitals to train for and take exactly the same examination as trained nurses, with the only difference being that subjects relating to male genito-urinary diseases replaced the midwifery subjects taken by the nursing students.

[147] 'Nursing Service, Indian Army', pp. 107–8.

develop a sustainable base for an Indian profession, but also Indian nurses were actively discriminated against throughout this period, with European and Anglo-Indian nurses consistently preferred. Borthwick writes that in Bengal in 1905 complaints were made against the European lady superintendent of the Calcutta Dufferin hospital on the grounds that she was substituting Eurasian nurses from Bombay for 'native nurses', who were dismissed.[148] Generally, government hospitals trained mainly Anglo-Indian and domiciled European nurses, leaving the missions to focus on training Indians. In 1923 Balfour reported with irritation that the Madras Maternity Hospital had trained 2,373 European and Anglo-Indian midwives, but only 72 Indians.[149] In 1945, Janet Corwin, nursing advisor at the Rockefeller Foundation, made a five-month tour of Indian hospitals. She found that government authorities still 'in certain places . . . tended to discourage those other than Anglo-Indians and domiciled Europeans from becoming nurses'.[150] Even in 1948, her successor, Anna Noll, found that the Nursing School at the Curzon Bowring Hospital in Calcutta still only admitted Anglo-Indians and domiciled Europeans, despite being a state-supported hospital. Noll's tour of Calcutta also included an interview with Ms Brough, the Matron of Medical College Hospital in Calcutta (at which the School of Nursing had 93 Indians out of a total of 186 students), who informed her of her dislike for Indian nurses due to their inadequacy as students and 'poor standards of living'.[151]

### Sporadic attempts at pragmatic reform

The 1930s saw a number of initiatives mounted by Indian politicians that attempted to rationalise and organise around the present needs of hospitals, in contrast to nursing leaders' preoccupation with building an empowered, educated nursing profession for the future. These attempts at pragmatic reform tried to come to grips with the reality of the Indian hospital system — a system that relied mainly on male carers, would clearly struggle for many years to provide a suitable working environment for 'respectable' middle-class girls, and which

---

[148] Borthwick, *The Changing Role of Women in Bengal*, p. 326.
[149] Balfour, 'Indian Nursing', p. 29.
[150] Corwin, 'Semiannual Report: Feb 11– June 30 1945', p. 2.
[151] Noll, Diary 1947–48.

desperately needed labour. These attempts at reform were the result of the 1919 India Act, which had shifted responsibility for health to Indian governments elected at provincial level. They reflected a desire to staff hospitals more effectively, but also to adjust the racial imbalance in the ranks of nurses.

Reforms in all cases were perceived by the Western nursing leadership as a serious threat to their professionalising agenda. In Sindh in 1938, the TNAI opposed a government initiative to reduce the standard of education required for nurse training so as to encourage more Indian women to become nurses.[152] In 1939, Indian legislators in Madras proposed a 50 per cent cut in nurses' salaries and a suspension of clothing and food allowances. The Madras government proposed reducing rather than increasing the educational requirements for nurses, giving widows first preference in recruitment to nursing institutions (which the nurse leaders felt would result in a much less educated pool of candidates), mandating teaching in the vernacular and banning women nurses from male wards entirely, in favour of creating a cadre of male nurses.[153] The plans were considered a disaster by the nursing leadership, as not only would they have lowered the standards nurse leaders sought to raise, they would also have meant the end of reciprocal registration with the General Nursing Council in England and the loss of India's place in the ICN.[154] The TNAI declared that:

> The Congress Government promised to raise the lot of the people but this Government Order will not only reduce the Nursing Service to the level of menials, but create an antagonistic spirit to all rules and demoralize the members of the honoured Profession of Nursing.[155]

---

[152] Hartley, 'Tour from Nagpur to Delhi', pp. 4–8, 13.

[153] Government of Madras (Education and Public Health Department), 'Order No. 3837 for the Reorganisation of the Provincial Nursing Service', *NJI*, vol. 30, no. 2, 1939, pp. 40–42.

[154] Anonymous, 'Resolution passed by the Members of the Trained Nurses' Association of India assembled at Conference and forwarded to The Hon. Mr Rajagopalachariar, the Hon. Dr. Rajan and the Surgeon-General with the Government of Madras on November 11th, 1938', *NJI*, vol. 30, no. 2, 1939, pp. 42–43.

[155] Anonymous, 'Resolution passed by the Members of the Trained Nurses' Association of India assembled at Conference and forwarded to The Hon. Mr Rajagopalachariar, the Hon. Dr. Rajan and the Surgeon-General with the Government of Madras on November 11th, 1938', *NJI*, vol. 30, no. 2, 1939, p. 43.

The deputation put together to approach C. Rajagopalachari, the Premier of Madras Presidency, indicated the anxieties this departure from Western-style female nursing occasioned in British and Anglo-Indian society, as Hartley was joined by a Mr Reid of the European Association and a Mr Bower of the Anglo-Indian Association in protesting the changes. Nurse leaders won some concessions — allowances were restored and the emphasis on the recruitment of widows lessened — but ultimately the resignation of the Congress government in 1939 meant that these reforms were not substantially implemented anyway. These attempts at reforms determined by local needs and the local socio-cultural context were a rare and interesting glitch in a broader history in which little thought was ever given by planners to how best a nursing service might be adapted to Indian needs. Ultimately, however, they faded away and were forgotten. There were clearly limits to the extent that any colonial government could reject the Christianised, feminised professional model of nursing that had emerged as a familiar pillar of medical modernity in the West.

## A late rush to reform

Crises caused by World War II combined with a rush to reshape the health legacy of colonialism meant that in the last, beleaguered years of colonial rule, nursing leaders finally found a central colonial administration open to their views. The first determinant of this new openness of the state to nursing reform was the severe scarcity of trained nurses that became starkly apparent during World War II. As British, Indian and other casualties poured into India from Asian and African battlefields, it became clear that the number of nurses available to care for them was vastly inadequate, let alone to cater simultaneously for the civilian population. In 1943, an army report recorded that the forces in India would have only 55 per cent of the British nurses allocated as essential (meaning 1,503 British nurses in India, instead of 2,720). Only 41 per cent of the entitlement of Indian nurses would be available (meaning 2,061, instead of 5,049).[156] Only 14 per cent of the available Indian nurses were fully qualified trained nurses, with the remainder composed of 'auxiliary Nurses with very

---

[156] L. G. Wilkinson, 'Statement Re Nursing Situation', 16 October 1943, OIOC, L/WS/1/876, 'Nurses and V.A.D.s India', p. 185.

little nursing experience'.[157] Meanwhile, recruitment became even more difficult than usual, as better paid and socially more highly regarded employment opened up for educated Indian, Anglo-Indian and domiciled European women in the Women's Military Services.[158] At the CMC Ludhiana Nursing School, during the war the average number of probationers dropped from 64 to 37.[159] In 1943, the combined total of probationers for all the Dufferin Fund hospitals of India was 364. The Vicereine Lady Wavell commented that 'this number in view of the urgency of the need is pathetically low'.[160] Civil hospitals were reported to be desperate both for students, who were in most cases the base of their labour force, and for qualified nurses who could teach the students they did manage to enrol.[161] This critical nurse shortage became a serious embarrassment for the Government of India and a matter of political sensitivity, as it was clear that the nursing provisions for white soldiers were much superior to those for Indian soldiers.

Rapid action was mandated and the chief available source of expertise was the TNAI, which was well prepared for this long desired moment in the planning spotlight. Hartley regularly observed that during the 1940s, the Government was routinely consulting the TNAI and seeking the advice of senior nurses. According to Janet Corwin, the leaders of nursing in India felt that as a result there had been as much progress between 1940 and 1945 as in the preceding 20 years.[162] Hartley recorded that the 'awakening' of the state and population during wartime had been so profound as to signify 'a new era' for the profession in India.[163] In 1942, E. E. Hutchings, formerly matron of the Dufferin hospital in Calcutta, was appointed as the first nursing advisor to the Government of India, the first step

[157] Wilkinson, 'Statement Re Nursing Situation', p. 185.

[158] Corwin, 'Semiannual Report: Feb 11–June 30 1945', p. 2.

[159] Francesca French, *Miss Brown's Hospital: The Story of the Ludhiana Medical College and Dame Edith Brown, O.B.E. its Founder*, London: Hodder and Stoughton, 1954, p. 85.

[160] Hilda Lazarus, 'Countess of Dufferin's Fund: Women's Medical Service News', *Journal of the Association of Medical Women in India*, vol. 32, no. 2, 1944, p. 68.

[161] Wilkinson, 'Statement Re Nursing Situation', p. 185.

[162] Corwin, 'Semiannual Report: Feb 11–June 30 1945', p. 3.

[163] Hartley, 'Nursing in India'.

in establishing an institutionalised voice for the profession in government and a development long promoted by the TNAI. In 1943, commissioned rank for army nurses was instituted.[164]

Some actions taken to address the wartime nursing crisis were a blow to TNAI leaders, but at the same time they were at least considered worthy of consultation. One dimension of the government strategy was to expand the training and employment of junior nurses, including auxiliary nurses and army orderlies — a move unpopular with the TNAI, which was averse to further erosion of nurses' professional territory. Detachments of Voluntary Aid Detachment nursing assistants (VADs) were also hastily recruited in Britain and sent to India.[165] This caused significant angst among the local leadership, who opposed the measure on the grounds that it was obvious to everyone that VADs, in a climate of extreme shortage, would be undertaking duties they were not qualified for and which had been defined as duties of trained nurses alone.[166] Protest was also raised on the grounds that the conditions under which VADs were appointed demonstrated the contempt of the state for the years nurse leaders had invested in attempts to raise the status of the profession. VADs were to be paid more than fully trained nurses educated in India. Moreover, at all times they were to be employed under the British sisters of the Queen Alexandra's Imperial Military Nursing Service (QAIMNS), and never under Indian Military Nursing Service (IMNS) employees (who might include Anglo-Indians or Indians). This stipulation, its author proposed, 'would not (repeat not) be contained in any official documents for reasons which will be obvious to you', but nevertheless the Government of India (War Department) was warned to be on its guard against a possible 'cry of racial discrimination'.[167]

---

[164] Anonymous, 'Calendar', *NJI*, vol. 49, no. 10, 1958, p. 344.

[165] The initial draft was 769 VADs and three liaison officers. The first batch of 250 left for Poona in June 1944, with the rest following soon after. They were then dispatched to field hospitals within the South East Asia Command Area, with many sent to the North East to receive troops and POWs coming from Burma (Hilda Nield, 'A Short History of the V.A.D. Unit, India, 1944 to 1946', Imperial War Museum, Department of Documents, Misc 183 [2751]).

[166] 'Record of a Meeting held at Hobart House on 25th November, 1943, to consider the Forecasted Requirements of India in Medical Officers and Nurses, and the Possible Extent to which Contribution towards these Requirements can be made from the U.K.', OIOC, L/WS/1/876, 'Nurses and V.A.D.s India', p. 182.

[167] G. N. Molesworth to Government of India, War Department, 9 June 1944, OIOC, 'Nurses and VADs India', L/WS/1/876, pp. 155–57.

The war, therefore, was in some ways damaging for a leadership that hoped to decrease reliance on untrained or junior personnel, and to increase respect for nurses trained in India. Even these less popular initiatives, however, involved extensive consultation with the TNAI and its members, as eminent TNAI nurses were called on to plan and regulate the training of the new auxiliary services. Among these were E. E. Hutchings, the nursing advisor to the Government of India, and Constance Wilson, the superintendent of the Minto nurses, who were given the task of forming the ANS.[168]

One of the most significant outcomes of the wartime crisis was the opening of the School of Nursing Administration in Delhi in 1943, which was designed to rapidly prepare desperately needed Indian nurse administrators. According to Adranvala, the war was the catalyst that finally motivated the government to provide post-certificate education for Indian nurses.[169] The school provided post-diploma courses in administration and, in response to the manifest inadequacy of nursing in general and the recommendations of Hutchings, it also ran a short sister tutor course for civilian nurses.[170] This represented an acknowledgement by the government that the TNAI had long hoped for: that post-diploma education for nurses needed to be provided in India. At the opening of the school, the Marchioness of Linlithgow commented that it was entirely due to TNAI research that such a school had been opened.[171] Wilkinson's reflections on the activism of the TNAI from the 1920s to the 1940s illustrate the extent to which the war brought the TNAI into the spotlight and refashioned it into an organisation of greater standing and impact than ever before:

> Then one thinks of the various Council Meetings — one when discussing the appalling shortage of Sister Tutors — when I pointed out the necessity of India establishing her own school for the training of such. Then followed meetings, deputations to Government, disheartening frustrations — when one was met with fair words

---

[168] Anonymous, 'Greetings and Messages', *NJI*, vol. 49, no. 10, 1958, p. 320.

[169] T. K. Adranvala, 'Developments in Nursing 1947–57', *NJI*, vol. 49, no. 10, 1958, p. 327.

[170] Adranvala, 'Nursing Profession in India', p. 173; 'Major-General Hance's Speech', in TNAI, 'Annual Report of the TNAI 1942–43', RCS, Indian nursing collection of Diana Hartley, RCMS 77/4/2, p. 8.

[171] The Marchioness of Linlithgow, 'The School of Nursing Administration, New Delhi', *NJI*, vol. 31, no. 2, 1943, p. 71.

but *no help, no deeds* — until finally the War with the tremendous need of more trained personnel, produced action, and a School for Post-graduate training in Hospital Administration and Teaching was established in Delhi, and from this grew the College of Nursing. Another was the establishing of Registration Acts and an All-India Nursing Council — hours of real hard work, perseverance, resolute courage, but all full of joy and great fun, working together and in the end some achievement for the nursing profession in India [italics original].[172]

New openness to the voices of nurses was also determined by what Arnold describes as 'a crisis of political legitimation' in the dying years of colonialism, which involved new attempts at 'defining the positive contribution Western medicine had to make to the material progress of the new India and distancing the medical services from the failures of the colonial past'.[173] In its last years, as Sugata Bose describes, 'colonialism under siege turned to development as an ideology of self-justification'. Nurses were able to present their plans as an essential dimension of projects of medical modernity and developmentalism, and nursing professionalism found its way into the planning agenda of the new state.

The chief manifestation of this rush to restructure and modernise the public health system that would be the inheritance of an independent India was the 1946 Report of the Health Survey and Development Committee (known as the Bhore Report after its chairman, Sir Joseph Bhore, an Indian doctor who had worked in England and came out of retirement in Jersey to chair the Commission). The Bhore Report was commissioned in 1943 by the Government of India to provide a detailed survey of health conditions and recommendations for future health planning. The Report was highly influential, as the Congress Party government that took power in 1947 adopted it as a blueprint for the development of the national health system. The Bhore Report highlighted many areas of neglect, but one of the most heavily emphasised was the failure to provide nurses. In the recommendations section of the report, it was recorded that:

> The conditions under which nurses have hitherto been required to carry on their profession in this country are recognised by all thinking

---

[172] Wilkinson, *A Brief History of Nursing*, p. 341.
[173] Arnold, 'Crisis and Contradiction', p. 349.

persons to be deplorable . . . It will be noted that in all cases it is within the power of Governments, if they so wish, to remove these obstacles which cause many aspiring candidates to refrain from undertaking this work which is of such prime importance to the welfare of their country.[174]

The recommendations of the Bhore Report reflected the main focuses of the leadership in India and confirmed the acceptance of their agenda. It advocated the institution of two degree colleges for Indian nurses, one in Delhi and one at the Christian Medical College, Vellore. It recommended that trained nurses with advanced qualifications in public health should be viewed as integral to the delivery of rural and urban public health programmes. It supported the creation of an All India Nursing Council, which would superintend the standardisation of education and curb the widespread exploitation of students. Ultimately, the late colonial state support for nursing reform, the supportive recommendations of the Bhore Committee and the development of advanced education for trained nurses reflected the success of the leadership in presenting professionalised nursing as an essential aspect of the modernisation of India's health system. Professional nursing was perfectly positioned for a place in Jawaharlal Nehru's post-1947 drive to modernise India. Anne Witz comments that the history of nursing shows that 'changes deriving from an agenda set by nurses have been successful only when they have been synchronised with wider organisational and governmental concerns'.[175] Nursing leaders were able to ally their own goals with those of a state on the brink of ceding independence and keen to refashion its legacy, thus ensuring the perpetuation of their vision (if not the reality) of a well educated, empowered and autonomous nursing profession for India.

## Conclusions

At Independence in 1947, the legacy of British rule was an education system run almost entirely by missionaries, a modus operandi in which the state substantially ignored the need for trained nurses,

---

[174] Bhore Report, p. 386.
[175] Anne Witz, 'The Challenge of Nursing', in Jonathan Gabe, David Kelleher and Gareth Williams (eds), *Challenging Medicine*, London: Routledge, 1994, p. 39.

and a rush of last-minute initiatives stemming from a late recognition of the underdeveloped state of the profession. Although professional infrastructure had been erected and the goal of high educational standards established, the reality on most of the hospital wards of India was grim and the nursing system to be inherited by independent India was grossly inadequate to the needs of the population. The numbers produced by the nursing schools of India were still extremely small. In 1947, there were only 7,000 trained nurses working in India, with a ratio of approximately one nurse to between 50 and 60 thousand people.[176] Even at this late stage, the Indian hospital system was substantially functioning without trained nurses, and with almost no Indian leadership. In 1943, there were eight Indian women qualified as sister tutors.[177] Gradually, more educated recruits were entering nursing schools, especially the better-run missionary institutions. Nonetheless, there was still a pervasive stigma attached to the profession, as Lazarus suggested in 1945, and nursing still did not attract 'women of education, culture and of good social status'.[178]

As the Bhore Report critically recorded, this situation had by no means been inevitable. The problem of nursing had awaited solution, but none had been found. Neither the state nor nursing leaders proved able to improve substantially the status of and conditions for nurses. On the one hand, leaders, with little support from any quarter, proved unable to do a great deal. The professional leadership, although steeped in imperialist notions of cultural, religious and racial superiority and seeing themselves as the bearers of shining, vivifying lamps that would illuminate the 'darkness' of India, were genuinely committed to the promotion of nursing as an autonomous, stimulating profession, in which Indian students would be assured of a challenging and well-rounded education and career. Disappointingly, in pursuing this professionalising vision they did not transcend the safety of their Western models. They were entirely inflexible in their commitment to 'standards', did not seek to include India's nurses on equal terms and did not focus on the welfare or the promotion of the rights of vernacular nurses — 'B' grade nurses, *ayah*s, *dai*s or one-year trained midwives. Rather, they remained committed to the distant

---

[176] Wilkinson, *A Brief History of Nursing*, p. 96.

[177] Major-General Hance's Speech', in TNAI, 'Annual Report of the TNAI 1942–43', RCS, Indian Nursing Collection of Diana Hartley, RCMS 77/4/2, p. 7.

[178] Lazarus, *Our Nursing Services*, p. 14.

prospect of replicating an idealised version of metropolitan nursing in the hospitals of India. Serious attempts to adapt this self-view so that Indians could participate as equals or as serious contributors were not made. The consequence was that organisational structures were weak and unrepresentative and nurses were not left with a strong infrastructure for nursing advocacy. John B. Grant, Director of the All-India Institute of Hygiene and Public Health, Calcutta, wrote in 1943 that 'there are less than 4,500 nurses throughout the country as compared with 42,000 doctors, and this is a measure of the present backward status of the profession . . . the problem now chiefly awaits leadership from Indian women'.[179] The problem was that space had not been created in representative institutions for Indian women, and it would not be until the early 1960s that they were capably and independently leading the profession.

The state, meanwhile, had persistently ignored the plight of nurses and the underdevelopment of nursing. It made cosmetic concessions in terms of instituting nurse registration and creating a few positions of authority for nurses, but it continued to tolerate terrible hospital conditions and the widespread exploitation of nurses. It was only the crises of the 1940s that finally opened the ears of the state to nurses' voices. In a late rush to leave a better health legacy, an audience was finally given to the nursing community. This meant that the work of the leadership in researching and promoting their vision of professional nursing became identified with the agenda of a state on the cusp of a massive modernising project and ensured that, at least rhetorically, the ethos of professionalism became a dimension of health planning over the succeeding decades. Nonetheless, these concessions were late, rushed and theoretical. This mode of interaction between profession and state — long years in which nursing leaders were ignored, followed by sporadic bursts of opportunistic interest — has also been the post-colonial pattern and has formed a problematic legacy for the nurses of India. The next chapter explores the attempts after Independence of an entirely new cadre of Western nurses to promote a similar but better resourced professionalising agenda, in the face of this continuing absence of state support.

---

[179] J. B. Grant, *The Health of India*, London: Oxford University Press, 1943, p. 25.

# An *Illustrious* Career
# Aleyamma Kuruvilla

I went to interview ALEYAMMA KURUVILLA in the home
to which she has retired after a lengthy career spanning
Vellore, Delhi, the US, and Britain.[1] She lives in a village
near the Kerala town of Thiruvalla, which houses a large
Syrian Christian community and has supplied workers
of all kinds to the Gulf and the West. The landscape is
dotted with enormous concrete mansions, many of which
are empty, waiting for their owners to return from the
Gulf or the West. Others are occupied only by elderly men
and women whose children have made good overseas.
The trend of nurse migration has had its effect here, as
in many Kerala towns and cities, and the opportunities
nurse migrants have found can, in part, be traced to the
work of Kuruvilla, one of India's most eminent nursing
leaders.

Kuruvilla, who never married, is now in her 80s. She
lives alone in a cool, pleasantly shaded house on a small
landholding, selling milk and other produce in order to
remain engaged with the local community. She continues
to work two hours each day for a newly constructed
Christian hospital near Thiruvalla, which has found it
impossible to get teachers for its nursing school and has
not been able to find a nursing superintendent. Although
she does not teach, she enjoys talking to the students
about the status of nursing. Working in this small town
school, she had been shocked by the dearth of resources,
the poverty of the library and the lack of opportunities
for further education and refresher courses, which form
a stark contrast to the facilities at the elite nursing college CMC Vellore, where she worked for much of her
career.

---

[1] Thiruvalla, 9 December 2005.

Kuruvilla's own interest in nursing developed as a teenager at a Syrian Christian boarding school in this same Kerala town. Her father was the headmaster of the school, which was handed over to the Syrian Christian church by the Congregationalist missionaries who established it. A British nurse worked there as a manager, and she talked a great deal about nursing to the girls. Many pupils asked Kuruvilla's father what he thought they should do after graduating. He often advised nursing, but none thought it a good idea. Observing this, Kuruvilla resolved to be different. Before studying as a nurse, however, under her father's advice she completed her BA degree at the Women's Christian College, University of Madras, from 1941–43, with a major in sociology. In 1944, she went as a student to CMC Vellore, and in 1947 qualified as a registered nurse. Kuruvilla was part of a dynamic and motivated generation of CMC graduates who went on to form the elite of nursing leadership in India (Meera Abraham records that by the late 1960s, 20 out of the 40 nursing colleges in India were headed by a CMC graduate[2]), but hers was possibly the most distinguished career.

With her aptitude for study and her Arts degree, she was identified as a promising leader by the nurses working for the international agencies in India. After working at CMC Vellore as a lecturer of sociology and a field supervisor in public health education, she was sponsored by the Rockefeller Foundation to complete a Masters degree in public health at the Teachers College, Columbia University. Her subjects there included supervision of public health agencies, interpersonal relationships and rural sociology and economics. She was highly successful in this study programme. Elizabeth Brackett, at that time Assistant Director for Nursing at Rockefeller, recorded that Kuruvilla and her two co-students, G. Chandramathy and K. Paulose Aleykutty, 'made outstanding records and have won the affection of all those who have gotten to know them well'.[3]

---

[2] Abraham, *Religion, Caste and Gender*, p. 110.
[3] Excerpt from the diary of Elizabeth W. Brackett, 6 July 1953, RF, Series 2.1 (Post-war Correspondence), R.G. 6.1 (Paris Field Office), Box 44, Folder 403, 'DMPH India, Nursing'.

A Rockefeller file-note records that in her early days at Columbia, Kuruvilla did not set foot outside Columbia's International House without a companion, finding New York terrifying.[4] Later, however, she became an experienced traveller, undertaking study tours and conference visits all around the world.

Kuruvilla has a unique record of leadership. She was Dean of CMC Vellore through the 1960s and 1970s and contributed to its reputation as the best nursing school and college in India. As dean, she launched an MSc programme in Nursing. She was the first woman and the first nurse to become the President of the Board of Nursing Education, South India branch, between 1972–74 and 1978–94. She served as the President of CMAI for four years — the first nurse to occupy this position of authority over the Christian doctors, nurses and allied health workers of India. She was also President of CNL and TNAI during the 1970s, positions which she used to vigorously lobby for the appointment of nurses not doctors as the heads of state nursing councils, the better representation of nurses in government and the development of nurse education.[5]

Kuruvilla's commitment to professional nursing has always been very strong. At a 1971 conference on the future of nursing education, she argued for an end to nursing's image as all about 'tea and sympathy', and suggested that only university education could give nurses sufficient skill in problem-solving and provide the intellectual maturity that would allow them to think for themselves. She wrote, 'for the complex role of the nurse we require a person with above-average intelligence, a deep sense of purpose and commitment and a sound understanding of the social sciences'.[6]

---

[4] Excerpt from the diary of Elizabeth W. Brackett, 29 September 1952, RF, Series 2.1 (Post-war Correspondence), R.G. 6.1 (Paris Field Office), Box 44, Folder 403, 'DMPH India, Nursing'.

[5] Anonymous, 'Abortion Act: Nurses' Rights on Moral Grounds Defended', *NJI*, vol. 62, no. 11, 1971, p. 352.

[6] A. Kuruvilla, 'Phasing of Diploma to Degree Programme', *NJI*, vol. 62, no. 6, 197, p. 192.

She described to me her pride in abolishing the system of stipends for nursing students at CMC. She implemented this policy in opposition to other missionary leaders, who argued that it would deter poor students. She felt that this step had dramatically raised the status of nursing as a career, and told me that, although the school offered generous scholarships, few applied for them. Students gained confidence knowing their education was worth paying for, and the nursing superintendent had been forced to reduce the hospital's demands on the students, as the justification that they must earn their stipend had been removed. The success of Kuruvilla's initiative led to the abolition of stipends in all CMAI schools.

Aleyamma Kuruvilla embodies all that Rockefeller, WHO and the other international agencies hoped for in their work in India. She has dedicated her life and work to nursing education and the evolution of higher standards of professional nursing in India.

◼

# 3

# 'Seeds That May Have Been Planted May Take Root'

## International Aid Nurses and Projects of Professionalism, 1947–65[*]

■

Upon the creation of an independent India in 1947, a cadre of international nurse advisors was dispatched to the new state, bringing ambitious plans for remaking the local profession.[1] These women, among the most highly qualified nurses in the world, worked for powerful international government and non-government organisations (NGOs), including the Rockefeller Foundation, USAID and the WHO. This chapter examines the impact of their work in India. Although they perceived themselves as marking a radical break from the practices of the colonial leaders described in Chapter 2, their agenda makes it clear that there were important continuities. There were three main focuses in international nursing programmes — support for university-based nursing programmes, the encouragement of a strong public health role for nurses and the education of Indian nurses overseas. These programmes clearly reinforced the professionalising, internationalist nursing culture espoused during the

---

[*]A version of this chapter was published as '"Seeds That May Have Been Planted May Take Root": International Aid Nurses and Projects of Professionalism in Post-Independence India, 1947–1965', *Nursing History Review*, vol. 17, 2008.

[1] Healey, 'Seeds That May Have Been Planted'.

colonial period. Randall Packard argues that post-colonial states were often inhibited from making a definitive break with their colonial medical systems by the renewal of Western dominance represented in the interventions of the international health agencies.[2] In the case of nursing, the work of international agency nurses dramatically strengthened the somewhat weak professionalising agenda of the colonial leadership.

This chapter draws on Rockefeller and USAID records, as well as secondary literature on other organisations, to examine international nursing programmes from 1947–65. Although international nurses made significant contributions — institutionalisation of degree education for the elite, a better infrastructure for the preparation of teachers and administrators, a broader awareness of the importance of public health among nurses — their projects were ultimately flawed by a passionate commitment to North American educational models insufficiently tempered by awareness of the socio-cultural context in which they intervened. International nurses encountered a local profession that was numerically small, almost without leadership, subject to dire working conditions, and stigmatised in wider Indian society. It was felt that the answer to these problems lay in the preparation of a small elite, who would be broadly educated and skilled as leaders. This would produce a 'trickle-down effect', raising teaching standards, elevating the profession in the public eye and eventually producing large numbers of more empowered nurses. This solution, however, was beset by a range of difficulties. With overcrowded wards, under-equipped hospitals, a frequently hostile medical profession and unsupportive governments, nursing degree programmes struggled to function at all. The view that high-level projects of professionalism were the best way to make use of the considerable resources and expertise invested in nursing is ultimately questionable. International programmes, in their attempts to institutionalise the values and infrastructure of the nursing professionalism that had evolved in early 20th-century North America, left a problematic cultural legacy for nursing leadership in India.

---

[2] Packard, 'Postcolonial Medicine', p. 98; Randall Packard, 'Malaria Dreams: Postwar Visions of Health and Development in the Third World', *Medical Anthropology*, vol. 17, 1997, pp. 279–96.

# International Nurses
# and Their Work in India

Post-colonial India welcomed a bevy of overseas nurse experts, who were sponsored by a range of international organisations to assist in the development of Indian nursing. Nursing was thus a small dimension of the massive cold-war commitment to liberal developmentalism. India, as Gary R. Hess writes, attracted a large proportion of the attention of international development agencies, because it was a 'critical test of the capacity of a democratic state to address the challenge of economic and social development'.[3] This was also the period of a new spirit of internationalism in health and medicine. The WHO, as Sunil Amrith writes, 'brought into a common institutional sphere the health policies of diverse, post-colonial, political entities'.[4] Along with this came, according to Joan Lynaugh, a new era in nurse internationalism, involving more emphasis and a wider application than ever before of the key values of 'internationalism, professionalism and standardization of nursing'.[5] This involved a strong focus on assistance in the development of nursing in former colonies. In India, this new spirit of internationalism was manifested in the establishment of nursing assistance programmes by most of the major international organisations. The WHO ran 22 nursing projects between 1948 and 1958, 15 per cent of all its projects in India.[6] The Colombo Plan provided considerable assistance throughout this period in 'raising the standard of nursing education', with the participation of the United States, Australia and New Zealand.[7]

---

[3] Gary R. Hess, 'The Role of American Philanthropic Foundations in India's Road to Globalization During the Cold War Era', in Soma Hewa and Darwin H. Stapleton (eds), *Globalization, Philanthropy and Civil Society: Toward a New Political Culture in the Twenty-First Century*, New York: Springer Science and Business Media, 2005, pp. 51–52.

[4] Amrith, 'Development and Disease', p. 217.

[5] Joan E. Lynaugh, 'From Chaos to Transformation', in Barbara L. Brush, Joan E. Lynaugh, Geertje Boschma, Anne Marie Rafferty, Meryn Stuart, and Nancy J. Tomes (eds), *Nurses of All Nations: A History of the International Council of Nurses, 1899–1999*, Philadelphia: Lippincott, 1999, p. 111.

[6] Central Health Education Bureau (CHEB), *International Organisations and India's Health Programmes*, New Delhi: Government of India, 1961, p. 1.

[7] CHEB, *International Organisations*, p. 15; Anonymous, 'Colombo Plan Nurses', *NJI*, vol. 44, no. 8, 1953, pp. 204–5.

USAID also invested in nursing projects. It initially focused on developing the mechanisms of nurse representation to government and providing specialised training, but from the late 1950s instead provided financial aid and personnel to support three new degree colleges of nursing.[8] The involvement of the Rockefeller Foundation was less extensive but still influential. It focused on providing expert assistance to the Colleges of Nursing in New Delhi and Vellore and the School of Nursing in Trivandrum, as well as sponsoring Indian nurses for advanced education in North America, especially in teaching, administration and public health.[9]

Only Rockefeller had significant previous exposure to nursing in India, although this was limited. Shirish Kavadi records that Mary Beard, as Associate Director for Nursing, was dispatched to conduct a survey of nursing in 1933. She reported the 'absence of modern nursing education, lack of qualified teachers in nursing schools and the universal understaffing of wards in hospitals'.[10] From the late 1930s, John Black Grant, director of the Rockefeller-sponsored All India Institute for Hygiene and Public Health in Calcutta, became increasingly concerned with the underdevelopment of public health nursing and advocated the appointment of a public health nursing advisor in India. Mary Tennant, associate director of nursing at Rockefeller's International Health Division toured India in 1941 to survey conditions, and as a result of her findings, Janet Corwin was appointed as the first public health nursing consultant at the Foundation's office in Delhi in 1945.[11]

The context into which the international agency nurses initially arrived seemed conducive to their work. In 1946, the government-appointed Health Survey and Development Committee, or Bhore Committee, published its report, which had extensive and ambitious recommendations for the future of nursing. It proposed an enormous numerical expansion to the nursing service, but also focused heavily on qualitative improvements. It recommended the creation

---

[8] CHEB, *International Organisations*, p. 19.

[9] Ibid., p. 26.

[10] Shirish N. Kavadi, *The Rockefeller Foundation and Public Health in Colonial India 1916–1945: A Narrative History*, Pune and Mumbai: Foundation for Research in Community Health, 1999, p. 128.

[11] Ibid., pp. 126–35.

of a corps of public health nurses, who would be trained with additional qualifications in public health and midwifery. Importantly, it extended strong support to university education as a means of preparing desperately needed leaders. It seemed, therefore, that in taking the Bhore Report as its template for the development of a national health system, the independent state of India would accord nursing a new level of importance, in both resources and status. The late colonial developments described at the end of Chapter 2 increased this optimism, as nurses had recently benefited from an expanded role in government, the institution of post-certificate qualifications, and the opening of the School of Nursing Administration in Delhi. At the same time, as Roger Jeffery suggests, there were also early indications of an incapacity to support ambitious health projects, as both central and state governments faced the serious financial and bureaucratic strain caused by the partition of colonial India, and the resulting enormous refugee flows and the rapid political change and tumult occasioned by the handing over of power.[12]

International nurses, however, were ambitious, confident and backed by the considerable resources of powerful international agencies. Nurses working for these organisations were highly qualified and articulate representatives of the profession, with extensive experience in nursing at home and abroad. Lillian Johnson is a relatively typical example. Johnson was a Rockefeller nurse and advisor to the School of Nursing at Trivandrum from 1952–56. She was 50 years old when she left for India. She had a master's degree in Public Health and had worked in New Guinea, in South American mining hospitals, as an army nurse in the Philippines, with Puerto Rican families in New York City, and as a medical social worker. A recommendation from the New York Community Service Society praised her as a 'singularly interesting person, refined and cultured', as well as a 'conscientious, patient, untiring worker' who 'writes extremely well and has poise and ability as a speaker in groups'.[13] Anna Noll,

---

[12] Roger Jeffery, 'Toward a Political Economy of Health Care: Comparisons of India and Pakistan', in Monica Das Gupta, Lincoln C. Chen and T. N. Krishnan (eds), *Health, Poverty and Development in India*, Delhi: Oxford University Press, 1996, p. 276.
[13] 'Reference for Lillian Alice Johnson from Community Service Society, New York, 25 November 1952, RF, Series 2.1 (Post-war Correspondence), RG 6.1, Box 44, Folder 402, 'DMPH India, Lillian Johnson, 1952–54'.

advisor at the Delhi College of Nursing and Rockefeller's nursing representative in India from 1947–58, was similarly highly qualified. In addition to her nursing training, she had a BA and a postgraduate teaching qualification. She had worked as a public health nurse for the East Harlem Nursing and Health Service, the Henry Street Visiting Nurse Service and the Army Nurse Corps, with two years of foreign service.[14] Ellen Wren, sent from New Zealand under the Colombo Plan in 1953, had specialised training in midwifery, childcare and public health, and had worked for the New Zealand Department of Health. Her colleague, Jean Taylor, sent to run the postgraduate teaching and administration training at the Delhi College of Nursing, had midwifery and child care training, a postgraduate qualification in Advanced Nursing Education from the University of Toronto and had undertaken a study tour of the United States and Europe, sponsored by Rockefeller.[15] International nurse advisors, therefore, were in general a group of exceptionally well-educated, experienced nurses, with a strong commitment to education and the ethos of professionalisation.

Their commitment to education and professionalisation was also strongly reinforced by the organisational context in which they worked. In general, the international organisations viewed themselves as the bearers of progressive, scientised medical practice, and emphasised public health and a high standard of medical education and research in their work.[16] Rockefeller, particularly, had a history of support for advanced nursing practice, having funded a number of seminal committees in the US during the first half of the 20th century. Anne Marie Rafferty writes that the findings of these committees supported university education for nurses, the development of a stronger leadership and the promotion of a curriculum that emphasised public health and social service.[17]

---

[14] Anna Noll to Mary Elizabeth Tennant, 13 March 1946, RF, RG 2, Series 100, Box 320, Folder 2168.

[15] Anonymous, 'Colombo Plan Nurses', *NJI*, vol. 44, no. 8, 1953, pp. 204–5.

[16] Ann Yrjala, *Public Health and Rockefeller Wealth: Alliance Strategies in the Early Formation of Finnish Public Health Nursing*, Tavastg: Abo Akademi University Press, 2005, p. 9.

[17] Anne Marie Rafferty, 'Internationalising Nursing Education During the Interwar Period', in Paul Weindling (ed.), *International Health Organisations and Movements, 1918–1939*, Cambridge: Cambridge University Press, 1995, p. 269.

International nurses were allowed considerable responsibility and autonomy by their employers, reflecting growing recognition in the international health community of the need to increase the quality and quantity of nurse involvement in overseas programmes. Elizabeth Brackett, assistant director for nursing at the International Health Division (IHD) at the Rockefeller Foundation, commented in a reference for Noll that her reporting skills were excellent. She reflected that this was important, given that 'it was on the basis of such analyses that our program in nursing in these countries was developed'.[18] Tehmina K. Adranvala, the first nursing advisor to the Government of India, wrote in 1958 that the presence of highly qualified, motivated international nurse advisors and the 'stress laid on nursing by the international health teams' had been significant in raising the social status of nursing in India.[19] It is important, however, not to exaggerate the extent to which international nurses presented an ideal of professional autonomy. It is also true that they answered to the doctors who were ultimately in charge of Indian programmes, and at times were mocked by these men as eccentric or emotionally erratic 'spinsters'. Yet to some degree the presence of international nurses did seem to create a visible, practical awareness that nurses could assume considerable responsibility and might adopt a leadership role outside the hospital.

International experts arriving after Independence were somewhat shocked by the lack of progress achieved by their mainly British colleagues who had led nursing under colonial rule. North American nurses' analysis of the situation in India reflected what Rafferty characterises as a longstanding and increasingly accepted view that American nursing, particularly in public health, represented the progressive future, compared to outdated British practices.[20] The new expert advisors thus perceived their own presence in India as marked by a profound discontinuity with the colonial era; as Juliette Julien (the Chief Nurse Advisor for the Health Division of USAID in India in the early 1960s) wrote: they understood their role in India to be

---

[18] E. W. Brackett to Ann C. Deeds, 3 July 1952, RF, RG2, Series 100, Box 5, Folder 28.

[19] T. K. Adranvala, 'Nursing Profession in India', p. 178; T. K. Adranvala, 'Developments in Nursing 1947–57', p. 328.

[20] Rafferty, 'Internationalising Nursing Education', p. 277.

'revolutionising nursing in all its phases'.[21] They often commented that nursing education and practice in India displayed the worst features of the British system. Brackett toured India in January 1952. The parlous state of education in the nursing schools of Madras was described as 'the British system of nursing education practiced at a very low level', and the Indian and Anglo-Indian matrons staffing the city's hospitals were said to 'bear the stamp of the British matron under whom they have been trained'.[22] Nurse training in India was felt to exhibit the worst tendencies of the English system in comparison to more progressive American education, especially in its greater reliance on nurses as hospital labour. In 1949, Kathleen Russell, director of the School of Nursing at the University of Toronto, wrote to Tennant, 'I think you and I will agree that, if there is to be any significant help given to India, they had better keep away from the traditional English methods'.[23]

Despite the American nurses' perception that they represented a new era, there was not significant conflict between the pre-Independence British and American nurses who remained in India and these new emissaries of Western nursing. International nurses arriving after Independence were mainly met with enthusiastic cooperation from the existing TNAI and mission leadership. Hostility to the nurse advisors' projects was common among the matrons and staff nurses working on the wards they used for clinical teaching, but the professional leadership in nursing organisations was supportive and enthusiastic. Although colonial leaders had not been able to affect much the practical transformation of nursing education, Chapter 2 highlighted that for many years they had promoted and supported the ethos of professionalism in nursing and had been researching the possibility of university education in India from the mid-1930s. Thus they welcomed an injection of funding and personnel from

---

[21] Julien, 'Case History on Nursing College Development Project No. 386-AF-54-AB-5', 1963, NARA, Box 157, Folder 'HLS 1-2 Nursing Schools (General)' pp. 22–23.

[22] Excerpts from Elizabeth W. Brackett's diary, January 1952, RF, RG 6.1, Series 2.1 (Post-war Correspondence), Box 44, Folder 403, 'DMPH India, Nursing'. This distaste was typical of the more general discourse of development prevalent in American aid projects of the era, which was marked by a rejection of colonialism and the projection of an idealistic new egalitarianism among nations. For a discussion of this discourse and the structural inequalities it disguised, see Gilbert Rist, *The History of Development: From Western Origins to Global Faith*, London: Zed Books, 1997, pp. 72–74.

[23] E. Kathleen Russell to M. E. Tennant, 4 June 1949, RF, RG 2, Series 464C, Box 461, Folder 3094.

international organisations that was designed to advance these aims. A 1946 policy statement by the Nurses' Auxiliary of the CMAI stated, for example, that there was a need to 'seek the best from every land, adapt it to India's needs and conditions and weld it into an integrated whole', and to 'give to nursing and nursing education the place which the International Council of Nurses advocate'.[24] Although the fact was not much recognised by post-Independence nurse advisors, colonial nurses had laid some of the ground for their projects and thus there was continuity in the direction of the Indian profession. International nursing advisors in effect entrenched and solidified the professionalising plans of the colonial leaders, ensuring a strong focus on the recreation of Western nursing models and standards and providing essential support in the construction of long hoped-for nursing degree programmes.

## International Interventions for the Development of a Professional Nursing Community

International nurses pursued their objective of promoting professionalism through three main policies: sponsorship of degree education for nurses, overseas education programmes for Indian nurses and promotion of public health nursing. The first of these, the development of university education, was enthusiastically supported by all of the international organisations. This was a highly ambitious and progressive project, given that few university programmes existed outside North America at the time and in India the hospital-based system for the three-year education of trained nurses was immensely troubled. Despite the low level of basic education, nurse advisors felt it best to aim high, in order to supply a well-qualified corps of leaders and educators, while also 'developing the status of nursing in India to that of a real profession'.[25] It was felt that by offering a high-status educational programme, nursing might be dissociated from the low-status widows and orphans who had made it their livelihood. Julien stated of the USAID degree programmes that 'candidates

---

[24] CMAI Committee, 'A Survey of Nursing', p. 19.
[25] Julien, 'Case History on Nursing', pp. 20–21.

were to be recruited from higher income groups and would have the
necessary educational and social background to raise the profession
to a respectable and honourable status'.[26] Similarly, Noll hoped that
degree education might win over 'parents in homes of better educational and social background' and to reduce the numbers who 'tend
to come from homes under economic stress and to choose nursing
not because the work appeals to them but because it offers them a
chance to earn a small stipend'.[27] International nurses, like the colonial leadership, were thus animated by an often expressed desire to
distance Indian nursing from its low class and low caste roots.

The Delhi College of Nursing, associated with University of Delhi,
was seen as the flagship of degree education for nurses in India and
received a large proportion of international nurses' attention and
resources. It was provided with substantial assistance, consultation, teaching expertise, and targeted scholarships for faculty by the
Colombo Plan, the Rockefeller Foundation and USAID. The other
of the two degree colleges established in the late 1940s was located
at CMC Vellore, awarding a degree from Madras University.[28]
The Delhi College of Nursing was viewed as the main source of a
hoped-for demonstration effect, with this example of progressive
education seen as likely to provide evidence of the efficacy of new,
modern ways of teaching. This was to be achieved through both
its BSc (nursing) course and its six-month Sister Tutor course, for
which nurses were sent from all over India. The BSc course at Delhi,
established by its American principal Margaretta Craig, was partly
based on the courses offered by the University of Toronto (one of
the most elite metropolitan centres of nurse professionalism, which
had been a focus of Rockefeller assistance).[29] Indian nurses at the
College of Nursing, who through the 1950s and early 1960s moved
into the higher ranks of the college faculty, had almost all received

---

[26] Julien, 'Case History on Nursing', p. 8.

[27] Anna M. Noll, 'Report on Nursing in Mysore State', 23 August 1949, RF, RG2, Box 461, Series 464C, Folder 3094, pp. 2, 4.

[28] The college of nursing at Vellore also received significant attention, but as it was part of a mission hospital it was serviced by international mission nurses and therefore required less advice and consultation, and was also politically more difficult to assist.

[29] Janet D. Corwin, 'India: Nursing: Second Semi-Annual Report for 1946', RF, RG 5.3, Series 464C, Box 204, Folder 2494, p. 8.

scholarships for advanced training in the best international nursing schools. They were thus as committed as their international colleagues to the project of advanced education in India.

The early fortunes of the Delhi College of Nursing illustrate both the strengths and the weaknesses of the Western nurses' professionalising project in India. The College of Nursing almost immediately met with some success in its plan to attract more educated and socially acceptable candidates and to recruit Indian women from outside the Christian community. The first intake of 13, although advertised late due to uncertainty about the availability of buildings and faculty, boasted in its ranks seven Hindus (of whom three were Brahmins), four Christians, one Muslim, and one Sikh. Corwin, Rockefeller's nursing consultant in India at the time, triumphantly added to this list the final note: 'Widows = none'.[30] Of these, two had two years of college education in science and arts, five had undertaken the University of Delhi's higher secondary examination and two had one year of college work. This was exceptional, given that most schools of nursing struggled to find candidates who had studied up to the 10th standard in high school. Although the quality and quantity of teaching at the College were often dubious, the educational focus was ambitious. The post-certificate course in administration devised by New Zealand nurses working for the Colombo Plan included subjects such as Nursing Legislation and Professional Problems, Public Speaking and English, Sociology, and Physics and Chemistry.[31] In 1959, when the College of Nursing had somewhat stabilised after its troubled early years, Edith Buchanan (a Canadian nurse employed by the Government of India as a founding member of the College of Nursing faculty) launched a master of nursing degree, attempting to introduce a culture of research into Indian nursing.[32]

The College of Nursing, however, experienced a set of problems that illustrate some of the constraints on the project of professionalism in Indian nursing in general. The decision to concentrate heavily on the education of an elite, rather than to address hospital conditions or the empowerment of working nurses or diploma students,

[30] Corwin, 'India: Nursing: Second Semi-Annual Report for 1946', p. 7.

[31] Brackett's diary, p. 80.

[32] Adranvala, 'A Review of Post-basic and Post-graduate Training of Nurses', *NJI*, vol. 56, no. 9, 1965, p. 248; 'Obituary: Dr (Ms) Edith Buchanan', *NJI*, vol. 94, no. 11, 2003, p. 258.

limited the quality of the courses that could be delivered. In short, while there was a desire to teach a high standard of nursing and even a pool of able candidates, hospital conditions, state apathy and the animosity of the medical profession made it difficult to impart this level of education. Conflict developed between faculty and the nursing staff in the designated sites for clinical instruction, the Lady Irwin and Lady Hardinge hospitals, where superintendents and ward sisters were unsupportive of the degree programme. Providing adequate clinical experience and clinical teaching in this context proved impossible. Doctors were frequently obstructive and unsupportive. Brackett reported attitudes of 'thinly veiled hostility' from a high-up doctor in the Ministry of Health, and often encountered the opinion that the college offered a programme of study that was overly sophisticated for nurses' needs.[33] The disdain of doctors has, of course, been a problem for university nursing programmes in every country. In India, however, it seemed to be expressed particularly destructively. The medical lecturers who had been assigned to teach science subjects at the Delhi College, for example, often did not bother to attend the classes they were paid to teach.[34]

One of the most serious problems the College of Nursing faced was that, despite strong assurances of state support, in general there was a lack of support from a beleaguered and under-resourced Ministry of Health. The minister, Rajkumari Amrit Kaur, offered strong moral support and always made herself accessible to College of Nursing faculty leaders.[35] The Union Ministry of Health had agreed to support the College of Nursing, and had initially promised an annual budget of ₹115,000, buildings to house the school, and six scholarships for the BSc course.[36] In practice, however, the ministry continually

---

[33] Brackett's diary, p. 84. Similarly, Aleyamma Kuruvilla, BSc graduate of CMC Vellore and, from 1960 onward, its Dean, wrote that she encountered 'painful comments and destructive criticism' from the rest of the medical team, who suggested that the BSc was an 'academic exercise and would be lacking in practical experience which was needed for any nursing course and hence would certainly not be suitable for India' (Aleyamma Kuruvilla, 'Letter from Miss A. Kuruvilla', in *College of Nursing, Christian Medical College and Hospital: Golden Jubilee Souvenir 1946–1996*, Vellore: College of Nursing, Christian Medical College, 1996).

[34] Anna M. Noll, 'Semi-Annual Report — Nursing (India and Ceylon), July 1 to December 31, 1948', RF, RG 5.3, Series 464C, Box 204, Folder 2496, p. 8.

[35] Alice Forman to Douglas N. Forman, 22 September 1949, RF, RG2, Series 464C, Box 461, Folder 3094.

[36] Corwin, 'India: Nursing: Second Semi-Annual Report for 1946'.

reneged on its promises of equipment and funding and failed to provide suitable accommodation.[37] As late as 1974, the College of Nursing was still housed in 'war-time hutments'.[38] In 1949, Noll described a request from a ministry official that the degree students should offer more assistance to cover the wards if they wished the provision of buildings to be expedited. This showed a minimal comprehension of the aims of the degree programme, which rested on the premise that students were not to be regarded as part of hospitals' labour forces.[39] At the same time, however, the College of Nursing was useful to an Indian government that wished to be seen as taking action to improve nursing, which was often commented on as something of a national embarrassment. Corwin described the College of Nursing as 'Exhibit A of the Health Department of the GOI', and government officials frequently brought visitors there.[40] Even for international nurses allied with influential, prestigious agencies, it seemed that the pattern of interaction between profession and state remained much the same as that described in Chapters 2 and 4 — theoretical, opportunistic support combined with egregious practical neglect.

Some of the problems documented by the Rockefeller representatives were related to the youth of the Delhi College of Nursing and the general context of post-Independence upheaval and resource scarcity. The experiences of the USAID nurses a decade later, however, confirm similar basic limits. Again, a strong focus on elite education was limited by a failure to co-opt ward nursing and medical staff and by the foundering of educational programmes in the context of an under-resourced, struggling hospital system. USAID became heavily involved in the development of degree colleges in the states of Andhra Pradesh, Madhya Pradesh and Rajasthan. The cost of these colleges of nursing project from 1961–65 was US$ 795,000.[41]

---

[37] Richmond K. Anderson to K. C. K. E. Raja, 12 April 1949, RF, RG2, Series 464C, Box 461, Folder 3094.

[38] Planning Commission of India, *Draft Fifth Five Year Plan 1974–79*, vol. 2, New Delhi: 1973–74, p. 247; Anonymous, 'New Building to House College of Nursing', *NJI*, vol. 62, no. 9, 1971, p. 295.

[39] Anna M. Noll to M. E. Tennant, 25 July 1949, RF, RG2, Series 464C, Box 461, Folder 3094.

[40] Corwin, 'India: Nursing: Second Semi-Annual Report for 1946', p. 9.

[41] Eugene Campbell, J. Heires, C. Pease, and Blume to Walter Wilson, and Richard C. Parsons, 'Recommended Deletion of Nursing College Development Project', 7 November 1962, National Archives and Records Administration, College Park,

The Hyderabad College of Nursing, launched in 1959 at Osmania University, was the most successful, as it received relatively strong support from the state medical director, who ensured provision of buildings, a library and a bus for transport (an essential and often lacking requirement that allowed nurses to do night work and visit clinical and public health sites in places where it was difficult and dangerous for them to use public transport). In 1963, there were 68 students studying in the college and it was anticipated that by 1966 USAID staff would not be required.[42] Project nurses reported to USAID headquarters that in Hyderabad, where 'young women from the higher economic groups' were entering nursing, it might even be possible that university education for nurses would bring 'equal status with the medical, engineering and other professions'.[43]

This hopeful analysis, however, is undermined by records of local conferences among USAID staff. In 1963, it was reported by the Hyderabad nurse consultants, Meral Loewus, Alice Hagelshaw, and Margaret Keller, that there had been no support from the medical profession or other nursing staff on the wards. Degree students were treated with 'hostility and resentment by the three-year graduates and supervisors who feel that these girls represent a threat to them'. Doctors were actively obstructive, to the extent of removing props for the support of broken limbs put in place by nursing degree students. It was commented that the college had started 'as an emergency with little in the way of sound planning, both for curriculum and administrative details . . . a pattern has now been set which is inadequate and yet may be difficult to change'.[44]

At the Indore and Jaipur colleges of nursing sponsored by USAID, problems were even more serious. The Indore College of Nursing, opened in 1958, from the outset received minimal state support, and was not provided with any facilities — accommodation, faculty or

---

MD (henceforth NARA), State Department Records, USAID, Record Group no 286, entry 385, Box 157, Folder 'HLS 1-2 Nursing Schools (General)'. All USAID archival material is from the same Record Group and entry, so henceforth I have only given the box number.

[42] Julien, 'Case History on Nursing', p. 13.

[43] Ibid., p. 20.

[44] John T. Gentry, 'Nursing Education and Nursing Care: Conference with Miss Meral Loewus, Miss Alice Hagelshaw, Miss Margaret Keller, and Dr and Mrs Carlyle Jacobsen, on January 26, 1963, Hyderabad', 11 February 1963, NARA, Box 157, Folder 'HLS 1-2 Nursing Schools (General)'.

classrooms — that were not shared with the pre-existing School of Nursing. In 1961, 14 BSc students shared three bedrooms in the attic of a dilapidated building. State support at both Indore and Jaipur was sporadic and unreliable and communication with the government difficult. The hospital administration at Indore was particularly unsupportive of the degree programme and the School of Nursing principal and staff were hostile to the USAID advisors and the college faculty.[45] A major dimension of the problems there was the struggle of the American advisors to provide university-level nursing education in a radically under-resourced and overcrowded hospital system. Arline Heath, advisor at Indore, reported to Julien:

> Conditions at the initiation of her activities included use of the same used needle and syringe for 20–30 patients without sterilization; patients' relatives on the ward at all times, sleeping in bed with patient or under the bed; up to five patients using the same dish for meals, and rice being served by hands from kitchen container to plates; no sterile forceps for dressing burns (fingers used!); no waste receptacles (soiled dressings were thrown on the floor); no screens to put around patient's bed during bathing or treatment procedures; 50% burn patients untreated and left to die; burn patients precipitated into shock and death by radical debridement within 24 hours (all blisters opened and stripped, with no sedation or fluid replacement, etc.); nurses giving doctors unsterile syringes because sterile equipment was not available and the nurse did not want to have to tell that to the doctor and then the doctor would have to wait for one to be prepared; generally dirty condition of patients; dirty and smelly latrines; no hot water, etc.[46]

USAID had withdrawn all support from Indore by June 1962. Nonetheless, it was hoped by Julien that 'contact with well qualified American nurses' would have meant that state and university officials 'learned of the type of educational programs nurses should receive', and that 'seeds that may have been planted may take root'.[47]

---

[45] John T. Gentry, 'Conference with Dr G. L. Sharma, Director of Medical Services, Madhya Pradesh', May 1962, NARA, Box 157, Folder 'HLS 1-2 Nursing School (College of Nursing — Indore)'.

[46] John T. Gentry, 'Conference with Miss Arline Heath, Aid Nurse Advisor, Nursing College, Indore; Conference With Dr Bhattacharya, Hospital Superintendent, Indore; And a Hospital Visit, on February 2, 1962', NARA, Box 157, Folder 'HLS 1-2 Nursing School (College of Nursing — Indore)'.

[47] Julien, 'Case History on Nursing', p. 19.

Degree and post-certificate programmes of this period at least partly fulfilled the hopes of the international nurses and their Indian counterparts. Sister tutor and administration courses developed at the colleges of nursing in Delhi and Vellore were used as a resource throughout India and as far as Ceylon, Thailand and Burma for training teachers. By the mid-1960s, teaching shortages had become less acute and it was clear that the post-certificate courses and BSc training were reducing reliance on foreign teachers. The early degree courses had also created considerable regard for university education programmes, which steadily expanded each decade after Independence. Julien wrote that the early college projects influenced the decision by the University of Bombay in 1959–60 to open a college of nursing and, in July 1963, the opening of an Indian Army College of Nursing at the University of Poona. Rockefeller and USAID were approached by several state governments, including Kerala, Mysore and West Bengal, for assistance in starting local degree colleges.[48] It is certain that when the international nurses left, India had a well-established system of university education for nurses, the development of which had relied to a significant degree on their finance and expertise. While initially the educational content was dubious, these courses at least established the ideal that nurses deserved a broad education. Alumni of international nursing projects emerged as the first generation of Indian leadership and perpetuated their teachers' professionalising focus as the theoretical basis for nursing education in India.

The difficulties that beset early degree programmes, however, are instructive. In establishing nursing colleges, the chief obstacles were the lethargy and inconsistency of state authorities, a severe lack of support from the medical profession, dire working conditions in the hospitals, conflict with diploma-trained nurses and matrons who opposed degree education and difficulty in establishing public health practice fields. Degree education created a strange duality. On the one hand, the BSc nurse's education promoted principles of autonomy and decision-making, expressed the importance of rich scientific and sociological knowledge, presented a vision of the nurse as a member of a 'health team' with a right to consultation and inclusion in her work environment, and suggested that the nurse could perform a meaningful role in community health. On the other

---

[48] Julien, 'Case History on Nursing', p. 21.

hand, the experience of clinical nursing on the hospital ward was entirely different: doctors were dominant, nurses were not consulted and there was little respect from patients or staff for them, regardless of their qualification. Not surprisingly, few BSc nurses stayed long on the wards, the majority quickly able to secure teaching or administrative posts removed from grim hospital conditions. Due to the ubiquitous scarcity of trained leaders, they were easily able to find such positions, with minimal clinical experience.[49] This entrenched an enduring problem in Indian nursing: the elevation of administration and teaching positions over bedside and practical nursing.[50] International nurses' emphasis on advanced education for a minority of nurses continually collided with the wider, systemic problems that they often elected not to address in their programmes. Creating an effective and high quality system of degree education that incorporated good clinical training was virtually impossible in the context in which they worked. Instead, what was constructed functioned more as a pathway out of clinical nursing, an outcome unlikely to address the serious and persistent problems of the majority of nurses. The leaders prepared by elite degree programmes often had comparatively little clinical experience and, predictably, a gulf later formed between leaders and working nurses. As Chapter 4 highlights, a leadership schooled in Western-style professionalism with relatively little experience of the grind of everyday ward-work was neither very representative nor very effective.

International nurses working on degree education projects struggled not just with this demanding practical context, but also with the difficulty of understanding the cultural context in which they worked. Intensely frustrated by the complexity of their new surroundings

---

[49] In 1961, the then CMC Director, Dr John Carman wrote of the difficulty even at CMC of finding sufficient teachers and administrators, due to 'the large demand for our graduates to go to the many new hospitals and schools of nursing which have been growing up in this state and all over India' (John Carman to Joyce Miller, 24 June 1961, CMC Archives, CMC-D/24/58, Box 18, Director's Office File, Folder 'Nursing Staff, Correspondence, 1958–1965'). See also Adranvala, 'A Review of Training of Nurses', p. 248.

[50] For discussion of the elevation of teaching and administration over bedside nursing, see Anonymous, 'Graduate Nurses', *NJI*, vol. 59, no. 6, 1968, pp. 179–81; Adranvala, 'Developments in Nursing 1947–57', p. 327; Harji Malik, 'Planning for Nursing Services — A Must: A Report on a Workshop', *NJI*, vol. 59, no. 7, 1968, pp. 206–7, 226.

and clinging strongly to the American system as a template, their programmes were at times characterised by a strong disdain for the local. The Indian nursing system was regarded almost as a blank canvas upon which not only models of better nursing, but also better womanhood, could be constructed. In a manner remarkably similar to and often less sympathetic than that of the pre-Independence mission nurses, much that was Indian was denigrated. Julien wrote in 1963:

> It appears to be a general fundamental trait within Moslem and Hindu groups that service to other human beings is not a personal responsibility. There is little if any of the 'good Samaritan' concept. This is a serious deficiency in the medical and nursing profession where the primary incentive for entering should be service to others . . . In India a physician will pass by a patient who appears to be in a hopeless condition, with no effort to do all in his power to save that patient . . . There seems to be a tragic lack of responsibility by both professions toward saving the lives of their fellow men.[51]

It was often implied that Indian women lacked strength of character. Loewus, one of the USAID nurses posted in Hyderabad, commented in 1963 that the Indian graduates sent from Vellore and Delhi to staff the new college of nursing were socially inadequate and struggled to interact with other staff. They had 'a limited capacity for self-direction', 'no understanding of psycho-social matters', minimal 'insight into human behavior', and could not successfully cope with problems. She went on, 'another factor in the nurse personality deficiency of faculty members was a considerable level of selfishness and ego-centeredness'.[52] USAID nurses planned to correct these traits through a programme of intensive re-education in workplace relations, designed to impart the assertiveness and team spirit that they associated with Western nurses. The Indian educational system was thus imbued in its early years with a pervasively outward focus, presenting the West as the site of better social relations as well as of better professional practice. As was characteristic of many programmes of development, the objects of international

---

[51] Julien, 'Case History on Nursing', p. 22.
[52] Gentry, 'Nursing Education and Nursing Care'.

nursing projects were forced to remake their social relations 'in order to enter the promised new world'.[53]

Although degree education programmes were purportedly designed to prepare Indian leaders, nurse advisors struggled to interact with the few existing Indian leaders on equal terms. The outstanding Indian nurse of this period was Adranvala, first Indian president of the TNAI, ICN vice-president, and nursing advisor to the government from 1948–66. Adranvala was generally very supportive of professionalism, but she also voiced the opinion that the international organisations paid insufficient attention to living and working conditions for students, focusing too exclusively on curriculum.[54] This was interpreted as aggressive professional competitiveness, and Julien retaliated with the accusation that Adranvala had routinely stolen USAID nurses' ideas and presented them as her own. Julien was quick to present conflict with Adranvala in terms of essentialised racial characteristics: the finale of her lengthy 1963 report on USAID nursing programmes involved a comparison of American nurses' 'know-how' and ability to get things done to Adranvala's weakness and inability to forcefully attack problems. It was clear that the policy of encouraging Indian leadership had its limits, and that conflict could arise when implicit hierarchies of race and culture were challenged. The 'alliance strategy' that Ann Yrjala describes as definitive of Rockefeller's nursing work in Finland in the 1920s and 1930s — in which Finnish and Rockefeller nurses 'shared a professional project' and had 'common visions' which they worked harmoniously to achieve — seemed missing in such interactions.[55]

## 'We need a great family of public health nurses in India'

The second platform of international nursing projects was the promotion of nurses' involvement in public health. This arose from an increasing awareness that the major health problems for the new nation mainly centred on the large, poor and ill-educated rural population. In 1953, Tennant wrote that 'if all Indian hospitals were closed, it would have little effect on the health situation in India,

---

[53] Rist, *The History of Development*, p. 2.
[54] Julien, 'Case History on Nursing', p. 24.
[55] Yrjala, *Public Health and Rockefeller Wealth*, p. 163.

because preventive measures are so needed in that country'.[56] There was thus a feeling that if nurses were to play a role in improving the national health profile they would need to move outside hospital walls and create a nurse role at the primary health care level. Also, the international nurses had come from the American system, in which a strong role in public health had been crucial in the development of nursing autonomy and professionalism.[57] They felt pride in and commitment to a system in which nurses played important health roles outside the hospital environment and hoped that this could be reproduced in India. Julien wrote in 1964 that American nurse expertise had been highly valued in India because 'our country has taken a leading role in the world in . . . the techniques of incorporating subjects such as public health in the nursing education'.[58] Corwin wrote in 1945 of the complete absence of public health nursing in India and felt that this was clearly linked to the failure to make headway in 'establishing or recognising nursing as a profession'.[59] The organisations for which they worked in general heavily emphasised public health as an important dimension of their nursing work. As Yrjala documents, for example, the Rockefeller Foundation vigorously promoted the professionalisation of public health nursing in both the US and numerous other countries, in harmony with the similar focus of the WHO.[60]

Creating a tradition of public health nursing in India was an ambitious goal, given that in 1947 there were fewer than a dozen nurses

---

[56] Mary Elizabeth Tennant to Elizabeth W. Brackett, 10 December 1953, RF, Series 2.1 (Post-war Correspondence), RG 6.1, Box 44, Folder 403, 'DMPH India, Nursing'.

[57] For accounts of this, see Melosh, *The Physician's Hand*; Karen Buhler-Wilkerson, *No Place like Home: A History of Nursing and Home Care in the United States*, Baltimore: Johns Hopkins University Press, 2001; Celia Davies, 'A Constant Casualty: Nurse Education in Britain and the USA to 1939', in Celia Davies (ed.), *Rewriting Nursing History*, pp. 102–22; Kalisch and Kalisch, *The Advance of American Nursing*.

[58] Juliette M. Julien to Richard C. Parsons, 'Nursing College Development Project, India', 6 November 1962, NARA, Box 157, Folder 'HLS 1-2 Nursing Schools (General)'.

[59] Anonymous, 'Public Health Education, Schools of Nursing, Far East, India and Ceylon: Developmental Aid to Nursing Education', 26 October 1945, RF, RG 1.1, Series 464 C, Folder 82, 'Developmental Aid (Nursing Education) 1945–1949'.

[60] Yrjala, *Public Health and Rockefeller Wealth*, pp. 3, 11.

in India with a public health qualification.[61] Significant effort and funding were thus put into to the difficult project of institutional-ising public health nursing programmes. International organisations provided targeted scholarships for Indian nurses to take public health nursing courses overseas, and attempts were made to develop a community health curriculum at the colleges of nursing in Delhi and Vellore. A post-basic course in public health nursing was begun at the Delhi College of Nursing in 1952; it moved out of direct nurse control in 1953, when it was transferred to the All India Institute of Hygiene and Public Health in Calcutta. International nurses were strongly involved in the development of the course of study at the Institute. Evelyn Davis, posted there by the WHO, wrote in 1953 that 'we need a great family of Public Health Nurses in India'.[62] In 1954, she supervised the instruction of 10 graduates, most from Bombay and Calcutta, with two Thai students. She felt that their 14 weeks of field training had helped them to 'gain a new respect and understanding of the family and its many social and health problems'.[63] In 1953, the WHO began a nursing project in Bombay, Calcutta and Hyderabad, as part of which a public health nursing specialist was sent to develop public health training for Indian nurs-ing students. As was usual in WHO projects, each of these nurses worked intensively with a specific Indian counterpart.[64] When the Shetty Committee of 1954 recommended the nationwide incorpora-tion of public health nursing into the undergraduate curriculum, the international organisations provided advice to schools and colleges on how to implement the new policy.[65]

International nurses felt that Indian women would be willing to take up public health nursing if they could be educated in its social role and philosophy during their training, so they set about institu-tionalising such a focus. They however neglected to address the enormous social constraints that limited the involvement of the nurse in work outside the hospital system. Davis wrote of her students'

---

[61] Adranvala, 'Developments in Nursing 1947–57', p. 328.

[62] Evelyn Davis, 'The First Public Health Course', *NJI*, vol. 44, no. 8, 1953, p. 197.

[63] Evelyn Davis, 'Ready to Begin', *NJI*, vol. 45, no. 7, 1954, p. 14.

[64] Brackett's diary, p. 54.

[65] Saroj Khaparde (Minister of State for Health and Family Welfare), 'Meeting the Needs of the Community', *Social Welfare*, vol. 35, no. 10, 1989, p. 6.

fieldwork as a thrilling adventure. She commented of their time in a Bengali village that it was

> a new World for most of the students; not like any hospital, town or city they had ever lived in. There were no electric lights or water taps and they had to adjust to the dust, and the many housekeeping problems.[66]

This was essentially the problem when it came to encouraging nurses to work outside the hospital system. Relatively protected women, they were not able to work easily or safely in remote villages without amenities, and there were no salary or promotional incentives to persuade them to do so.

It became clear that the theory and teaching methods associated with American public health nursing were inadequate in the Indian context. An Indian nurse academic working in the US, Amaravathy Bachu, in 1970 identified some of the reasons for the foundering of public health nursing in India over the preceding decades. She wrote that 'in spite of having up-to-date knowledge and skills' the Indian public health nurse would often feel 'hopeless, dejected, disappointed and defeated'. This was due to a range of difficulties, including the lack of transport and infrastructure that might allow public health nurses to travel safely outside cities, the absence of resources needed to fund public health projects and a general societal perception that 'the woman's place is in the home', meaning the public health nurse experienced stern moral disapproval, harassment and even violent attack.[67]

The generally troubled state of public health nursing was graphically illustrated to the USAID nurses when in 1961 they sponsored a promotional film to be used for recruitment purposes. At Adranvala's suggestion, the film was to have focused on nurses working in public health in the Bombay area. This plan failed, however, because interviews on the field at the unit selected for the film revealed public health nursing to be a manifest disaster, with unhappy nurses unable to articulate any coherent opinion about the meaning of public health. The film's director, Miriam Bucher of Art Films of Asia, commented

---

[66] Davis, 'Ready to Begin', p. 14.
[67] Amaravathy Bachu, 'Public Health Nursing: How They Are Different in the United States', *NJI*, vol. 61, no. 11, 1970, p. 361, p. 373.

on 'the failure of public health nursing programs' and the 'maladjustment of the young nurses'. The initial film was scratched and the project reconceived as a study of nursing at the JJ Hospital in Bombay. Bucher asked pointedly whether she needed to remove all reference to public health nursing from the new film, *The Call*, given that the desired effect was a film that 'glorifies nursing'.[68]

The establishment of a role for trained nurses in public health was perhaps too ambitious a task to be achieved at this stage. It would have required overcoming the limits of poor infrastructure, providing financial incentives for nurses to work in rural areas and educating the public on the role of the trained nurse. The complex nature of such a task unsurprisingly defeated the international advisors' approach. Their promotion of public health, however, ultimately contributed to a conflicted occupational culture, in which community health is emphasised by leaders and in nursing curricula, while in practice nurses play only a limited role in the national public health system.

## International education programmes for Indian nurses

The third pillar of international nursing work was the policy of sending Indian nurses to the West to take postgraduate courses, chiefly in education, public health and administration. As with the other international nursing programmes, this policy involved the injection of large quantities of funds into the preparation of an elite minority, with a trickle-down effect that never really turned into the hoped-for torrent. The programme was designed so that Indian nurses sent overseas would return and contribute to the improvement of local nurse education and practice. Narender Nagpal, a former TNAI president, described the years from the late 1940s to 1970 as a period of 'renaissance' for Indian nursing, with WHO, the United Nations' Children's Fund (UNICEF), USAID, and the Colombo Plan all providing funding for education abroad.[69] During 1949 and 1950, the WHO awarded 71 fellowships in the Southeast Asia region, of

[68] Miriam Bucher to Robert R. Blake, 20 May 1961, NARA, Box 157, Folder 'HLS 1-2 Nursing Schools (General)'.

[69] Narender Nagpal, 'Development of Nursing and Health Care: 1947–2000', in *History and Trends in Nursing in India*, Delhi: TNAI, 2001, pp. 96–97.

which 34 went to Indians.[70] In 1959, Rockefeller gave two nursing fellowships and the Colombo Plan sent 29 nurses abroad for higher training.[71] In 1961, USAID had seven students studying on fellowships in North America, at a total cost of US\$ 60,000.[72] In 1962, 45 nurses were sent for training in public health in the United States by USAID. Between 1959 and 1961, the WHO gave nine fellowships to Indian nurses.

Given the size of the Indian population, these were small numbers. Nevertheless, the impact of the programmes was large because, as was the plan, most returnees went on to play important leadership roles. The majority of eminent post-Independence Indian leaders received some form of sponsorship for study abroad, and until at least the 1980s, time spent overseas was viewed as an essential component of a leader's resume. In 1972, for example, out of 11 candidates nominated for election as TNAI officers for Maharashtra, nine had an international qualification.[73] International nurse education programmes ensured successful and influential careers for their participants, who rendered valuable professional service in the Indian health system. Mehra Doctor, sponsored by UNICEF for a study programme in New Zealand, became the first Indian nursing superintendent in Bombay. According to Brackett, she was able to raise the minimum standards set by the Bombay Nursing Council for teacher qualifications, syllabus content and nurse–patient ratios.[74] International organisations collectively groomed a new professional leadership for nursing in Kerala — Lucy Peters, C. Chandramathy, C. Chandrakanthi, and Chellamma George all returned from fellowships to play a major role in establishing professional education in the state.[75] Aleyamma Kuruvilla, whose career has been described earlier, emerged after her time abroad as one of the most influential post-Independence leaders.

---

[70] Anonymous, 'WHO Fellowships', *NJI*, vol. 42, no. 4, 1951, p. 125.

[71] Julien, 'Case History on Nursing', p. 9.

[72] Anonymous, Office Memo, 29 April 1961, 'General Nursing Project — Participants cost', NARA, Box 159, Folder 'General Nursing — General Participants, FY 61'.

[73] Anonymous, 'Candidates for TNAI Elections October 1972 — Bombay', *NJI*, vol. 63, no. 9, 1972, pp. 317–19.

[74] Brackett's diary, pp. 55–56.

[75] Abraham, *Nursing History in South India*, p. 107; author interview with Professor C. Chandrakanthi, Thiruvananthapuram, 4 December 2005.

Overseas education for Indian nurses exposed them to the most contemporary Western thinking about public health, education and specialised nursing. It imparted some of the skills and the confidence needed to the large percentage of candidates who returned to India to take up positions of responsibility in very new institutions. It is questionable, however, to what extent overseas programmes were tailored to provide training that could easily and usefully be applied to the Indian context. Fellows of the various programmes experienced considerable problems of adjustment when they returned to India. They were often full of enthusiasm about the task of setting up independent and autonomous nursing schools and promoting better standards in nurse education. They faced an inflexible, often unsympathetic medical profession, as well as a set of colleagues unfamiliar with their new ideas about nursing. They could thus become isolated and lonely. Daisy Charles, a US-trained Rockefeller beneficiary, returned to Mysore in south India in 1949 in an attempt to develop public health nursing. She left in disgust after a couple of years of frustrating inaction due to conflict with local bureaucrats, returning to the safer and more sympathetic environs of the College of Nursing in Delhi. Marshall C. Balfour, assistant director at Rockefeller's Division of Medicine and Public Health, reported that local doctors felt that she had returned from her fellowship inclined to complain frequently and displaying 'a superior air'. Balfour felt that fellows needed to be made aware that their study abroad did not 'automatically transplant them to a position of respect and equality'.[76] As Kavadi records, Richmond Anderson, field director in India, questioned the value of fellowship programmes for nurses. He commented in 1948 of returning graduates: 'Training abroad appears to have given these nurses a belief they can speak with authority plus a zeal to put their American type of nursing into effect more rapidly than local conditions will permit, leading to frustration and antagonism'.[77] There was a common and rather unpleasant sentiment that fellows returning to India were likely to think rather too much of themselves and their position in health hierarchies. As individuals, they were frequently not in a position to achieve the kind of sweeping professional change their overseas tutors had envisaged.

---

[76] Extract from the diary of Marshall C. Balfour, 1949, RF, RG2, Series 464C, Box 461, Folder 3094.

[77] Quoted in Kavadi, *The Rockefeller Foundation and Public Health*, p. 133.

It is also questionable to what extent Western nursing, public health and educational knowledge were straightforwardly transferable to the Indian context. Fellows of USAID programmes struggled with the requirement to write detailed reports about the possible application of their expensive American education to the hospitals, schools and clinics to which they returned. While letters from fellows abroad frequently mentioned that their study programme and the associated travel had expanded their horizons and developed their confidence, they spent little time writing of radical challenges to their ideas about nursing itself. Annamma K. M., a CMC Vellore graduate sponsored for study in Australia in 1963, wrote honestly about finding little to learn in Melbourne hospitals, given that the patient load was so much smaller and so different from what she had worked with at home. She wrote that 'I haven't learned much from the nursing point of view. I don't think I can learn anything more ... I haven't seen a busy hospital like CMC'.[78]

The sponsorship of nurses for education in the West was a policy implemented in numerous developing countries during this period. In 1959, the WHO held a conference on the design of Western programmes for developing world nurses, motivated by the many problems that had arisen in the delivery of such programmes. In the American nursing schools, to which many fellows were sent, it was pointed out that the faculty needed to be better prepared, because overseas nurses had proven to need 'about three times more faculty time than the national students'.[79] It was suggested that fellows were being prepared for positions that did not exist in their home countries and that participants and home employers held different understandings of the purpose and content of overseas education. In many cases, fellows became frustrated on their return by the relative scarcity of resources and lack of time to spend caring for individual patients. The report concluded with the statement that 'in view of the readjustment difficulties which face many returning students more thought and planning might be needed'.[80] It is clear that graduates

---

[78] Annamma K. M. to Sister Jacob, 24 October 1963, CMC Archives, CMC-D/24/58, Box 18, Director's Office File, folder 'Nursing Staff, Correspondence, 1958–1965'.

[79] WHO, 'Postbasic Nursing Education Programmes for Foreign Students: Report of a Conference, Geneva, 5–14 October 1959', World Health Organization Technical Reports Series 199, Geneva: WHO, 1960, p. 11.

[80] Ibid., pp. 37–39.

of international education programmes, in India and elsewhere, struggled with the task of transferring Western nursing knowledge into a very different local socio-economic health environment. As with in-country degree programmes, there was an implicit desire to demonstrate the superiority of Western social and gender relations through international education, with the assumption that Indian women would be empowered by life abroad. Witnessing interactions between Western nurses and the medical profession would, it was felt, impart to Indian nurses the confidence to reorder the Indian medical workplace according to the vision of Western professionalisers. Comments about potential overseas scholarship applicants frequently specified that they must be exposed to administrative forums so that they could witness American nurses interacting with the medical profession, displaying instructive professional and personal assertiveness.[81] The WHO study discussed earlier pointed out that on her return a student might find difficulties stemming from the fact that her home country accorded 'a less gratifying status to women' than did the United States. Ideally, however, her American education would have provided an understanding of the 'evolution of cultural change' that would equip her with patience in handling her fellow nationals. The end of the report suggested the need for an evaluation of the policy of overseas education for nurses, in which one of the main questions was to be whether there had been 'any effect on the wide-range problems associated with status, including the role of women in public life?'[82] It was clearly felt that promoting professionalism in India would require challenging local gender roles, a challenge that was felt could partially be achieved by providing nurses with a year or two of exposure to Western health systems and Western society.

## Different Approaches

A minority of international nursing programmes took different approaches, with a less ambitious focus and a less pronounced commitment to replicating Western-style professionalism. In 1964,

---

[81] See, for example, 'Project Implementation Order', 17 April 1961, NARA, Box 159, Folder, 'Miss V. Purushotham — Indore — General Nursing FY 61'; and 'Project Implementation Order', 17 April 1961, NARA, Box 159, Folder 'Miss M. Sosamma — Indore — General Nursing FY 61'.

[82] WHO, 'Postbasic Nursing Education Programmes', pp. 37–45.

for example, Katherine Feisel, a WHO nurse educator, launched the project of an independent nursing school for the state of Goa. She ensured that the project was administered by the Directorate of Health Services and was not allied to any one hospital, reserved Sundays and public holidays as free days and made a rule that the entire student body was to be present on campus between three and six in the afternoon every day. In 1971, Sister Delphine, a local nurse educator, described the programme as highly successful — students had time to study, their results were excellent, there were better than usual relations between patients and students and the students were happy.[83] The success of this programme seemed to lie in the strong and direct identification of main local obstacles — the likelihood that hospital administrations would sabotage educational objectives, the tendency for students to be radically overworked — and a willingness to confine the programme to realistic goals, delivering a high quality general nursing education rather than attempting the vastly more complicated and ambitious project of setting up a degree school. Sister Delphine in 1971 recognised that 'the desire for college study is the craze of today's youth; if it is true that we are shaped by our environment we cannot deny that nurses also have this in-born desire of being called a College Graduate'.[84] She felt that a transition to degree programmes was thus inevitable, but proudly held up the independent school of nursing project in Goa as an example of the excellence that could be achieved in non-degree schools.

Similarly, Rockefeller assistance to the school of nursing in Trivandrum was shaped by a more realistic assessment of potential local achievements. In 1952, Rockefeller assigned Lillian Johnson to assist with upgrading the Trivandrum School of Nursing, which had until then been run by Swiss nuns who had taught only a basic nursing course. Johnson seemed to deal capably and happily with the local medical profession, a skill less common among the nurses working on degree programmes. Encountering the belief of the medical superintendent of the new medical college hospital that the roles of nursing school principal and hospital nursing superintendent could

---

[83] Sister Delphine, untitled paper given at a conference on nursing education in Chandigarh, April 1971, *NJI*, vol. 62, no. 6, 1971, p. 193.
[84] Ibid., p. 193.

economically be combined (because all the superintendent had to do, he felt, was take a morning roll-call), she discussed the issue with him and carefully prepared a paper that described in detail the role and responsibilities of the different roles.[85] Johnson also focused very strongly on the need to address hospital administration. In 1953, she wrote to Robert Watson, Rockefeller's director for the Far East, that it was not the content of nurses' education that was the main problem for nursing in Trivandrum, but the 'complete lack of organisation in the whole set up in relation to the care of patients'. Accordingly she set about improving basic conditions in the Trivandrum General Hospital.[86] Work at the Trivandrum School of Nursing was viewed as very successful; in 1955 the Government of Travancore-Cochin requested that Rockefeller extend Johnson's posting. The request was signed by the Surgeon General V. R. Narayanan Nair, and the Director of the General Hospital R. T. Kesavan Nair.[87] In 1976, Lucy Peters, the Kerala nurse who became the principal of the school of nursing at the end of Johnson's time in Trivandrum, remembered Johnson's work as an important contribution to the raising of standards in Kerala.[88] Support for better standards at the school of nursing seemed to lay appropriate grounds for the later founding of the BSc in Nursing in Trivandrum in 1972. In 1955, a Rockefeller memo recorded that Trivandrum represented 'a good opportunity to make some fundamental improvements in the teaching of nursing in India within the confines of a hospital nursing school'.[89] It seemed that if the other projects had been similarly guided by such realistic appraisals of existing needs rather than by ambitious plans for development along professionalising lines, the international aid investment might have proved more productive.

---

[85] Lillian Johnson to Mary Elizabeth Tennant, 15 February 1954, Series 2.1 (Postwar Correspondence), R.G. 6.1 (Paris Field Office), Box 44, Folder 402, 'DMPH India, Lillian Johnson, 1952–54'.

[86] Lillian Johnson to Robert Watson, 23 January 1953, RF, RG 2 (1953), Series 100, Box 4, Folder 22 (Lillian Johnson).

[87] Memorandum by Mary Elizabeth Tennant, 5 January 1955, RF, RG 2 (1955), Series 100, Box 6, Folder 40.

[88] Lucy Peters, 'Nursing Education in Kerala', in *A Quarter Century of Caring: Medical College Trivandrum, 1951–76*, Trivandrum: Medical College Trivandrum, 1976.

[89] 'Grant in Aid for the Purchase of Equipment and Supplies, in Addition to those Provided Under Ga-Mph 5343, Needed by Miss Lillian Johnson, Temporary Employee

# Conclusions

International nurse advisors during the 1950s and 1960s sought to recreate in India the pillars of the system that they considered had brought status, fulfilment and increased autonomy to nurses in their home countries. They provided considerable assistance in the establishment of university-based colleges of nursing, which they hoped would provide generations of confident, skilled Indian leaders. Promising Indian nurses were sponsored for education abroad and returned as committed as their teachers to professionalism in nursing. Vigorous attempts were made to institutionalise a focus on public health work for nurses, in the hope that this would ensure a sphere of more autonomous nursing work, as had happened at home, and that nurses would find ongoing relevance in a new nation that was struggling with massive rural health problems.

The results of their projects were not what nurse advisors optimistically envisaged. Execution of all these projects encountered serious difficulties. Hostility from the medical profession, lack of practical state support, opposition from nursing staff in the hospitals, and incomplete understanding of the local socio-cultural context, all restricted the extent to which international nurses were able to encourage high quality education and practice through their programmes. Rather than addressing these issues of conditions and context, however, a strong focus was maintained on improving nurses themselves. It was felt that well-educated confident nurses would be the source of a 'trickle-down effect', improving standards of practice among their colleagues, and that this would inevitably effect a transition in negative state and societal attitudes toward nursing.

It may be suggested that the strong and sustained focus on professionalisation, promoted so enthusiastically by international nurses, was not the most effective path to have taken in the Indian context. Given the troubles that constantly attended international professionalising projects, this focus might sensibly have been adapted or revised, so as to extend the benefits of overseas funds and expertise to a larger number of nurses, or to attempt a more sustained assault on

---

of DMPH in Connection with her Assignment to the School of Nursing in Trivandrum, India', RF, RG1.2, Series 464C, Box 53, Folder 493, 'India, Trivandrum School of Nursing, Equipment, 1953–1958'.

poor living and working conditions. The professionalising approach, however, unsurprisingly came to occupy a central place in Indian nursing culture. Indian leaders modelled their organisations and plans for professional development on those that Western leaders had promoted so vigorously. The result, as Chapter 4 will show, was a professional leadership that struggled to meet the challenges of the local health environment and to engage successfully with the state.

# Nursing the Community
## Evelyn Khannan

EVELYN KHANNAN is Assistant Secretary at the TNAI headquarters in Delhi. When I met her in January 2006, she spoke knowledgeably and comprehensively of plans to expand the organisation's capacity for advanced education and of its role in creating and maintaining a professional community in India.

She commented with evident sadness on the inadequacy of accommodation for India's nurses, the low salaries they received and their unscrupulous treatment in many private hospitals. At the same time, although she felt there were many problems with so many nurses leaving India, she thought that rapidly expanding opportunities for nurse emigration had raised the social status of the profession and brought greater assertiveness to the student body.

At one point in the interview, a nurse interrupted us with a letter for Khannan to sign. It was explained to me that this nurse had upgraded her diploma to a BSc (nursing) degree, but had been refused the pay rise it mandated. The TNAI had helped her to write an initial letter of protest, to which the Medical Superintendent of the hospital had replied 'we don't need BSc nurses', suggesting that she should resign. Khannan expressed the feeling that this reflected a widespread lack of support from the medical profession.

The topic of greatest interest for Khannan, however, was that of community health. She was the daughter of a Christian family; both her parents were teachers, who, she emphasised, had 'strong values of compassion'. Her father had run welfare projects in the small village in which they lived. Her career in community health nursing practice had allowed her to practise this central family ethos of social service.

She had taken her GNM course at the Christian Fellowship Hospital in Oddanchatram, Tamil Nadu, after that a post-certificate course in community health nursing at CMC Vellore, and then a post-basic BSc in Nursing from the Indira Gandhi National Open University. She had 15 years' experience in teaching community health. She described preventive public health work as the most interesting job a nurse could do, requiring a much broader knowledge than other fields of nursing. She emphasised, however, that the community health nurse needed enormous commitment, because the success of her work depended on living in villages so as to truly understand the issues of village life. As an example, she told me the story of an NGO which had sent her clinic an expensive refrigerator, which then sat unused in a corner because the village had no reliable source of electricity.

Sadly, she told me that there was no infrastructure to allow those other than the passionately motivated to work in rural health, and most nurses, she felt, preferred towns. Nursing education gave the students a good theoretical grounding in public health work, but not an awareness of the realities of rural communities and their needs.

Khannan gave up her work in community health only when her husband, who worked for the Planning Commission, unexpectedly died at a young age, leaving her with two children to raise alone. The job with the TNAI clearly represented a source of security. Somewhat forlornly, however, she wondered if her work as a leader in Delhi would bring the same benefits to the nation as her work in the villages of Tamil Nadu.

◼

# 4

# From Green Park
# to Bollywood

## The Development of
## Nursing Organisation, 1947–2006

▣

This chapter describes the Indian leadership that emerged from the projects of professional development described in Chapters 2 and 3. I trace the culture of early organisation, suggesting that it was heavily determined by nursing's colonial and Western heritage and little suited to mobilising the growing ranks of Indian nurses. The TNAI, the INC and the Christian nursing organisations remained substantially wedded to a professionalising agenda based around the identity of nursing as an international sisterhood and the lifting of standards in education. This agenda, however, found little resonance with a constituency struggling to care for patients in understaffed wards, to sleep in dangerous and dilapidated accommodation and to keep themselves physically safe in hospitals. Dissatisfaction with organisational culture was evident even in the early post-Independence years and reached critical levels by the late 1970s. Ultimately, this dissatisfaction combined with a new, more gender-sensitive social and political environment to produce more militant and creative experiments in organisation. Conditions for nurses remain woeful and organisations still struggle to exact small concessions from an obdurate state, but these new trends at least suggested a new and more locally grounded generation of nursing leadership.

# The Persistence of
# Poor Working Conditions

The central challenge facing the Indian leadership from Independence through to the present day has been poor working conditions. Hospital administrators faced with scarce resources have consistently economised by reducing numbers of nurses employed, making the maximum possible use of student labour and spending little on salaries and benefits for nurses. Although the severity of poor working conditions has lessened in some parts of India over this period, in general the same problems have been repeatedly identified. In 1952, a USAID nurse described 'deplorable living conditions in nurses' hostels; poor quality and insufficient food . . . gross lack of equipment in hospitals . . . overcrowding and unsanitary conditions in hospitals . . . Long working hours and extremely low salaries'.[1]

In 1957 Rajkumari Amrit Kaur, the first health minister of independent India and a woman highly sympathetic to the problems of nurses, lamented the fact that nurse trainees in hospitals were treated as 'sweated labour'.[2] In 1958, Adranvala listed some of the problems the profession faced — the exploitation of students as cheap labour, the failure to provide adequate accommodation, the lack of safe transport facilities, and the gross understaffing of wards.[3] In 1963, Juliette Julien recorded that in an average week, student nurses worked between 52 and 64 hours on day duty and between 72 and 84 hours on night duty, which rendered them 'physically incapable of studying'.[4] In 1973, an SNA meeting proposed that student nurses' 'clinical experience' should be limited to 48 hours per week.[5] In 1982, T. Stephens, touring north Indian hospitals as TNAI secretary, discovered that nursing students at a hospital in Kanpur (which he considered typical of the Uttar Pradesh hospitals he visited) worked consecutive 12-hour night shifts for an entire month, during which

---

[1] Julien, 'Case History on Nursing', p. 3.

[2] 'The Indian Nursing Council (Amendment) Bill, 1957', in Rajkumari Amrit Kaur, *Rajkumari Amrit Kaur*, New Delhi: Lok Sabha Secretariat, 1992, p. 214.

[3] T. K. Adranvala, 'Developments in Nursing 1947–57', pp. 326–28, 334.

[4] Julien, 'Case History on Nursing', p. 3.

[5] Anonymous, 'Business Session: Problems of Student Nurses', *NJI*, vol. 64, no. 12, 1973, p. 412.

time they were left in sole charge of two large wards. In the BHW Hospital in Bareilly, 166 students shared a single classroom with 14 desks.[6] Even by the 1990s, it seemed that radical change had not ensued. Nirmala Mehan, J. P. Gupta, and R. S. Gupta wrote in 1992 that nursing schools still generally regarded their students as a 'source of cheap labour'.[7] Many of India's private hospitals continue to practise the exhausting double-shift system (in which nurses work 12-hour day or night shifts rather than three eight-hour day, evening and night shifts) that was rejected by the ICN in the 1920s.

Throughout India, understaffing, inadequate accommodation and overcrowding remain issues for most hospitals. In Delhi, union leaders and TNAI representatives concurred in estimating that in most of the city's hospitals the nurse to patient ratio was one to 50 or 60. During night shifts, this could rise as high as one to 80 or 90.[8] Estimates for Thiruvananthapuram given by the nurses I interviewed there were similar. To put such figures in context, an ICN fact sheet states that the optimal ratio is one nurse to four patients. Research showed that if this increased to one to six, patients were 14 per cent more likely to die within 30 days of admission. If it rose to one to eight, there was a 31 per cent increase in mortality.[9]

Nurses have not found protection from violence against women in their workplaces. They have worked without even basic guarantees of personal safety and, moreover, have watched as the perpetrators of attacks against their colleagues have gone unpunished, while the victims' careers have been ended by the stigma attached to rape. Frequent understaffing (often determined by a desire to economise, rather than by shortages) has not only resulted in lower standards of care, but in a working environment characterised by danger for the nurse, who is often the sole female employee on the ward. Patients and relatives have frequently harassed nurses, who have also been

---

[6] T. Stephens, 'TNAI in Uttar Pradesh', *NJI*, vol. 73, no. 8, 1982, pp. 216–17.

[7] Nirmala Mehan, J. P. Gupta and R. S. Gupta, 'Development of Nursing Education in India', *Health and Population*, vol. 15, nos. 3–4, 1992, p. 130.

[8] Author interview Mrs G. K. Khurana, All India Government Nurses' Federation, 6 February 2006; author interview with Evelyn Khannan, assistant secretary at the TNAI, 27 January 2006; author interview with Nanthini Subbiah, Deputy Secretary General at the TNAI, 27 January 2006.

[9] International Council of Nurses (ICN), 'Nurse: Patient Ratios', Nursing Matters Fact Sheets, 2003, http://www.icn.ch/matters_rnptratio_print.htm (accessed 21 September 2006).

viciously attacked by fellow hospital employees.[10] In 2004, a Delhi ward nurse spoke at a public meeting of the recurrent harassment of nurses by relatives and staff. She said that Class IV employees (usually ward servants and cleaners) and security guards frequently reported to work 'in a drunken state' and posed considerable danger to night nurses, who were often posted on wards alone.[11]

There have been numerous documented cases of rape of nurses. In Mumbai, the particularly violent rape of a nurse in November 1973 drew significant public attention and was the subject of a book by a local journalist, Pinki Virani.[12] The nurse was attacked at King Edward Memorial Hospital (KEM) by a ward boy, Sohanlal Bhartha Walmiki, who was not tried for rape because no one was willing to act as the complainant in the case (Aruna Shanbaug, the victim, currently remains comatose due to the effects of the brutal attack). He was imprisoned only on charges of assault and was freed after seven years. KEM nurses, who held the first strike in the hospital's history after the attack, demanded the employment of new, better-trained security guards, better discipline of ward boys and lighting in all areas of the hospital.[13]

Public health nurses, ANMs and staff nurses working in isolated areas in the primary health system have also worked without basic guarantees of safety. In 1972, a Bombay public health nurse spoke at a seminar of frequent cases of rape and molestation of public health nurses in the villages and recounted the story of a widowed nurse

---

[10] Sapna Dogra, 'Delhi has a long way to go in ensuring security of nurses', *Express Healthcare Management*, 16–31 January 2004, http://www.expresshealthcaremgmt.com/20040131/nursingspecial02.shtml (accessed 9 July 2004). See also this account of violence against nurses over 1986–87: Anonymous, 'Victims of Male Aggression', *Hindustan Times*, 11 January 1987, Sunday Magazine, p. 7.

[11] Anonymous, 'Florence Nightingale Anniversary: Nurses Air their Grievances', *The Tribune*, Chandigarh, 13 May 2004, http://www.tribuneindia.com/2004/20040513/ncr3.htm (accessed 14 April 2012). 'Class IV' refers to the pay scales for employees of the government.

[12] Pinki Virani, *Aruna's Story: The True Account of a Rape and its Aftermath*, New Delhi: Viking, 1998.

[13] Virani, *Aruna's Story*, pp. 29, 38. The Supreme Court of India recently rejected a case brought by Virani, a journalist and friend of Aruna Shanbaug, to allow euthanasia for Shanbaug. The nurses who continue to care for Shanbaug welcomed the verdict ('Rebirth for Aruna, say joyous Mumbai hospital staff', *Deccan Herald*, 7 March 2011, http://www.deccanherald.com/content/143798/rebirth-aruna-say-joyous-mumbai.html [accessed 25 February 2012]).

who had been constantly harassed, until she moved to a different village. There she took to wearing 'man's attire' to prevent attack.[14] In the same year, the TNAI reported that 'the nurses posted in villages are exposed to dangers for want of personal security threatening the chastity of the traditional Indian woman and the honour of the nursing profession'.[15] A 2005 survey of conditions in public health nursing in six states found that, in general, staff nurses working in public health reported a total lack of security, felt that answering night calls was a threat to their safety, were harassed by 'people who were drunk', and suffered from the absence of safe, well-maintained living quarters in the primary health centres. Overall, it was felt that 'authorities did not pay attention to the security of staff nurses at PHCs (primary health centres) and CHCs (community health centres)'.[16]

This is, of course, a generalised discussion of nurses' working conditions. There is certainly a variation dependent on the state and sector in which hospitals function. At the same time, there are relatively few exceptions with regard to the problems of low salary, understaffing and exploitation by the management. The Indian private sector has developed rapidly in the recent years. In a few cases, this has brought benefits to nurses. In some high-level 'super-speciality' hospitals, nurses have received good training, benefits and sought-after access to migration through international partnerships. These elite institutions, however, are few in number compared to the thousands of small private hospitals, and even the most prestigious hospitals do not invariably give nurses a better deal than they find in the government sector. In my interviews with nursing principals in Thiruvananthapuram, it was universally agreed that every nurse's preference would be for work in a government hospital, as these paid a better salary and observed the three-shift system. In contrast, private hospitals, even the mushrooming 'super-speciality' variety, paid less and usually practised the double-shift system. The majority of the private sector, moreover, is constituted by small hospitals and nursing

---

[14] Anonymous, 'Brain Trust on the Theme: Family Welfare', *NJI*, vol. 63, no. 12, 1972, p. 414.

[15] Anonymous, '6th Biennial Conference: Resolutions', *NJI*, vol. 63, no. 12, 1972, p. 421.

[16] Academy for Nursing Studies, Hyderabad, 'Situational Analysis of Public Health Nursing Personnel in India: Based on national review and consultation in six states', Hyderabad: Academy for Nursing Studies, 2005, p. 30.

homes, not by large, modern 'five-star' institutions. In many of these smaller hospitals, nurse exploitation is endemic, and conditions are significantly worse than in government hospitals.[17]

Some Christian hospitals have provided more support for the development of nursing, more nurse autonomy and better conditions. CMC Vellore, in particular, made this a founding principle. Its school and college of nursing have both experienced autonomy and budgetary control, independent of the hospital administration (although, according to Aleyamma Kuruvilla, former Dean of the CMC College of Nursing, this was regularly challenged).[18] Other mission hospitals, however, are unable or unwilling to practice these high standards, and all mission hospitals, CMC included, pay very low salaries. Michelle Kermode's study of injection safety practices and occupational safety in the Christian, north Indian, Emmanuel Hospital Association's (EHA) hospitals found nursing to be a 'liminal and dangerous' occupation. The EHA hospitals have more resources and a better standard of medical care than government hospitals operating in the same rural regions in Uttar Pradesh and Bihar.[19] Yet nurses worked in unsafe conditions with minimal enforcement of injection safety, low levels of staffing, and the expectation that they would work long hours for little money. Although nurses in these hospitals were frequently doing the work of doctors, they were subject to a harsh disciplinary regime, and were expected to show complete submission to doctors and surgeons.[20] Kermode's study examined only a few, relatively well-resourced hospitals, yet it is a powerful representation of the most commonly cited problems faced by Indian nurses.

These persistently poor conditions have represented the key challenge for nursing organisations to confront. Yet, as the following

---

[17] Purba Kalita, 'Nursing System in Poor Health', *The Times of India*, 9 September 2003, http://timesofindia.indiatimes.com/cms.dll/html/uncomp/articleshow?msid=174084 (accessed 3 March 2004); Syed Falaknaaz, 'India faces Acute Shortage of Teaching Staff in Nursing Colleges', *Express Healthcare Management*, 1–15 December 2003, http://www.expresshealthcaremgmt.com/20031215/focus01.shtml (accessed 20 February 2005).

[18] Author interview, Thiruvalla, December 2005.

[19] Michelle Kermode, 'Safer Injections, Fewer Infections: Management of Needles and Sharps and Occupational Blood Exposure in Rural North Indian Health Settings', unpublished PhD Dissertation, University of Melbourne, 2004.

[20] Kermode, 'Safer Injections', pp. 127–28.

analysis will show, the culture of professionalism bequeathed to India by Western nurses did not equip them to confront it effectively.

## Nursing Organisations in Independent India

Since Independence, a group of organisations have represented the nurses of India. The Indian Nursing Council (INC), constituted in 1949, and the state-level nursing councils were established as the professional regulators. They are responsible for nurse and ANM registration, the setting of curricula and examinations and the inspection of schools and colleges, but have no remit for advocacy or representation. The Council is composed of representatives from the state-level councils, central and state health departments, the military nursing services, the Indian Red Cross, schools and colleges of nursing, the TNAI, the Medical Council of India, the Indian Medical Association, and the Lok Sabha. There are 55 members, of whom 31 are nurses and 19 are doctors. Its educational work has reflected the professionalising orientation of most nursing leaders during this period, and thus its curricula have emphasised the importance for nurses to keep themselves up to date with new scientific and technological developments in medicine, and have also stressed a public health role for the nurse. In general, however, the INC is a weak organisation, hamstrung by a lack of political support and medical dominance.

Christian nurses in India have long been represented by the CNL, a wing of the CMAI. The CMAI has also maintained its Boards of Nursing Education (BNEs), which oversee examinations and curricula for Christian hospitals. The CMAI shares some of the powers of the nursing councils, in that it is recognised by all state governments (except for Kerala) as a professional regulator, entitled alongside the INC to conduct school inspections and administer examinations.[21] The influence of CMAI nurses has been evident in the affiliation of the organisation with the INC and in the fact that its leaders have also often held senior positions in the TNAI and the INC.

---

[21] This examination system is generally viewed as superior to that of the INC, as it has an institutionalised practice of external examination, whereas the INC sets examinations but does not administer them.

The CMAI in general inherited a relatively higher esteem for nurses and nursing, institutionalised in the programmes set up by well-educated and often assertive mission nurses and their Indian pupils. Several Christian hospitals, for example, have continuously maintained the separation of nursing schools from hospital administrations and have allocated entirely separate budgets, meaning that nurses themselves have had greater control over the direction these schools have taken. The CNL has often proved relatively assertive, particularly given that it exists as a wing of a wider organisation of other medical and health workers. In 1964, it changed its status and name from that of an auxiliary to that of a league, suggesting a rejection of medical dominance.[22] During the 1970s, the nursing leader Aleyamma Kuruvilla became president of the CMAI, an outstanding instance of a nurse occupying a position of authority over the medical profession.[23] Although most Christian hospitals have to some extent experienced the poor working conditions described earlier, it can still be stated that CMAI nursing leaders, sharing in the professionalising aims espoused by most post-Independence leaders, have experienced relatively more room to pursue them.

The TNAI remains the largest national, non-religious representative body and is strongly defined by its focus on nurse professionalism. Although not a powerful organisation, it has wielded some influence. Mehan states that it is 'accepted as the voice of nurses in India', and it is true that when the government has sought nurse opinion it has consulted the TNAI. Government nursing advisors at state and national level have typically been enthusiastic TNAI members and there is a TNAI representative on the INC. The TNAI has never, however, been a strongly representative professional body. Raghavachari briefly touches on the issue of the TNAI's relevance in her 1990 study of Delhi nurses, which found that only 35 per cent of the sample read the *NJI*, whilst 55 per cent of those who did read it only did so occasionally.[24] Mohan wrote that most of her interviewees in Delhi were 'either passive members or dead [lapsed] members'.[25] The TNAI has not achieved the membership levels to which it aspired. During the 1960s, the leaders aimed to recruit

---

[22] Abraham, *Nursing History in South India*, p. 18.
[23] Ibid., p. 110.
[24] Raghavachari, *Conflicts and Adjustments*, pp. 194–95.
[25] Mohan, *Status of Nurses in India*, p. 96.

60 per cent of Indian nurses, the percentage required, they felt 'to become an effective negotiating body'.[26] In 1998, a generous estimate would have put membership at 12 per cent.[27]

In recent years, a challenge has emerged for the traditional modes of organisation represented by the TNAI and the CNL, in the form of new nurse-led unions. These are discussed at greater length later in the chapter.

## Organisational Culture in Indian Nursing

Professional organisations have unfortunately in general proved to be ineffective and easily marginalised. This can be understood as a product of both the youth and immaturity of organisation in India, and also of the problematic, conservative and insufficiently adapted culture left to nurses by early Western leaders. On the one hand, professional organisation is only in its early stages. Leadership has only been substantially in local hands from the early to mid-1960s, meaning that there has thus been only about half a century of complete local control. Mehan and her co-authors write that the current stage of development of nursing in India is similar to that of American nursing in the 1950s.[28] This suggests that while the structures of organisation and elite leadership are firmly in place, Indian nursing is only at the beginning of the process of confronting demands for a more representative and democratic leadership. At the same time, the cultural legacy of colonial modes of organisation has also been problematic. Organisation in India has mainly been defined by timidity, conservatism and a preoccupation with professionalisation. Leaders

---

[26] Anonymous, 'Resolutions: The Trained Nurses' Association of India in session at Jaipur from September 26 to October 1, 1960, adopted the following resolutions', *NJI*, vol. 51, no. 11, 1960, p. 9.

[27] This is based on TNAI membership figures provided for 1999 in Satish Chawla, 'As Nurses We are One', *NJI*, vol. 96, no. 12, 2005, pp. 270–72; and on the figures for the number of nurses in 1998 in Ministry of Health and Family Welfare, 'Annual Report 2001–2002', New Delhi: Government of India, 2002, http://mohfw.nic.in/reports/Annualpercent20Reportpercent202000-01.pdf/Partpercent20-I-6.pdf (accessed 6 May 2004).

[28] Mehan et al., 'Development of Nursing Education', p. 131.

have struggled to reflect the ordinary lives of working nurses; their preoccupations have not been those of their constituency.

A definitive feature of the leadership has been a pervasive emphasis on education and on the belief that better educated nurses might transcend and ultimately remedy the poor conditions in which they have worked. According to this view if, as a textbook recorded in 1990, a nurse who was disciplined, honest, loving, courageous, gentle, intelligent, efficient, resourceful, and well-balanced could be produced by the schools of India, society must ultimately accord nurses the respect they deserved.[29] Adranvala was one of the most significant and successful proponents of this approach. In 1957 she described what she saw as the positive effects that had already accrued from the redefinition of nursing as a fully-fledged profession:

> From being an occupation, not too well favoured, nursing is now being looked upon as a career worth considering by intelligent and ambitious young women. This change reflects, in part, the general change in the position of women and the increasing opportunities open to them in public life. But the main reason for the changed attitude is recognition that nursing is a calling based on educational as well as moral requirements.[30]

The strong commitment to professionalism has in part been a generational phenomenon. The Indian leadership that developed during the 1950s and 1960s was a group of rare and exceptional women, produced by a very specific moment in history — encouraged and cultivated by an extensive international health presence, inspired by the new task of constructing a national health system and often defying their families to pursue what they saw as an exciting career of service. Their motivations for joining nursing tended to revolve around strong conceptions of duty to religion and society. As Meera Abraham notes: 'A burst of ability and leadership characterised the first post-independence group of Indian nurses'.[31] The illustrious careers of Kuruvilla and Adranvala have already been discussed. Another such leader was Durga Mehta, who was superintendent of

---

[29] Joglekar, *Hospital Ward Management*, p. 87.

[30] T. K. Adranvala, 'Trends in Nursing Education', *Journal of the Christian Medical Association of India*, vol. 32, no. 5, 1957, p. 255.

[31] Abraham, *Nursing History in South India*, p. 111.

nursing at the King Edward Memorial (KEM) hospital in Bombay and TNAI president in the early 1990s. Mehta was interviewed by the journalist and author Pinki Virani, who recorded that Mehta was the niece of the first chief minister of Gujarat, Jivraj Mehta. She was inspired to join nursing in 1951 by a speech she had heard as a young girl, delivered by Sardar Vallabhbhai Patel on women's special contribution to the freedom struggle. She was also motivated by her uncle:

> Whenever he would be touring peri-urban and rural Gujarat, the people would turn to her uncle and ask for hospitals. Fine, he would say, I will give you the four walls and the doctors. Will you make your daughters the nurses? The people would shy away. But when articles began to appear about Dr Jivraj Mehta's own niece becoming the first nurse in the entire Gujarati community, it made a lot of difference to their perception. The men of Gujarat grew less sceptical about their daughters training as nurses.[32]

Altruistic, religious and nationalist motivations were frequently found among this generation of leaders, and women such as Mehta, gifted with talent and privileged backgrounds, were not unusual. Almost all of this generation of leaders received sponsorship to study abroad, and all were strongly committed to the ethos of professionalism. Relatively few married. The leaders who emerged in the 1970s and 1980s to take on roles in the TNAI and the INC, however, were different. They were often married and had less extensive experience abroad. Their commitment to the ethos of professionalism was solid, but their understanding of it was less developed. Early leaders either retired or moved to work in the Christian or private sector, and their replacements tended to pursue the same goals, but with less conviction.

The professionalising agenda pioneered by early leaders and inherited by their successors has had important achievements in India. This is evident in the now extensive presence of degree colleges and an educational programme that in theory recognises the intellectual training needed for a nurse. The INC won some victories in the attempt to promote higher educational standards. Even in 1957, when it had only been established for eight years, it could be said

---

[32] Virani, *Aruna's Story*, p. 113.

that the level of nurse training had significantly improved. Adranvala wrote to Hartley that there were 'many more tutors, good teaching equipment and a better educational standard of entrants'. The overcrowding of hospitals led her to question 'whether the patient is really better off', but she nonetheless hoped that better education would ultimately improve outcomes for all concerned.[33] The INC emphasised the need for nurses to keep pace with scientific and technological change and promoted research, viewed as crucial to the attainment of professional status. The 2007 nurse educated according to their curriculum should gain a good foundation in science, community health, midwifery, and the key fields of clinical nursing.[34] The INC's curricula have preserved the theoretical belief, at least, that there is a crucial role for nurses in public health delivery and that nurses require and deserve a broad, empowering education.

The TNAI has consistently advocated educational development and professionalisation as the best means of advancing the interests of the Indian profession. It has a strong history of providing opportunities to nurses for further education, as far as its budget has allowed. In 1951, Adranvala described the success of recently instituted TNAI refresher courses for practising nurses.[35] In 1960 the TNAI participated in an ICN conference held in Delhi on the need to foster a research ethic among nurses. The president that year was Edith Paull, a Eurasian nurse who was one of the first Indian faculty members at the Delhi College of Nursing and who later worked for the Indian Red Cross. She stated in her welcoming address that 'no progress can be made without research' and that the development of a stronger research focus would mean 'that nurses may achieve both personal and professional growth'.[36] The TNAI consistently provided scholarships to enable nurses to access further education.

---

[33] T. K. Adranvala, Christmas card to Diana Hartley, 22 November 1957, Cambridge University Library: Royal Commonwealth Society Library, Indian nursing collection of Diana Hartley, RCMS 77/6.

[34] Indian Nursing Council, 'Syllabus and Regulations: Diploma in General Nursing and Midwifery', New Delhi: INC, 2001; and Indian Nursing Council, 'Syllabus: Basic B.Sc. Nursing', New Delhi: INC, 2004.

[35] T. K. Adranvala, 'President's Address', *Nursing Journal of India*, vol. 42, no. 1, 1951, pp. 6–8.

[36] ICN, 'Learning to Investigate Nursing Problems: Report of an International Seminar on Research in Nursing', London: ICN, 1960, p. 19.

In 1971, for example, it awarded scholarships to 29 nurses, three for studies in England and 26 for further qualifications in India.[37] It has continuously emphasised the need for nurses to keep pace with scientific progress and development, publishing many articles in the *NJI* espousing a more scientific nurse education and the establishment of a stronger research component in nursing.[38]

When I asked her in 2006 what the main achievements of the TNAI had been, Evelyn Khannan emphasised the holding of professional conferences, the provision of scholarships for further study and the running of continuing education workshops.[39] The most recent TNAI project, ongoing in 2007, is the construction of a Central Institute of Nursing (CIN), which will run professional training courses and host conferences. The project reflects the TNAI emphasis on the notion that better educated nurses are the key to progress; as the constituting committee stated:

[T]he overall objective is based on the principle that progress in Nursing and Health fields depends to a considerable extent on enhancing the abilities of nurses who are in service so that they can more effectively meet the demands of the health care system.[40]

The Christian nursing organisations have also been animated by a professionalist ethos expressed through the desire to improve nursing education. In the case of the South India BNE, courses in public health, family planning, mental hygiene, sociology, and economics were added to the curriculum in 1960 (although many schools found it difficult to cater for the additions).[41] In 1974, it launched a new nursing school curriculum, that provided for two years of intensive classroom work with limited clinical work, followed by a one year internship on the wards, in an interesting attempt to solve the

---

[37] Anonymous, 'TNAI Scholars — 1971', *NJI*, vol. 62, no. 6, 1971, p. 202.

[38] L. M. Bischoff, 'This I Believe', *NJI*, vol. 59, no. 11, 1968, pp. 372–73; K. C. Aggarwal, 'Research in Nursing II — It's High Time to Act Now', *NJI*, vol. 67, no. 12, 1967, pp. 263–64.

[39] Author interview, New Delhi, 27 January 2006.

[40] Anonymous, 'A Preliminary Blueprint: Central Institute of Nursing', *NJI*, vol. 81, no. 8, 1990, pp. 235–36.

[41] Aleyamma Kurian, 'Study of the Implementation Phase of a Curriculum Change in Christian Schools of Nursing of South India', 1976, doctoral dissertation, Columbia University Teachers College, p. 24.

eternal problem of the overworking and under-instruction of nursing students on the hospital ward.[42] CNL and CMAI nurses also made a vital contribution to the preparation of textbooks. In 1947, the CMAI's survey of mission nursing schools had found that:

> One of the significant factors in retarding the progress of Nursing Education in India is the dearth of literature in English and the Indian languages which is suited to the background and experience of students and nurses. The translation of foreign materials is of assistance to some extent, but does not fill the basic need. India requires the development of a body of nursing knowledge based on her own conditions of life available in English and in the Indian languages in which Nursing is taught.[43]

CMAI nurse leaders maintained a strong emphasis on the production of these desperately needed local nursing textbooks. A large range of local texts was not available until the 1980s, but in 1961, Lois Marsiljie and Vera K. Pitman published *A New Textbook for Nurses in India*, updated by Ann Zwemer in 1968 and K. V. Annamma in 1986.[44] The BNE also sponsored the publication of *An Introduction to Community Health Nursing (with Special Reference to India)* by Kasturi Sundar Rao (the daughter of a male mission nurse who became an expert in public health, heading public health nursing at CMC Vellore during the 1960s).[45] A British Methodist nurse, A. M. Chalkley, wrote the first textbook for ANMs in 1967, which was published in English, Tamil and Telugu.[46]

The strong educational focus of the INC, the TNAI and the CMAI also involved enthusiastic support for degree education and its expansion in India. In 1957 Adranvala wrote of troubling issues in nurse education that 'the only sound solution is for the student

---

[42] Aleyamma Kurian, 'The '2 + 1' Nursing Curriculum: An Evaluation', *NJI*, vol. 73, no. 10, 1982, pp. 260–61.

[43] CMAI Committee, 'A Survey of Nursing', p. 22.

[44] Lois M. Marsiljie, Vera K. Pitman, Ann Jansma Zwemer and K. V. Annamma, *A New Textbook for Nurses in India: Volume 1: The Foundations of Nursing*, Madras: B. I. Publications, 1986.

[45] Kasturi Sundar Rao, *An Introduction to Community Health Nursing (with Special Reference to India)*, Chennai: B. I. Publications, 1997.

[46] A. M. Chalkley, *A Textbook for the Health Worker (ANM): Volume II*, New Delhi: New Age International Publishers, revised edn., 1985.

to be a student, freed from the obligation of hospital service' and praised the strong educational focus of the existing BSc programmes and their provision of a grounding in sociology, English and history as well as in science and medicine.[47] Kuruvilla felt that the expansion of collegiate education was a major factor 'in attracting more educated young women from good families into the nursing profession'.[48] According to her, this would address the problem that India had a preponderance of 'rule-of-thumb' nurses, who were incapable of acting independently and assertively. In 1971, the TNAI sponsored a conference in Chandigarh at which those present (including the secretary of the INC and nursing advisor to the Government of India, Annamma Cherian, and a large number of school and college principals) endorsed the need to move nursing education into the university system.[49] The TNAI continued to espouse the phasing out of GNM degree programmes through the 1990s and 2000s, and in 2005 the INC decided that all of India's nursing schools should be upgraded to colleges as soon as possible.[50] There has also been strong support for MSc degrees and more recently for the establishment of doctoral programmes in nursing.[51] The major nursing organisations of the post-Independence era have thus placed a profound faith in the liberating effects of continuing educational advances.

## The international orientation of the first-generation organisations

The source of the ideology of nursing professionalism was Western nurses, as discussed in previous chapters, and as an ideology it is characterised by the suggestion that it is international and universally applicable. The pursuit of professionalism in India has involved the

---

[47] Adranvala, 'Trends in Nursing Education', pp. 256–57.

[48] Aleyamma Kuruvilla, 'Status of Nursing in India', *NJI*, vol. 66, no. 5, 1975, pp. 99–100.

[49] Anonymous, 'Resolutions', *NJI*, vol. 62, no. 6, 1971, p. 198.

[50] Satish Chawla, 'Mrs Satish Chawla Addresses SNA Platinum Jubilee and Biennial Conference', *NJI*, vol. 96, no. 1, 2005, p. 9.

[51] Anonymous, 'Nursing Education', in TNAI, *Indian Nursing Year Book: 1996–97*, New Delhi: TNAI, 1998, pp. 17–18; Chawla, 'Mrs Satish Chawla Addresses SNA Platinum Jubilee'; Rajiv Gandhi University of Health Sciences, 'Application for PhD (Nursing)', www.rguhs.ac.in/noti/nurphd.pdf (accessed 28 November 2006).

retention of this pronounced outward focus among leaders. Jeffery writes of the medical profession that 'their source of legitimation has been their connections with the ex-imperial metropolis, and the neo-imperial powers, and they have few strong ties with the mass of Indian society, either socially or culturally'.[52] The same has largely been true of the nursing leadership. Disempowered in the workplace and struggling for state support, Indian leaders have continued to look to international nursing programmes and organisations for a source of legitimacy and resources for professional development.

Like South African professionalising leaders, India's nursing organisations have thus drawn heavily on 'the familiar language of international nursing'.[53] This is particularly true of the TNAI, which has often sought to compensate for the refusal of state endorsement by seeking international partnerships. In the 1950s and 1960s, the TNAI's general secretary, Kumari Lakshmi Devi, was a particularly enthusiastic exponent of internationalism. An Australian citizen whose immigrant family had raised her in New Zealand, she trained in New Zealand and was one of the most uncompromising supporters of professionalism. She pursued links with all of the international nurses, and at times exasperated them and her Indian colleagues with her fervour for educational improvement, which she often expressed immoderately and adamantly. In 1957, she wrote to Frances Goodall of the Royal College of Nursing (RCN) in London for advice and assistance in institutionalising TNAI's position as the main representative body for Indian nurses.[54] In 1958, she received a grant of US$4,300 from the Rockefeller Foundation to travel to the US to observe the activities of the American Nurses Association (ANA), in order to enhance her skills as a professional leader. She wrote that

[T]he TNAI is very close to my heart and that the Rockefeller Foundation have recognised it as worthy of assistance means a great deal to me; the travel grant to one of its officers will move it one step up the social and professional ladder.[55]

---

[52] Jeffery, 'Allopathic Medicine in India', p. 561.

[53] Marks, *Divided Sisterhood*, p. 200.

[54] Guildhaume Myrddin-Evans to J. S. P. Mackenzie, 1 August 1957, UK National Archives, Kew, LAB 13/1288.

[55] Kumari Lakshmi Devi to Virginia Arnold, 13 November 1958, RF, RG 1.2, Series 464, Box 53, Folder 491, 'India: Trained Nurses' Association, Devi, Kumari Lakshmi, 1958–1960'.

Links with the ICN have also been an important determinant of status for the TNAI. In 1960, the TNAI and the INC together hosted an ICN international seminar on nursing research.[56] Several TNAI officers served on the ICN, including Adranvala, who was vice-president, and Paull, who was on the membership committee. Close links were maintained with the Florence Nightingale International Foundation, the educational wing of the ICN. Despite the blow of disaffiliation from the ICN in 1995 (due to its prohibitively expensive affiliation fee), the TNAI continues to use international forums to emphasise its role as the representative voice of India's nurses, enthusiastically pursuing links with international nurse organisations. A flashing banner on its website advertises affiliation with the Commonwealth Nurses Federation (CNF), to which India has contributed several executive officers.[57]

The TNAI's enthusiastic support for the work of international development agencies in the 1950s and 1960s has continued. It has frequently sought to participate in the international development projects sponsored by foreign agencies. To some extent, it has been able to position itself to international donors as an effective 'local partner' organisation. In 2000, it jointly organised a conference in Delhi with McMaster University, Canada, on 'Women's Status: Vision and Reality'. In 2005 it participated in a workshop in Stockholm, sponsored by the Swedish International Development Agency, and was involved in a workshop jointly organised by the Government of India and the United Nations Conference on Trade and Development (UNCTAD).[58] Other projects were developed with UNICEF and European Union (EU) collaboration.[59] Nanthini Subbiah, assistant secretary at the TNAI, told me that such links with international organisations are viewed as crucial in raising professional status.[60]

For leaders, therefore, both nursing internationalism and affiliation with the agencies of international development have proved a central aspect of activity and identity. The ethos of nursing internationalism has animated the post-colonial TNAI as much as its colonial

---

[56] ICN, 'Learning to Investigate Nursing Problems'.
[57] TNAI website, www.tnaionline.org/about.htm (accessed 15 November 2005).
[58] 'News from TNAI Headquarters', *NJI*, vol. 97, no. 1, 2006, p. 3.
[59] Chawla, 'As Nurses We are One', pp. 270–72.
[60] Author interview, New Delhi, 27 January 2006.

incarnation, which also displayed a strong need to find recognition and esteem outside a society that seemed so often to dismiss its claims to professionalism and status.

## The search for a role in public health

It has unfortunately been a widely accepted orthodoxy that the Indian nursing profession is irremediably urban-oriented and has little potential to serve the cause of public health in rural areas. It is less known, however, that the leadership in nursing has fought this perception with vigour, albeit not with success. The professionalising culture of the leadership has included a strong emphasis on public health, which was strongly promoted particularly in the work of Western nursing advisors after Independence (as discussed in Chapter 3). Nursing leaders, motivated by this culture as well as by the increasingly important political role of rural health and community health in planning, have put considerable energy into the continuing search for a nurse role in the public health system. This search, however, has always been framed within the ideology of professionalism, which has ultimately limited its effectiveness.

The INC has ensured that public health has been a part of the curriculum for all nurses. In early 1957, it agreed to enhance the component of public health training for the GNM nurse, introducing an increased minimum component.[61] In 1965, the GNM curriculum was revised so that public health was emphasised more strongly.[62] In 1959, the TNAI's Jubilee Conference stressed 'that Nurses should rise above the lack of facilities and comforts in the villages, and take their skills to places where they were badly needed'.[63] The TNAI continuously tracked trends in public health policy through the pages of its journal, exhibiting an enthusiastic desire to locate a role for nurses within each new health discourse. Thus, as Indira Gandhi reoriented health programmes and health spending towards the frequently brutal promotion of family planning, the pages of the

---

[61] Adranvala, 'Trends in Nursing Education', p. 257.

[62] Marsiljie et al., *A New Textbook for Nurses in India*; C. Oonnie, 'Nursing Students of the 70's', *NJI*, vol. 64, no. 12, 1973, p. 410.

[63] Helen Cowan, *Health and Wealth*, No. 25 (March 1959): 1, from University of Birmingham, Church Missionary Society Collection, Papers of the Medical Department, M59/E2/2, 1959–63.

*NJI* instructed nurses to use their familiarity with patients to promote contraception and sterilisation as widely as possible.[64] The 1970s, in general, saw a much stronger focus on public health and on the provision of health care to rural areas; this reorientation was again enthusiastically reflected in the policy and writings of the TNAI. In 1972, the assistant director of health services (nursing) for Madhya Pradesh, Chellamma Oonnie, wrote in the *NJI* that:

> Nursing being one of the basic and highly practical professions, nurses have a great contribution in finding out new and workable methods of translating available knowledge into the reality of the local setting . . . The future of nursing in developing countries like ours, lies in the field of prevention of disease and promotion of health.[65]

In 1976 an *NJI* article proclaimed that 'we nurses have to come down from secure four walls of the hospital to serve the deprived masses', and lamented the irrelevance of nurses to definitive national health problems.[66] The *NJI* and the TNAI closely followed the emerging international consensus on the need to reorient national health systems to rural needs. The Alma Ata declaration of 1978 and its accompanying declaration of the goal of 'Health for All by 2000' were reported on, and members of the TNAI often posed the question of how nurses in India might benefit from and participate in the new health policy environment.

Plans for degree education for nurses were also infused with the principles of public health and presented as a means of encouraging nurses to work in this field. The BSc (nursing) courses at Vellore and Delhi both focused on community health issues, the role of preventive work and the potential for nurses to be leaders in rural health delivery.[67] The leaders fervently hoped that, through such courses,

---

[64] Swarnlata Arora and Germaine Krysan, 'A Look at Nursing and Family Planning', *NJI*, vol. 58, no. 11, 1967, pp. 281–84; S. Kamalamma, 'The Role of a Public Health Nurse in Family Planning Programme', *NJI*, vol. 59, no. 12, 1968, pp. 392–93, 397; V. Naraindas, 'Family Planning and Public Health', *NJI*, vol. 59, no. 5, 1968, pp. 149, 151.

[65] Oonnie, 'Nursing Students of the 70's', p. 411.

[66] K. C. Aggarwal, 'Some Suggested Structural Changes in Nursing Education', *NJI*, vol. 67, no. 7, 1976, p. 169.

[67] Margaretta Craig, 'The College of Nursing, New Delhi: Progress Report to the TNAI November 1946', *NJI*, vol. 38, no. 2, 1947, p. 72.

the role of the specialist public health nurse (with a degree and a postgraduate qualification) envisaged by the Bhore Report would become a reality. Despite an egregious lack of evidence that this was happening, the leadership continued to feel that the solution to getting nurses into the field lay in getting students into degree programmes. In 1976, an *NJI* article put forward this idea, suggesting that new university-based colleges could establish four-year degree programmes to prepare specialised public health nursing practitioners, who would be 'well qualified people who could serve diverse health needs in the rural community'.[68] How this would overcome the problems of low pay and poor infrastructure that prevented both ANMs and nurses from remaining in rural health work was not addressed. In general, the approach of the leadership to public health was impossibly grounded in their agenda for the professionalisation of nursing, as is suggested by the very fact that they could propose expanded university education for nurses as a solution to rural health problems.

The longstanding theoretical emphasis on public health among the leadership has thus borne little fruit. In 1974, a survey of the nursing profession in India was jointly conducted by the Coordinating Agency for Health Planning (CAHP) and the TNAI, in order to form policy recommendations for the voluntary sector. In the section of the report unendorsed by the TNAI, the CAHP strongly criticised the failure of public health education in nursing, reporting that 16 per cent of nursing schools entirely failed to provide public health experience, while in almost all of the remaining 84 per cent this experience was unplanned and vastly inadequate.[69] Overall, the survey reflected the shallowness of leaders' engagement with public health. The board and staff of CAHP found the nursing leaders who collaborated on the survey so exclusively focused on 'the uplift of the social, educational and economic position of the nursing profession' rather than on the needs of Indian citizens, that they published a separate set of recommendations at the start of the report. This, they felt, would 'rouse more interest in the neglected needs of the people, as distinguished from the needs of the profession'.[70]

---

[68] K. B. Kapadia and R. K. Julius, 'Nurse Practitioner Programme', *NJI*, vol. 67, no. 7, 1976, p. 173.

[69] CAHP, 'Report of a Nursing Survey in India', pp. x–xi.

[70] CAHP, 'Report of a Nursing Survey in India', Preface.

It should, however, be acknowledged that individual nurses and individual hospitals have served the cause of rural health with great effectiveness. In 1972, Pramila Shantaram Haldankar, a nurse at the V. S. General Hospital in Thana, was awarded the Maharashtra Chief Minister's Merit Award. She had played an active role in establishing a regional blood bank and, it was recorded, had 'carried out many social activities like organising a *mahila mandal* [a women's group], starting the milk scheme and arranging cultural programmes for the villagers'.[71] In the same year, Ms A. Simon, sister tutor at the Victoria Hospital in Jabalpur, was to be promoted to public health nursing educator and transferred to the public health training centre at Gwalior. This was in recognition of a three-year commitment to providing nursing services to a local refugee camp.[72] At CMC Vellore, a succession of nursing leaders have contributed to the establishment of a rural health programme now run entirely by nurses. In 1987, this programme catered to a rural population of 22,000 and a semi-urban population of 23,000. Such achievements, however, have been isolated victories in a larger story of crumbling infrastructure and an urban-oriented nursing education, problems which the professionalising leadership has failed to tackle.

## The limitations of genteel lobbying

The organisational culture developed under colonial rule has continued in many ways to determine the means by which professional organisations approached the state. Nurses, as members of the oft-praised dutiful and obedient 'noble profession', have been urged by leaders to avoid disruptive protest and industrial action and to focus instead on the genteel petitioning of the state. Leaders' actions over poor conditions, circumscribed by the desire to preserve 'respectability' and 'dignity', have tended not to be very successful. In 1959, Alice Zachariah described the approach generally favoured:

> We believe that if we stand together in making these demands, and if we approach the authorities with the dignity befitting our profession, surely we can expect to achieve those privileges enjoyed by other government employees. It is obvious that nurses have been and still

---

[71] Anonymous, 'Nursing World', *NJI*, vol. 66, no. 4, 1975, p. 81.
[72] Ibid.

are being exploited, but this can be remedied by our clearly stating the existing facts that surround the employment of nurses in India.[73]

The TNAI regularly noted issues of under-staffing, low salary and the mistreatment of students. In 1951, for example, it lobbied for adequate staffing ratios, salaries on par with 'other full-time professional workers' and better accommodation.[74] In 1960, priorities included advising governments to collect more statistical information about nurses' working and living conditions, support for better allowances for nurses working in rural areas and a stop to the common practice of delayed payment of salaries.[75] The 1970s saw an increased focus on working conditions as it became increasingly clear that things were not improving as it had been hoped they would. In 1972, the TNAI conducted a nationwide survey on 'the socio-economic status of nurses', receiving 2,121 responses from 13 states and highlighting issues such as the regular non-payment of salaries in some states and the drastic inadequacy of food and clothing allowances.[76]

In earlier years, the 'genteel lobbying' approach brought a modicum of success. Indira Dorabji, who led the Student Nurses Association from 1948–64 and then worked as TNAI secretary until her retirement in 1967, wrote of the pride felt during this period at the willingness of governments to receive and consider TNAI resolutions.[77] In August 1959, Zachariah recorded that the Andhra Pradesh branch of the TNAI had attained victory, persuading the state government to pay retrospectively the rations, *dhobi* (washerman) and uniform allowances that had been withheld since January 1958, when the government neglected to order their continuance.[78] TNAI submissions to the Mudaliar Committee on the treatment of students

---

[73] Alice Zachariah, 'News from the States: Andhra Pradesh', *NJI*, vol. 50, no. 8, 1959, p. 274.

[74] Anonymous, 'Policy of the Trained Nurses' Association of India', *NJI*, vol. 42, no. 1, 1951, p. 41.

[75] Anonymous, 'Resolutions: The Trained Nurses' Association of India in session at Jaipur from September 26 to October 1, 1960, adopted the following resolutions', *NJI*, vol. 51, no. 11, 1960, p. 312.

[76] Anonymous, 'Socio-Economic Status of Nurses in India', *NJI*, vol. 63, no. 12, 1972, pp. 405–6.

[77] Indira Dorabji, 'Greeting Message', *NJI*, vol. 59, no. 11, 1968, p. 366.

[78] Zachariah, 'News from the States', p. 273.

and nursing representation were reflected in the recommendations presented in the final report, as is discussed in Chapter 5.[79]

In general, however, there was frequent and increasing dissatisfaction among nurses with the cautious and conservative approach of the TNAI toward poor working conditions. It was felt that leaders mainly focused on the relatively easy work of publishing the *NJI*, compiling reports and holding conferences from Delhi, while neglecting the difficult task of invigorating state branches and taking meaningful and effective action to improve conditions. Members' dissatisfaction was expressed in the early and increasing tendency of nurses to join government or paramedical workers' unions in preference to the TNAI. Anna Noll of Rockefeller recorded as early as 1949 that Calcutta nurses were discontented and that 'some of them are looking to trade unions for help in improving working and living conditions as well as salaries'.[80] In 1959, Zachariah referred to individuals and small groups of nurses in Andhra Pradesh who were 'trying to discredit the TNAI' because it was perceived to be moving so slowly and cautiously in addressing the poor conditions nurses faced.[81] In the late 1960s, nurses in Rajasthan left the TNAI in bulk to join the general unions that represented paramedical workers. The Rajasthani unit of the TNAI did not actively function again until 1976, when the *NJI* claimed that the trained nurses returned due to 'disillusionment from the limited goals and shoddy means adopted by the unions'.[82] Similarly, in Punjab in the early 1970s many young nurses had become disenchanted with the TNAI. They had watched as the paramedical unions 'captured the consultative machinery' in the hospital, while employers ignored the TNAI. Many left to join these paramedical unions, to the extent that the TNAI in Punjab in 1972 had only 300 members left, of which 60 per cent came from three mission hospitals.[83] In 1982, Stephens, on his TNAI sponsored tour of north Indian hospitals, discovered a radical decline in

---

[79] Government of India, 'Report of the Health Survey and Planning Committee' (Mudaliar Committee), New Delhi: Ministry of Health, 1961, vol. 1, pp. 370–71.

[80] Anna M. Noll, 'Annual Report on Nursing in India, Pakistan and Ceylon 1949', RF, RG 5.3, Series 464C, Box 204, Folder 2497, p. 7.

[81] Zachariah, 'News from the States', p. 274.

[82] Narender Nagpal, 'It's Never too Late', *NJI*, vol. 67, no. 9, 1976, p. 209.

[83] U. Sapra, 'Punjab Nurses', *NJI*, vol. 63, no. 10, 1972, p. 363.

organisational fortunes in Uttar Pradesh, where less than 20 per cent of nurses were members — the rise of associations with 'pragmatic aims' was identified as the cause of a mass desertion.[84]

Union participation allowed nurses to become involved in strident activism directly aimed at improving conditions and salary, in contrast to the genteel work of the TNAI. In November 1970, a large percentage of nurses in Maharashtra joined a general strike of all Class III and Class IV government employees of the Maharashtrian government.[85] A significant nurse strike over poor working conditions occurred in Delhi in 1973.[86] In 1975, the health minister in Bihar, Bindeshwari Dubey protested the increased militancy of nurses in the state, calling on nurses 'to desist from agitations for getting their demands redressed'.[87] In the same year, Gyan Prakash, the secretary in the Union Ministry of Health and Family Planning, lamented the rise of nurse presence in trade unions, which he felt had undermined the public reputation of nurses for 'dedicated service to the humanity and nobility'.[88]

Witnessing the draining of their members into such unions, TNAI members expressed dissatisfaction with the relative passivity and politeness of their own organisation. A letter to the *NJI* in 1970 called for action in Maharashtra:

> We also feel that it is high time for the TNAI to step in and take measures to discourage the nurses from joining trade unions. The TNAI will have to make tremendous efforts towards this end . . . The TNAI which is the only recognised national body of nurses, which has been working for the betterment of nurses for more than 60 years now, should also take up the cause of nurses more effectively towards improving their working conditions.[89]

---

[84] Stephens, 'TNAI in Uttar Pradesh', p. 218.

[85] V. B. Purohit, S. G. Nitsure and A. Gunian, 'Nurses' Strike', *Nursing Journal of India*, vol. 61, no. 12, 1970, p. 412.

[86] A. K. Kisku, 'Nursing Education Needs Change', *NJI*, vol. 64, no. 12, 1973, p. 412.

[87] Anonymous, 'Branch Affairs', *NJI*, vol. 66, no. 8, 1975, p. 182.

[88] Narender Nagpal, 'Workshop on Trends in Health Care system and its Implications for Nursing', *NJI*, vol. 66, no. 5, 1975, p. 103.

[89] Purohit et al., 'Nurses' Strike', p. 412.

At the annual conference in 1972, members expressed dissatisfaction at the continuing practice of sending polite resolutions and
dispatches to governments. The secretary of the TNAI pronounced
that 'there was a general feeling that unless the Association gains the
status of a negotiating and bargaining body our system of despatch-
ing resolutions and reminders would be worthless'.[90] Zachariah,
a TNAI leader since before Independence, wrote in 1971 that the
leadership was complacent on the subject of the 'ghastly' conditions faced by nurses and were 'interested only in safeguarding their
"chairborne" positions'.[91] A letter to the editor in 1975 asked for
harder struggle from the TNAI, pointing out that 'in the present day
world, which is dominated by the sterner sex nothing is expected by
humble appeals'.[92] In 1975, Kuruvilla, a committed Christian and
eminent CNL and CMAI leader, felt that a stronger approach was
needed (although she eschewed the use of strikes) and called for the
strengthening and reshaping of the TNAI into a 'strong body capable
of collective bargaining'.[93] Adranvala wrote to the *NJI* criticising
strikes as the cause of 'unethical measures, undignified behaviour
and neglect of nursing care of patients'. She attributed the resort to
industrial action to a breakdown in the leadership, and lamented the
declining capacity and willingness of the TNAI to work effectively
with the government.[94] Letters to the TNAI continued throughout the
1980s to call for a better focus on working conditions, more activity
at state level rather than at the centre and a renewed emphasis on
producing material in regional languages.[95]

The desired reorientation and strengthening of the TNAI did not
really eventuate, although frequent nurse strikes during the 1980s
(discussed later) did prompt a more sustained focus on conditions.
At present, although the TNAI continues to recognise the oppression of nurses and to protest against poor working conditions, it

---

[90] M. Philip, 'Secretary's Report', *NJI*, vol. 63, no. 12, 1972, pp. 412–13.

[91] Alice Zachariah, letter to the editor, 'Wanted, a Criteria', *NJI*, vol. 62, no. 2,
1971, p. 63.

[92] G. Bhullar, letter to the editor, *NJI*, vol. 66, no. 8, 1975, p. 173.

[93] Kuruvilla, 'Status of Nursing', p. 100.

[94] T. K. Adranvala, 'Professional Behaviour: Some Aspects of Nursing Practice',
*NJI*, vol. 64, no. 10, 1973, p. 357, 363.

[95] See for example, Sindhu Tilak, 'Readers' Views: Nursing and the Role of the
TNAI', *NJI*, vol. 73, no. 12, 1982, p. 314.

maintains as its priority the preparation of better-educated, more confident nurses with skills in leadership. A strong focus remains on the model of an ideal nurse leader, who 'should be a visionary, critical thinker, an expert communicator, mentor and an achiever of goals', rather than on radical action to remedy the difficult and dangerous context in which nurses have worked.[96] Ultimately, India's nursing organisations preferred a safe, already established model of dignified, elite-led organisation around education and the idealisation of the international, rather than a creative approach to local nursing or an attempt to mobilise the support of the beleaguered ward nurses of India.

## Disunity and division: The neglect of auxiliary nurses

In India's tiered system of primary health centres (PHCs) and sub-centres, the 18-month trained ANM is intended to be the main health worker at the sub-centres, the first port of call for the rural population of India. Lady health visitors (later re-designated as 'Health Supervisors Female'), who usually have two years' training, are posted at the PHC level and have some supervisory functions. Whilst the role of the public health nurse has been sidelined, ANMs have emerged as the main personnel in the rural health system. In 1991, 76.2 per cent of ANMs worked in rural areas, compared to 9.7 per cent of trained nurses.[97] Organisational culture in Indian nursing has not encouraged the participation of these auxiliaries, leading to disunity and a situation in which nurses' less-educated colleagues have been left virtually unrepresented and consequently defenceless. This partly reflected a worldwide trend in nursing, which the WHO described in 1966 as 'an unfortunate tendency to underestimate the potential contribution of auxiliary workers and to regard their work as something the nurse could do better if only she had the time'.[98]

The leadership has not ignored auxiliaries; in fact their efforts to reach them have been sustained and regular, albeit unsuccessful and

---

[96] Chawla, 'Mrs Satish Chawla Addresses SNA Platinum Jubilee'.

[97] Lalita Manocha, 'Challenges for Nursing Profession: A Retrospection', in TNAI, *Indian Nursing Year Book 1996–97*, New Delhi, 1997, p. 114.

[98] 'WHO Expert Committee on Nursing: Fifth Report' Geneva: WHO, 1966, p. 14.

unpopular. Leaders have long recognised the problems facing ANMs and health visitors. In 1971, for example, the TNAI Council passed a resolution emphasising the disadvantages and dangers faced by ANMs and health visitors working in the countryside and planned to lobby the union government so that all nursing personnel working in public health received the same provision for accommodation and allowances as staff nurses.[99] The pages of the *NJI* at times acknowledged the lack of promotional avenues, insecurity and absence of accommodation that rural ANMs confronted.[100] The TNAI has maintained a grade of membership for ANMs and health visitors, but these auxiliary wings have generally not been popular. In 1960, the Health Visitors' League had only 226 members and their page in the *NJI* was not run due to the complete lack of contributions.[101] By 1971, things had not improved. Out of 22,000 ANMs in India, a mere 296 were members of the TNAI's ANM Association.[102] In 1982, D. S. Elisha wrote of finding her election to the post of secretary of the Health Visitors' League somewhat dispiriting, given that membership numbered 35 out of 20,000 registered health visitors.[103] Obstacles to auxiliary participation identified by the leadership at the time included the failure to produce vernacular language materials and the lack of any significant associational presence in rural areas.

Nurse leaders' inability to effectively create links with ANMs and health visitors was partly motivated by anxiety over the erosion of their own professional territory. The state did not implement in practice the supervisory structures of the public health system that existed on paper, which specified that ANMs and health visitors should work under the supervision of public health nurses. Instead, the role officially prescribed for the nurse in the public health system was substantially ignored. This justifiably led the nurses to feel that the need for trained nursing had been disregarded in favour of dependence on the cheaper labour of unsupervised auxiliaries.

---

[99] Anonymous, 'TNAI Council Meets', *NJI*, vol. 62, no. 3, 1971, p. 68.

[100] See, for example, P. P. Das, 'ANM Uniforms', *NJI*, vol. 62, no. 1, 1971, p. 29.

[101] K. Thomas, 'Report of the Health Visitors' League', *NJI*, vol. 51, no. 11, 1960, p. 311.

[102] Anonymous, 'Reports', *NJI*, vol. 62, no. 1, 1971, pp. 13–14, 29.

[103] D. S. Elisha, 'Readers' Views: An Appeal to Health Visitors', *NJI*, vol. 73, no. 11, 1982, p. 298.

Nirmala Mehan, J. P. Gupta and R. S. Gupta found that 'the nursing component of the health care delivery system especially at the peripheral level is being managed by semi-professionals and auxiliaries'.[104] This has continually motivated professional anxiety among nurses. K. C. Aggarwal, the chair of the TNAI's public health section in 1975, wrote that 'if we fail to live up to the expectations of the community, a new category of workers will take our place, and the position of a nurse will get extinct from the health care team'.[105] The TNAI suggested in 1999 that the 40-fold expansion in the number of ANMs between 1954 and 1990 had had grave ramifications for trained nurses, as 'the profession will not be in position to occupy its rightful place in the overall health manpower mix in the country'.[106] The threat posed by auxiliaries to nurses' professional terrain has not been confined to the public health field; further friction developed over the tendency of hospitals to economise or to solve nurse shortages by employing ANMs trained for community health work instead of nurses.[107] Motivated by anxiety over their displacement, nurse organisations have focused more on the need to develop a trained nurse role in public health and on providing routes for ANMs to upgrade to GNMs, than on engaging with or representing auxiliaries' concerns.

Similar problems evolved in relation to health visitors, who, given that they often worked as the supervisors of ANMs, seemed to pose even more of a threat to the development of a strong public health nursing cadre. A 1975 column written by Adranvala suggests some of the reasons that the TNAI was not popular with health visitors:

> Health visitors may feel that we do not support them because the TNAI has consistently recommended the closure of health visitor schools but, perhaps we have failed to make it clear that this is primarily in the interests of the health visitors. There are no career opportunities for an health visitor unless she becomes a nurse.[108]

---

[104] Mehan et al., 'Development of Nursing Education', p. 125.

[105] Anonymous, 'Nursing world', *NJI*, vol. 66, no. 4, 1975, p. 15.

[106] Anonymous, 'Development of Nursing Services Under Ninth Five Year Plan', in TNAI, *Indian Nursing Year Book, 1998–1999*, New Delhi: TNAI, 1999, p. 30.

[107] Jaiwanti P. Dhaulta, 'A Report on the Community Nurses' Meet', *NJI*, vol. 78, no. 1, 1987, pp. 17–18.

[108] T. K. Adranvala, 'A Point to Ponder', *NJI*, vol. 66, no. 5, 1975, p. 97.

The exclusion of auxiliaries from nursing organisations was also, however, largely determined by the state policy of establishing separate nursing cadres — an effective means of dividing and conquering the nation's nurses. Pay scales and conditions for public health nurses and auxiliaries were treated separately than those for hospital nurses. Although the INC supervised the curriculum and delivery of ANMs' education, it did not have authority over their employment and promotional avenues. The state also gave nurse leaders no authority over new grades of village level carers that emerged in the 1970s (discussed further in Chapter 5), giving nurses little motivation to advocate on their behalf.

Divisions in the ranks of nurses and auxiliaries have reduced the power and effectiveness of both. ANMs, often working alone and directly supervised by doctors, have been under-organised, seriously under-represented and easily exploited. Adranvala commented in 1975 that 'nurses have a special responsibility to speak for health visitors and ANMs as they do not have a say in regulating education . . . nor in identifying their own functions'.[109] It is difficult to argue that this special responsibility has been adequately discharged. ANMs have worked in dangerous, under-resourced conditions, have experienced a general decline in skill and capacity to function independently, often suffer from lack of supervision and an unclear understanding of their role, and have almost no avenues for promotion other than by training as GNMs, for which many lack sufficient education.[110]

At the same time, the bargaining power of nurses and their ability to participate in the nation's health debates has been reduced by the failure to develop meaningful links with junior public health nursing personnel. Indian feminists have often identified the challenge of inclusively organising across boundaries of class and caste as of definitive importance for the future of the women's movement.[111]

---

[109] Adranvala, 'A Point to Ponder', p. 97.

[110] Academy for Nursing Studies, 'Situational Analysis', p. 18.

[111] Mary E. John, for example, writes that 'if there is a common condition that feminism must address, it is one of unequal patriarchies and disparate genders. The imperative, then, is to recognise how asymmetries and structures of privilege may have prevented solidarities; and to fight on many fronts to enable the development of more viable feminisms' (Mary E. John, 'Feminisms and Internationalisms: A Response from India', *Gender and History*, vol. 10, no. 3, 1998, p. 544).

It seems that for nurses, organisation that includes auxiliaries remains an important challenge. Again, a culture centred on the professionalisation of nursing has reduced the ability of leaders to meet this challenge.

## Nurses and the problem of public relations

Narender Nagpal, editor of the *NJI* in 1976, commented that:

> For centuries we have lived a somewhat secluded and socially introverted existence. It was perhaps due to the low status assigned to nursing vis-à-vis other professions and partly due to the habit of living within the closed circle of the hostel or the hospital, and not caring much to mix up in the society.[112]

As Nagpal suggested, the organisational culture of Indian nursing has been characterised by a troubling degree of introversion. In the context of widespread stigmatisation, a society unfamiliar with the function of modern nursing, and a public sphere that anyway presented difficult challenges to women leaders, the extent to which nurses have been able to build a successful relationship with the public has been highly limited. The effects of this social context were magnified by the inheritance of a nursing culture defined by an ethos of service and self-effacement, which strongly discouraged self-promotion. T. K. Oommen, in his comparative study of nurses and doctors, wrote in 1978 that:

> The doctors' capacity to link patient-care with broader issues of nation-building and economic development seems to be anchored on their class background, high level of education, etc., and the *achievement ethos* associated with their profession. In contrast, the nurses look at patient care in a limited context of imparting services to the immediately vulnerable and down and out due to the *service ethos* characteristic of their profession and also because of their lower-middle class background and limited education which does not equip them to relate the meaning of their role activity to wider issues' [italics original].[113]

---

[112] Narender Nagpal, 'The Healing Hands', *NJI*, vol. 67, no. 3, 1976, p. 1.
[113] Oommen, *Doctors and Nurses*, p. 141.

Oommen's analysis highlights the problematic failure of the nursing leadership to effectively promote nursing to the public. Unlike allopathic doctors or even practitioners of indigenous medicine, who Jeffery describes as a 'vocal lobby . . . able to use the Gandhian images of *swaraj* and *swadeshi* to justify state support', nurses have not managed to promote their own indispensability.[114] This has proved a significant brake on plans for development. It is clear, as Sarah Elise Abrams points out, that the establishment of a strong and autonomous professional domain for nursing depends not only on a determined leadership but also on a supportive and engaged public.[115]

From the beginning, the underdeveloped relationship with the public was recognised as a problem by India's nursing leaders. In 1951, Alice Clark, an American mission nurse who had worked in India for decades, wrote that the responsibility to connect with the local community had been neglected by leaders:

> The hospital staff should be doing more to acquaint the local leaders of the community with the working of the hospital. We are a technical profession and people outside the hospital do not know what the duties of a nurse are; except when they have to come to the hospital as a patient, and then see it in an entirely critical manner . . . We need to work for a complete change in the attitude of the public towards nursing.[116]

By the early 1970s, the increasing neglect of nursing was becoming apparent, and it formed a stark contrast with the political success of the medical profession. In 1970, Cheriyan informed the CMAI that 'in their efforts to improve their professional status the nurses should more than before direct their attention to establishing and maintaining good public relations'.[117] In 1971, Muriel Wasi, the co-ordinator of a study of educated women in India, suggested that

---

[114] Jeffery, 'Toward a Political Economy of Health Care', p. 278.

[115] Sarah Elise Abrams, 'Seeking Jurisdiction: A Sociological Perspective on Rockefeller Foundation Activities in Nursing in the 1920s', in Anne Marie Rafferty, Jane Robinson and Ruth Elkan (eds), *Nursing History and the Politics of Welfare*, London and New York: Routledge, 1997, pp. 208–25.

[116] Alice M. Clark, 'Training for Leadership', *NJI*, vol. 42, no. 2, 1951, p. 67.

[117] T. Cheriyan, 'Future of Nursing', *Christian Nurse*, no. 230, 1970, p. 17.

nurses needed to focus on winning attention and stature in the public eye, so that it would be impossible, come the next Five-year plan, to again dismiss the profession in four lines.[118] Kuruvilla wrote that nurses needed to concentrate on reaching out to the community, taking steps such as joining women's organisations to broaden the support for nursing causes.[119] From the mid-1970s, leaders became more aware of the need for better engagement with the community, with the TNAI using occasions such as International Women's Day and International Nurses' Day to encourage its members to focus on public relations.

In general, however, the focus on education and professionalism remained far stronger in the TNAI and the CNL, at least, than the emphasis on constructing a more positive relationship with the public. Nurses' serious public image problem persisted, and they have continued to be a popular media scapegoat for the failings of Indian hospitals. A letter to the *Hindustan Times* in 1987 regretted the poor security provided in hospitals, but claimed that the typical nurse was harsh to patients, arrogant, conceited, and frequently stole from patients and the hospital.[120] Usha Rai wrote in a 2003 article published in the Chandigarh *Tribune* of 'a lack of professional care' and that 'being in a government hospital, even if it is one of the top ones in the country, can be a nightmarish experience. Nurses are never around to help you when you need them'.[121] Purba Kalita wrote in *The Times of India* in the same year:

> When a loved one is in hospital, you have enough to worry about. But what if the people who are supposed to help you through this trying time add to your woes? It's a story that's unfortunately being repeated all too often, in one hospital after another.[122]

---

[118] Muriel Wasi, 'Trends and Priorities: Training for Leadership', in Muriel Wasi (ed.), *The Educated Woman in Indian Society*, Bombay and New Delhi: Tata McGraw Hill, 1971, pp. 163–75.

[119] Kuruvilla, 'Status of Nursing', p. 100.

[120] T. T. Sakaria and A. K. Gupta, 'Plight of Nurses', *Hindustan Times*, 25 January 1987.

[121] Usha Rai, 'Forging a Bond in a Government Hospital', 16 December 2003, *The Tribune* (online edition), Chandigarh, http://www.tribuneindia.com/2003/20031216/edit.htm#7, (accessed 22 August 2006).

[122] Kalita, 'Nursing System in Poor Health'.

The poor public image of nursing, reinforced by working conditions that reduce the standard of care nurses are able to deliver, has certainly contributed to frequent verbal and physical violence against nurses in Indian hospitals. The professionalising leadership has not yet proved capable of contesting this image in the public domain.

## Nursing organisations, but not women's organisations

It is clear that the success of professional organisations has been to some extent limited by the difficulties of organising women in a society that features a particularly strong private patriarchy. Again, however, the conservative cultural inheritance of colonial nursing has circumscribed the ability of nursing organisations to respond to this challenge. In effect, leaders ensured that organisations represented nurses, without strongly or practically acknowledging that nurses were also women struggling with dual domestic and professional roles.

Nirmala Banerjee suggests that when women go to work, their family orientation is carefully retained and that they can pursue careers without necessarily experiencing emancipation from patriarchal structures at home.[123] According to Rajan, Indian women's strong ties with family and community make them difficult to organise:

> It is not clear whether women have associational tendencies with women in any social setting, belonging instead more 'naturally' to mixed-gender (and hierarchical) families and communities, an important fact (though not the only one) that makes any kind of separating out and mobilization of women acutely difficult.[124]

Research into the lives of nurses clearly shows how strongly circumscribed their working lives are by obligations to maintain an ideal domestic environment and to ensure that the status of the husband as chief breadwinner and patriarch is not challenged. George's study

---

[123] Nirmala Banerjee, 'Analysing Women's Work Under Patriarchy', in Kumkum Sangari and Uma Chakravarti (eds), *From Myths to Markets: Essays on Gender*, New Delhi: Manohar, 2001, pp. 330–31.

[124] Rajan, *The Scandal of the State*, p. 14.

of Malayali nurses in the US highlights the difficulty many Kerala nurses have faced in ensuring that their well-paid, stimulating work does not undermine their husband's identity and self-perception as the head of the family and that they conform to cultural expectations of wives and mothers.[125] Proshanta Nandi and Charles Loomis suggested in 1977 that nurses tend to construct identities around family, not work in the public sphere.[126] The general stigmatisation of nursing has often dictated that, in their private and family lives, nurses have tried to distance themselves from their working identities. Ann Zwemer, a missionary nurse in India during the 1950s and 1960s, in 1971 wrote of nurses' lack of involvement in professional activism:

> The image of the nurse within the Indian society creates a deep conflict for the married nurse. The husband, children and other relatives will seldom take pride in her work as a professional person. It takes a woman with very deep dedication to the nursing profession to remain active in it after marriage.[127]

Nursing organisations have thus always encountered the limitations of patriarchy, but they have not usually responded to them effectively. The TNAI has instead often chosen to view the non-involvement of nurses as lethargy. In 1951, Adranvala suggested that the main barrier to nurses taking on a more equal role in hospitals was their own apathy.[128] She reiterated this conviction in 1960, when her speech at the TNAI conference asserted that 'many of our problems were due to lack of loyalty to fellow nurses' and that 'nurses need to support each other in an effort to solve their problems'.[129] In 1953, Kumari Lakshmi Devi regretted Indian nurses' lack of interest in their national association, viewing it as likely to erode the status gains won in the late 1940s. She urged that 'they will have to be more courageous as their lack of firmness and resolution is surely

[125] George, *When Women Come First*.

[126] Nandi and Loomis, 'Professionalisation of Nursing in India', pp. 43–59. See also Joseph Kuruvilla, 'Occupational Stress in Nursing', *Social Welfare*, March 1989.

[127] Ann Zwemer, 'Letter to the Editor: Volunteer Service in Hospitals', *NJI*, vol. 62, no. 7, 1971, p. 237.

[128] Adranvala, 'President's Address', pp. 6–8.

[129] A. C. Chakrapani, 'Minutes of the 49th Conference — TNAI', *NJI*, vol. 51, no. 11, 1960, p. 306.

selling the profession into slavery'.[130] In 1975, Kuruvilla wrote that nurses needed to join together to strengthen the TNAI, as it would only be through a stronger ethic of associationalism that battles would be won.[131] All of these eminent and successful leaders were single women; it seems that they experienced trouble recognising and acknowledging the constraints of nurses' ties to home and family.

The tendency to view the lack of an associational ethic as evidence of apathy illustrates some of the limits of the professionalising culture of nursing organisation. Devaki Jain, in her 1980 study of programmes to liberate women workers, wrote that the successful organisation of women needed to account for the fact that it was often the household, not only the community or the workplace, in which women required emancipation.[132] The older nursing organisations, such as the TNAI and the CNL, have focused on nurses as professionals and not as professionals who are also women.

# A New Generation in Nursing Organisation

In 1995, the romantic comedy *Dil Ka Doctor* (the Heart's Doctor), the story of a love triangle between a middle-aged doctor, his receptionist and a young teenager, was released. It met with only moderate success, but it was notable in that it aroused the ire of an entirely new section of India's nursing leadership, who vocally and publicly protested against dance sequences depicting nurses in short skirts dancing between doctors' legs. These new leaders raised the funds to take the producers of the film through the courts, all the way to the Supreme Court of India, seeking as much media attention as possible along the way. Ultimately they won a historic victory, forcing the withdrawal of the offending scenes.

This successful flexing of nursing muscle in the glamorous world of films suggests that the organisation of nurses may finally be transcending its home in the peaceful Delhi suburb of Green Park,

---

[130] Kumari Lakshmi Devi, 'The Fruits of Freedom', *NJI*, vol. 44, no. 8, 1953, p. 188.

[131] Kuruvilla, 'Status of Nursing', p. 100.

[132] Devaki Jain, *Women's Quest for Power: Five Indian Case Studies*, Ghaziabad: Vikas Publishing House, 1980, p. 8.

whence the TNAI has long pursued its professionalising plans for nursing. While poor conditions persist and the state remains difficult to motivate into action, there are now indications of new approaches to nursing issues and new types of leaders, with concerns other than internationalism and professionalism. One such indication is the emergence of nurse-led unions as powerful negotiating bodies willing to take industrial action. They have identified themselves as feminist organisations and have distanced themselves from nursing's colonial inheritance. Whereas leaders' earlier victories were bestowed by a paternalistic, benevolent state, the new nursing unions have been able to exert power on governments, forcing unwilling concessions. In exploring this trend toward greater nurse unionisation, I have based my analysis partly on a case study of the Delhi Government Nurses' Union (DGNU), a government nurses' union that operates from the Ram Manohar Lohia Hospital in Delhi, where I conducted interviews in January 2006.

The beginnings of this shift in the organisational culture of nursing was in the 1980s, which saw an expansion of nursing unions. While many of the striking nurses of the 1970s had joined broader trade unions, which were often male dominated, these new unions differed in that they were set up exclusively by and for nurses.[133] In 1980, a nurses' union called the Rajkiya Nurses' Sangh presented a set of unusually ambitious demands to the Uttar Pradesh Third Pay Commission, requesting a tripling of board allowance, a doubling of the student stipend, a qualification allowance to be paid to graduate nurses, and the payment of overtime at double the current rate.[134] This was a sign of things to come; by 1999, the TNAI was writing with concern of the 'rapidly increasing number of Government Nurses' Service Associations formed in various states'.[135] Strengthened nurse unions had emerged all over India, including in Maharashtra, Uttar Pradesh, Haryana, Andhra Pradesh, and Punjab.

---

[133] Prior to the 1980s, nursing was incorporated into unions representing a group of occupations, with only a small number of nurses involved and few positive results for nursing.

[134] Government of Uttar Pradesh, 'Report of the Second U. P. Pay Commission', Allahabad: Government of Uttar Pradesh, 1980, vol. 2, pp. 114–15.

[135] Anonymous, 'Policy Statement on Strike', *Indian Nursing Year Book: 1998–1999*, New Delhi: TNAI, 2000, p. 9.

The emergence of strong and visible nurse unions can be viewed as the result of two factors. The first was the groundswell of dissatisfaction during the 1970s, described earlier, which suggested the distance of the existing leadership from nurses' everyday lives and their inability to achieve change, or, more simply, their failure to develop a strong presence at the local level. Second, the rejuvenation of nurse organisation was determined by a political and social context increasingly infused by awareness of developmental failures in relation to gender and the accompanying growth of a new wave of Indian feminism.[136] The seminal Committee on the Status of Women in India was appointed in 1974. It produced a report that identified a general decline in the status of women since Independence, providing a catalyst for a general reinvigoration of the feminist movement.[137] This resurgent women's movement formed part of a general growth in organisation around civil rights prompted by the Emergency, and represented a new generation of feminists, more focused on organising across caste and class boundaries. New women's groups tackled a wide range of issues including violence against women, dowry murders, working conditions for poor women, and the need for legislative reform. The feminist movement continued to grow and ensured the ongoing placement of women's issues on the political agenda (however disappointing the outcomes of this were). This general climate of heightened gender awareness informed the greater assertiveness that has emerged in nursing organisation and has created the social and cultural space for nursing leaders to present nurses' issues as women's issues. The DGNU, for example, is an overtly feminist group and maintains close links with the All India Democratic Women's Association (AIDWA). It views itself as an advocate of women's rights and draws heavily on feminist notions of women's empowerment in its campaigns. It reflects the increased emphasis of feminist organisations over the first decade of the 21st century on combating violence against women and increasing women's democratic participation.

---

[136] For accounts of new developments in Indian feminism from the 1970s, see, for example, Indu Agnihotri and Vinu Mazumdar, 'Changing Terms of Political Discourse: Women's Movement in India, 1970s–1990s', *Economic and Political Weekly*, vol. 30, no. 28, 1995, p. 1869; John, 'Feminisms and Internationalisms', p. 542.

[137] 'National Plan of Action' New Delhi: Government of India, 1976; 'Towards Equality: Report of the Committee on the Status of Women in India', New Delhi: Department of Social Welfare, Government of India, 1974.

## A *new style of nursing organisation*

The formation of the DGNU was an important signpost in the history of Indian nursing. It marked the emergence of a more radical and assertive style of leadership in the national capital that recognised many of the faults of the old. It was born from a powerful wave of nurse discontent that swept Delhi in 1987. The Fourth Pay Commission, convened to conduct a survey of government salaries and to evaluate which groups of workers required adjustments, recommended the acceptance of nurses' longstanding demands for increased food and uniform allowances and for revisions to pay scales that would adequately reward nurses in positions of authority.[138] To the outrage of India's nurses, its findings, published in 1986, were not implemented. As a result, a group of government nurses banded together to lead industrial action, calling themselves the Joint Action Committee (JAC). Several were august and longstanding members of the TNAI, who were angry enough to defy a longstanding anti-strike policy.

The resulting strike was lengthy and dramatic, lasting 17 days from 19 January until 4 February 1987. As it continued, it was joined by growing numbers of nurses and disabled all the major Delhi hospitals, including AIIMS, Safdarjung Hospital, Ram Manohar Lohia, and even the prestigious Postgraduate Institute for Medical Education and Research (PGIMER) Hospital in Chandigarh. On 28 January, *The Times of India* described the capital's health services as 'paralysed', with a small number of trainee and private nurses maintaining only scattered emergency services.[139] At AIIMS, it was reported that primary school teachers and social workers had been drafted to provide assistance on the wards.[140] By 23 January, 50 per cent of patients at AIIMS had been discharged and the strike had made the

---

[138] Government of India, 'The Fourth Central Pay Commission Report', New Delhi: Ministry of Urban Development, 1986; Anonymous, 'Pay Scales for Nursing Personnel as Recommended by the Fourth Central Pay Commission: Central Government, Union Territories and Armed Forces', *NJI*, vol. 77, no. 8, 1986.

[139] Anonymous, 'Striking Nurses Stage Rally at Nirman Bhavan', *The Times of India*, 28 January 1987, p. 3.

[140] Anonymous, 'No Solution Yet to Nurses Strike', *The Times of India*, 22 January 1987, p. 3; 'Govt Ignoring Nurses' new JAC', *Hindustan Times*, 22 January 1987, p. 3.

front page of the *Hindustan Times*.[141] The government was forced to post army nurses in its hospitals, as well as college students (who were encouraged by the TNAI to report for duty).

The strike made disastrously clear the disdain of the state and of hospital employers for nurses and the value of nursing in the health system. As Nagpal observed, 'one lesson of the strike was that the Government had succeeded in treating the cause of the nurses in a rather casual manner, as usual'.[142] On 1 February, the JAC issued a press note stating that the government had issued 'false propaganda' that the city's hospitals were functioning adequately without nurses.[143] The medical superintendent of Jayaprakash Narayan hospital, which was being run by orderlies, medical interns and doctors, publicly asserted that the hospital was managing well without its nursing staff.[144] After nine days on strike, nurses burnt an effigy of the Union Health Minister Saroj Kharpade, who had consistently refused to meet with their leaders, instead sending an official.[145] It was reported that the Delhi police sent to monitor the strike had been drunk on duty and had harassed and attacked nurses.[146]

More positively, the strike showed the efficacy of industrial action and its power to win the support of a wide range of social groups that had not allied themselves with nurses before. Teachers' unions, a range of women's organisations and the Centre of Indian Trade Unions extended their support and the strike was extensively covered in the media.[147] At the beginning of the strike, the health minister had not found time in her schedule even to meet with nurses; as events progressed, the government offered first ₹100, then ₹300 and finally ₹400 in monthly allowances for uniforms and living expenses. It also committed to refer pay demands to the Anomalies Committee, and to

---

[141] Anonymous, 'Plan to Recruit ad hoc Nurses', *Hindustan Times*, 23 January 1987, p. 1.

[142] Narender Nagpal, 'Was the Strike Worthwhile?', *NJI*, vol. 57, no. 3, 1987, p. 57.

[143] Anonymous, 'Nurses' Strike Enters 13th day', *Hindustan Times*, 1 February 1987, p. 5.

[144] Anonymous, 'Sack notice for 25 striking nurses?', *Sunday Observer*, New Delhi, 25 January 1987, p. 5.

[145] Anonymous, 'Striking Nurses Stage Rally', p. 3.

[146] Anonymous, 'Health Chief Ignorant of Nurses' Recruitment', *The Times of India*, 23 January 1987, p. 3.

[147] Anonymous, 'No Solution Yet to Nurses Strike', p. 3.

appoint a High Power Committee that would examine pay scales, the status of the profession and the nursing education system (the TNAI had been requesting the appointment of such a committee through its reports and memoranda for several years). Editorials in the *NJI* recorded disapproval at the sufferings of hospital patients in the capital, and described the government's concessions as 'meagre', but were reluctantly forced to concede that the High Power Committee's appointment was an important victory.[148]

Following the strike, several of the JAC leaders formed the Delhi Government Nurses' Union. The new nurses' union was ultimately led by Gurdarshan Kaur Khurana, a longstanding TNAI member. Khurana was one of the more moderate strike leaders, who had been in favour of calling an early halt. However, as a leader she has led the DGNU on a path of increasingly strident activism, and has been integral to the organisation's success. Khurana was a nurse and then a matron at the Ram Manohar Lohia hospital in Delhi for 38 years and was a well-regarded member of the TNAI. She was thoroughly schooled in the traditional, conservative ethos of nurse professionalism, and was even the student of Satish Chawla, TNAI president in the late 1990s and early 2000s. She emerged, however, as a leader who proved capable of acting effectively on the widely felt dissatisfaction with this style of leadership. The reasons for this, it can be suggested, are evident in both her personal and professional profile. Khurana typifies the popular stereotype of the Punjabi mother — confident, assertive and slightly terrifying. She speaks loudly, at great length, has a very useful cutting wit, and takes great pride in anecdotes of her victories over big names ranging from Bollywood producers to the Uttar Pradesh Chief Minister Mulayam Singh Yadav. She is married to an engineer from Ferozepur, whose support she told me, with evident emotion, had been the foundation of all her political successes. She has three children (a son in business, another son studying engineering and a daughter with a commerce degree, who is a housewife). These children were born relatively late in her life, and it seemed that this might in part have facilitated her very strong commitment to her career. A strong personality, an obvious enjoyment of power, and a supportive and

---

encouraging family allowed Khurana to push and support a new mode of nursing organisation that was defined quite strongly against her own background of involvement with more traditional styles of leadership, but which was informed by a long career of witnessing, as she told me, the painful humiliation of nurses.[149]

In contrast to a history of leaders' preoccupation with professionalism, the DGNU's central cause is the improvement of hospital conditions for nurses, with campaigns based on issues such as salaries, security, staffing norms, and the provision of crèches in hospitals.[150] Although Khurana says that the DGNU is slow to strike due to potential patient suffering, and has a policy of holding rallies and demonstrations before striking, the organisation has become a veteran of industrial action, conducting major strikes in 1989, 1990, 1995–96 and 1998, all of which were extensively supported.[151] In 1998, for example, the vast majority of the 12,000 government nurses in Delhi joined a DGNU strike, which caused chaos in the city's hospital system.[152] The achievements of these actions have been significant, albeit not revolutionary. A notable victory, following a strike in early 1990, was an agreement with the government that it would fund and build a large nurses colony to provide good quality accommodation for 400 to 500 Delhi nurses.[153] In January 2006 the building was finally dedicated and opened, after a series of protests over the slow progress of construction and the omission of a water supply for the building. In 1998, after a strike in May during which Khurana informed a BBC journalist that 'some nurses may choose self-immolation if their demands are not met', the DGNU signed an agreement with the Directorate-General of Health Services.[154] It provided for a large increase in the number of senior nurse roles,

---

[149] Author interview with G. K. Khurana.

[150] Anonymous, 'Florence Nightingale Anniversary'; author interview with G. K. Khurana.

[151] Author interview with G. K. Khurana.

[152] Satish Jacob, 'Delhi's nurses want strike to spread', BBC News Online, 10 May 1998, http://newsrss.bbc.co.uk/2/low/world/s/w_asia/90516.stm (accessed 12 April 2012).

[153] Delhi Government Nurses' Union (DGNU) and Government of India, 'Memorandum of Settlement', February 1990, 3. From the institutional files of the DGNU.

[154] Jacob, 'Delhi's Nurses want Strike to Spread'.

a raise in nurses' living and uniform allowances, and a commitment to work towards the establishment of a separate Directorate of Nursing.[155]

By the early 2000s, the DGNU had achieved a high profile, with its strikes regularly reported and its increasingly assertive leader often appearing in the newspapers and on television. Khurana claimed that as a result, when Uttar Pradesh nurses struck over their allowances in 2005, a telegram from her office to the Chief Minister Mulayam Singh Yadav, threatening a DGNU visit to his office, was enough to persuade him to accede to nurses' demands.[156] Like the first-generation organisations, the DGNU has been frequently ignored by the state and has suffered from the non-implementation of state promises. It has, however, often managed to vigorously protest this in a way that has caused political and financial damage to the interests of the state and has exacted some unwilling concessions.

Another important feature of the DGNU has been its willingness to protest against cases of rape and violence against nurses directly and publicly. This has placed the issue firmly in the public sphere. It has ensured that the mistreatment of nurses who have been victims of rape has been widely acknowledged, whereas in the past nursing leaders either tiptoed euphemistically around cases of sexual abuse or chose not to be associated with them at all. In 2003, the DGNU, in remarkable contrast to such timidity, brought its membership onto the streets to offer strident public support to a nurse who was raped and viciously attacked at Shanti Mukund Hospital.[157] It issued vehement statements to the media criticising hospital management and provided legal and moral support to the victim in court.[158]

UNESCO's 2000 'World Culture Report' emphasised that the continuing inequality of women rested in part on their unequal access to information and the media.[159] The DGNU's style of activism

---

[155] Jacob, 'Delhi's Nurses want Strike to Spread'.

[156] Author interview with G. K. Khurana.

[157] Anonymous, 'Delhi Rape Case: JMS Stages Angry Demo Against Hospital', *People's Democracy*, vol. 27, no. 39, 28 September 2003, http://pd.cpim.org/2003/0928/09282003_delhipercent20jms.htm (accessed 9 July 2005); Dogra, 'Delhi has a Long Way to go'.

[158] Sapna Dogra, 'Delhi Nurses' union seeks ₹10 lakh compensation for rape victim', *Express Healthcare Management*, 1–15 October 2003, http://www.express healthcaremgmt.com/20031015/hospinews02.shtml (accessed 27 November 2006).

[159] In Devaki Jain, *Women, development and the UN: A Sixty-year Quest for Equality and Justice*, Chesham: Indiana University Press, 2005, p. 137.

recognises this inequality, and takes the promotion of positive representation of nurses and nursing issues in the media as a central dimension of its work. According to Khurana, in the past a major failure of nurses was their unwillingness to engage with the public in this way. In 1991, the DGNU confronted the government television channel Doordarshan over a serial it ran showing careless nurses allowing patients to die. A letter was written threatening that a DGNU delegation would be sent to picket Doordarshan headquarters with black flags. The director, N. K. Rana, ordered an apology to be broadcast on the channel and took the serial off air. In 1995 an even more aggressive confrontation occurred with the producers of the film *Dil Ka Doctor*, with the successful results described earlier.

In a more positive sense, Khurana and the DGNU have also sought the support of media and journalists for their activism on behalf of nurses. According to Khurana, the impact of repeated strike actions has been enhanced by support from media organisations including the popular television channel Zee TV, and the national broadsheet *Hindustan Times*. Nurse organisers may be seen to have satisfied what Rajan identifies as a new media hunger for sensationalist 'women's issues' stories, which consistently present women as 'external and adversarial rather than as integral and ambivalent', but this seems preferable to a past in which their problems found no audience at all.[160] This new and creative willingness to engage with a variety of media, albeit often on the media's terms, shows potential to rework the problematic public image of the nurse in India.

The DGNU has also been increasingly characterised by a desire to localise the culture of nursing, deliberately and overtly defining themselves against what Khurana described as 'the missionaries'. One of the most interesting campaigns fought by DGNU was against an important legacy of Western nurse leadership: the wearing of white frocks, described by Khurana as 'a vestige of the colonial regime'.[161] Frocks were a longstanding bone of contention, disliked by many nurses. This was first because many Hindus associate the colour white with widowhood and mourning. Second, in India it is mainly only young girls who wear frocks. Third, as is common for patients and their relatives to sleep on the floor, short nurses' uniforms have historically caused discomfort and self-consciousness for some nurses.

---

[160] Rajeswari Sunder Rajan, *Real and Imagined Women: Gender, Culture and Postcolonialism*, London: Routledge, 1993, p. 137.

[161] Anonymous, 'Florence Nightingale Anniversary'.

The DGNU request to change the uniform was refused by the union government, with the comment that the white uniform was a 'symbol of purity and professional dignity'.[162] Doctors at Ram Manohar Lohia dispatched a memorandum to the government insisting that they preferred nurses to wear white frocks, in reply to which the DGNU sent a retaliatory memorandum stating their own preference for doctors in black trousers. Nurses changed their uniforms regardless of state opposition, and 99 per cent of the hospital's nurses purchased the new saris (which remain technically illegal) at their own expense.[163] According to Khurana, nurses and their parents enthusiastically welcomed the change. Whilst limited to one hospital, this campaign received considerable media exposure, including newspaper coverage, a televised debate and a public declaration by the health minister that he would see Khurana in a white frock (he did not).[164] Maithreyi Krishna Raj writes:

> [W]e in India not only have the task of uncovering 'male bias' in our institutions that have led to male dominance but have the additional task of unburdening our colonial legacy — a legacy that persists in the cultural and intellectual subordination.[165]

The casting off of a uniform that many saw as a source of shame and a cause of the questioning of nurses' morality is an interesting grassroots example of this.

In South Africa, increased unionism and radical strike action during the 1980s provoked 'a crisis of legitimacy' for the South African Nursing Association and a subsequent improvement in its collective bargaining machinery.[166] It seems that India's new nurse unions may similarly shape the priorities of the older nursing organisations. The TNAI was from the 1970s anxiously aware of the growing keenness of nurses for unions and watched the expansion of government

---

[162] Regunathan, Sudhamahi, 'Nurses don't Wear Short Frocks and Kiss Doctors', *The Times of India*, 20 January 1996, p. 11.

[163] Author interview with G. K. Khurana.

[164] See for example, Regunathan, 'Nurses don't Wear Short Frocks'.

[165] Maithreyi Krishna Raj, 'Why Women's Studies? Some Feminist Perspectives', *Women's Studies in India: Some Perspectives*, Bombay: Popular Prakashan, 1986, p. 41.

[166] Marks, *Divided Sisterhood*, p. 206.

unions with trepidation. It maintained its emphasis on education and professional development, but at the same time increasingly attempted to position itself as a more convincing defender of the average nurse. It has been forced, by clear evidence that strikes succeeded where their own policies failed, to adopt a more nuanced policy on industrial action. In 1990 the TNAI President, Durga Mehta, joined nurse unionists to negotiate an agreement with the Ministry of Health and Family Welfare. Reflecting on this, Nagpal wrote that 'it was thus the efforts of the agitating Nurses and the national Nurses' association in tandem that could bring about a satisfying way out of what seemed to be an impasse', suggesting an entirely less condemnatory attitude than was the case in the past towards striking nurses.[167] In 2004, the theme of the TNAI's biennial conference was working conditions, and in 2006, Nanthini Subbiah of the TNAI made a presentation for the 'Dialogue for a Safe Delhi' campaign in which she emphasised the ongoing failure to provide nurses with accommodation, low pay, the absence of transport, and the unavailability of toilet facilities.[168]

With the TNAI willing to talk toilets, it seems that cultural change has occurred in nursing organisation. On the other hand, many problems remain with leadership. One that suggests itself quite intensely is the continuing absence of any organisation that really strongly concerns itself with Malayali nurses. The professionalising TNAI has little to offer to young, vulnerable, freshly-trained Malayali nurses from rural backgrounds, who arrive in Delhi or other cities often with poor language and little experience of city life. Nair's work interviewing these nurses suggests they face a range of hazards in and outside the workplace.[169] The DGNU, which reportedly mobilises north Indian nurses more strongly, does not seem to address itself to Malayalis' particular issues (this dissonance is illustrated, for example, in the change to khaki uniforms; Kerala nurses indeed have no problem with white, in their home state it is a popular and

---

[167] Narender Nagpal, 'End of an Agitation', *NJI*, vol. 81, no. 3, 1990, p. 73.

[168] Anonymous, 'TNAI Attends Dialogue for "Safe Delhi"', *NJI*, vol. 7, no. 2, 2006, p. 27.

[169] Sreelekha Nair and Marie Percot, 'Transcending Boundaries: Indian Nurses in Internal and International Migration', Occasional Paper, Centre for Women in Developing Societies, New Delhi, 2007.

frequently worn colour without the same negative associations it has in the north). On the other hand, it does seem that the emergence of new nursing unions may suggest an important and potentially productive point of departure from an old and tired culture of nursing organisation.

## Conclusions

In a society where working women have continued to experience discrimination, harassment and exclusion, the older nursing organisations have maintained a long record of promoting high-quality education for a non-elite group of working women. Their vision of nursing as a skill that ought to be more highly valued, and of nurses as deserving autonomy and a broad education in the humanities and the social and physical sciences, is in many ways admirable. In a context of subordination and prejudice against nursing, they provided the structures of a professional community and continued to promote the idea that nursing should be much more than it was allowed to be.

This was an idea that took strong hold. In 1975, an article published in the *NJI* discussing the legal definition of a nurse specified that the doctor–nurse relationship was one of 'master to servant'.[170] For months afterwards the journal received a flurry of letters of protest. M. N. Holkar wrote that the 'nurse is a co-worker of the physician, you may call her as an "assistant" but in no case is she a servant to the physician'.[171] Saramma K. V. wrote 'there is no question of "Master-Servant" relation between a doctor and a nurse'.[172] Maya Sengupta pointed out that 'the scientific, educated nurse is competent to save the life of a patient before the arrival of the doctor'.[173] Sindhu Tilak began a lengthy protest with the exclamation that 'really it is striking to me and touches my heart. I will never be servant of any doctor in my life'.[174] This debate reflected a generally strong Indian internalisation through education of the professionalising nurses'

---

[170] J. D. Powar, 'Nursing Functions and Law in India', *NJI*, vol. 66, no. 1, 1975, p. 4.

[171] M. N. Holkar, Letter to the Editor, *NJI*, vol. 66, no. 5, 1975, p. 107.

[172] Saramma K. V., Letter to the Editor, *NJI*, vol. 66, no. 5, 1975, p. 107.

[173] Maya Sengupta, Letter to the Editor, *NJI*, vol. 66, no. 4, 1975, p. 79.

[174] Sindhu Tilak, Letter to the Editor, *NJI*, vol. 66, no. 3, 1975, p. 58.

view of nursing as a separate and equal field of expertise (even though the chance to practise this view was another matter entirely).

Although limited by a Christian heritage defined by service, obedience and an opposition to industrial action, the TNAI frequently made representations to the state protesting against the dreadful conditions under which nurses worked. It is true that in practice their suggestions were frequently ignored, but they were also regularly consulted and it was through them that a reasonably strong nursing perspective was incorporated into each of the major health planning committees of the period (although the practical results of these were disappointing).

In general, however, successes have been moderate. Their intensive espousal of the ideology of professionalism and educational development, strongly determined by their colonial heritage and determinedly internationalist focus, has continually encountered a hostile reality. The INC, the TNAI and the CNL all hoped that by advocating for and developing better nursing education, they would create empowered professionals, who would inevitably win the respect of colleagues and society. Melosh writes that as a strategy, professionalising is bound to fail and as an ideology it weakens and divides.[175] This contention seems borne out by the experience of the first-generation organisations, which largely failed to bring any substantial improvement in the treatment of nurses. Throughout this period, India's nurses have been underpaid, overworked, often endangered by their workplace, and have failed to claim the public health role that health planners defined for them. Professionalism did not win the enthusiastic support of the majority of India's nurses, who seemed to find it distant from the everyday difficulties of their work. Chattopadhyay wrote that women leaders in general, up until the 1970s 'forged no links with the wider mass of women, who are only approached briefly at voting time to secure their ballot papers'.[176] Similarly, nursing leaders advertised their strong commitment to professionalism and educational development, while doing little practically to connect with their constituency. As Oonnie (assistant director of health services in Madhya Pradesh in 1973) identified,

[175] Melosh, *'The Physician's Hand'*, p. 16.

[176] Kamaladevi Chattopadhyay, 'The Women's Movement: Then and Now', in Devaki Jain (ed.), *Indian Women*, New Delhi: Publications Division, Ministry of Information and Broadcasting, Government of India, 1975, p. 33.

nurse leaders often failed to come to terms with an often hostile and uncomfortable 'world of reality', instead remaining confined to a 'fantasy world of resolutions'.[177]

In recent years, however, new types of nursing leadership have emerged. These have challenged the conservative approach of the older organisations. It is perhaps the case that the profession has reached a new stage of maturity, with a broader national representation of women in its ranks, a better level of education among its recruits and a slowly increasing self-confidence. As a result, a productive although often traumatic reshaping of identity, purpose and cultural location can be seen to have begun. The emergence in Delhi and elsewhere of nurse-led organisations willing to venture outside the hitherto heavily circumscribed sphere of nursing activism is exciting. With intensive media engagement, emphasis on a very high public profile, well-established links with other feminist organisations, and a strong concentration on local culture and local issues, it is at the very least clear that the new organisations are defined in radical opposition to the old.

Like their forebears, however, these new leaders face the challenge of engaging with a state peculiarly disengaged from and unaware of the need for the services of nurses. The next chapter addresses this issue, sketching the contours of what has historically been a limiting, damaging and contemptuous relationship between the profession and the state.

---

[177] Oonnie, 'Nursing Students of the 70's', p. 411.

# A *Parsi Nurse in* UP
## Gool Pestonji Kapadia

GOOL PESTONJI KAPADIA qualified as a nurse at the King Edward Memorial (KEM) hospital in Bombay in 1937. After working as a staff nurse, she took her Sister Tutor's diploma at the Lady Reading Health School in Delhi.[1] Her colleague and friend of many years, Alice Zachariah, an eminent nursing leader who worked in Andhra Pradesh, remembered their time together as students in Delhi. Reminiscing about her friend's enthusiasm for current affairs, she wrote 'Gool would have me read out the entire daily newspaper after breakfast'.[2]

Kapadia was sponsored to study in London for her diploma in nursing administration. Later, the UP government selected her as the national counterpart to the WHO's nursing representative in the state, and in 1957 she was appointed as the Superintendent of Nursing Services. She served in this position (which later became the Deputy Director of Health Services) until 1972.

She was a member of the TNAI Council from 1947–74 and President of the UP State branch, as well as chair of the TNAI's education section and economic welfare committee. Her obituary in the *NJI* recorded that she had worked on several projects to collect more accurate data on the economic situation of nurses. When she died on 11 February 1975, she had been working on suggestions for the revision of rules on nurses' pensions and dearness allowances, as well as preparing the blueprint for a college of nursing for UP.[3]

---

[1] Anonymous, 'Candidates for TNAI Elections October 1972 — Bombay', *NJI*, vol. 63, no. 9, 1972, pp. 317–18.

[2] Alice Zachariah, 'A Tribute to a Departed Friend', *NJI*, vol. 66, no. 5, 1975, p. 107.

[3] Anonymous, 'Obituaries', *NJI*, vol. 66, no. 3, 1975, p. 59.

Zachariah wrote of her friend that '"Good bedside nursing" was an endearing and favourite theme of her life, herself being a down-to-earth bedside nurse as well as an excellent teacher'. She had visited Kapadia during her initial hospitalisation, and remembered that:

> When I visited her in Lucknow after her first illness she expressed great disappointment and remorse at the low standards of nursing care in the hospitals. The fact that she was not spared from the difficulties caused by these conditions pained her very much. She said that if another chance were given in her life, she would labour for a revival of nursing.[4]

Her obituaries in the *NJI* recorded that Kapadia, who never married, worked all her life for the betterment of nurses' education and their economic welfare. One author wrote 'it was mainly through her efforts that Nursing Education had made great strides in U.P. She was the pioneer of planning a College of Nursing for U.P. nurses' and also that she 'devoted her life in doing humanitarian service for her country'.[5] Zachariah sadly wrote that 'in the untimely death of Miss Gool Kapadia the TNAI members have lost the most inspiring friend and the most industrious leader'.[6]

■

---

[4] Zachariah, 'A Tribute', p. 107.
[5] R. N. Singh, 'In Memoriam', *NJI*, vol. 66, no. 4, 1975, p. 79.
[6] Zachariah, 'A Tribute', p. 107.

# 5

# The Indian State and
# the Disappearing Nurse

◼

In 1965, the Indian government sponsored a seminar in Madras on the role of voluntary agencies in public health and family planning. Of 123 participants, only one, Tehmina K. Adranvala, was a nurse.[1] This illustrates the extent to which the association between the state and the nursing profession has been radically underdeveloped. This rocky relationship has to a large extent determined the problematic post-colonial experience of Indian nurses, who have continually suffered dangerous workplaces, low salaries, stagnant careers, and an inadequate and exploitative educational system.

The orientation of the state towards nursing has undergone important shifts since Independence. Until the mid-1960s, professionalising plans in nursing found resonance with both the ambitious plans of the Congress government to improve health standards, and the influential new developmentalism that was having a profound impact on health planning. At the same time, practical inaction and a federal health setup imbued with many of the flaws of the colonial system were disastrous for nurses. Ambitious promises were not fulfilled, and when sweeping realignments occurred in politics and health from the mid-1960s, nursing was in a position of such weakness that it was completely marginalised. Until the mid-1980s, the concerns of nurses were swept aside in a health system caught up in

---

[1] Andhra Mahila Sabha, 'National Seminar on the Role of Voluntary Agencies in the Implementation of Public Health, Medical Care and Family Planning Programmes under Five Year Plans', Madras: Andhra Mahila Sabha, 1965.

enthusiasm for family planning on the one hand, and an increasing national and international realisation of the neglect of rural health on the other. Recent decades have seen some increase in attention to nursing, mandated by the perception of nurse emigrants as a lucrative export, a more gender-sensitive socio-political environment and a more assertive profession, but such improvements are easily overstated. In general, the state continues to recognise nurses' problems through committees and on-paper initiatives, while in practice allowing violence and exploitation to carry on unchecked. Throughout this post-colonial period, there has been a consistent refusal to recognise the role of nursing in any meaningful, practical way. As women's work, nursing has been rendered mostly invisible. This confirms feminist analysis of the difficulty of engagement with a patriarchal state and suggests the futility of expecting the state to strongly address the root causes of nurses' problems.

## Health, Women and the Post-colonial State

The post-colonial Indian state in general has promised much to women and delivered little. Rajeswari Sunder Rajan writes that in its orientation to women's issues it has been characterised by a difficult duality: on the one hand it is a violent, patriarchal, exclusionary entity, and on the other, it can also be motivated by its self-consciously liberal, democratic, modern and social-justice oriented character.[2] Flavia Agnes' account of the women's movement and the state during the 1980s also has resonance for nurses. She describes the eager rhetorical support of the state for anti-violence legislation, which was defeated by its own practical inaction. The legislature, she records, was 'over eager to portray a progressive pro-women front by passing laws for the asking', while the 'executive and the judiciary did not reflect even this token concern at the level of interpretation and implementation'.[3] The state was ultimately incapable of tackling the

---

[2] Rajan, *The Scandal of the State*, p. 25.

[3] Flavia Agnes, 'Protecting Women against Violence?: Review of a Decade of Legislation, 1980–1989', in Partha Chatterjee (ed.), *State and Politics in India*, Oxford: Oxford University Press, 1997, p. 522.

root causes of violence against women, and it proved impossible to translate the pro-woman rhetoric of some branches of the state into effective action by others.

The case of nursing reinforces such analysis and replicates some of the women's movement's encounter with the state. Nurses have on the one hand received endless promises, presented to them in the fashionable developmental language of the day, whilst in practice being subject to a perplexing and damaging disengagement which has suggested the most thorough-going contempt for their work, their role in the modern hospital and their safety.

The post-colonial politics of health allowed little room for nursing leaders. The history of the health system in India, according to Roger Jeffery, records the dominance of two groups: doctors and planners.[4] The post-Independence history of health in India shows on the one hand an over-concentration of resources in urban hospitals, and on the other a strong health discourse emphasising the importance of improving rural health and focusing on public health outside the cities. Neither phenomenon has benefited the nursing service weakened by state inaction.

The neglect and exclusion of the nursing profession is to some degree the result of medical power. Jeffery validly argues that the professional power of doctors in India has been relatively less than is usually the case in the West, as they have faced administrative control, the lack of a strong colleague-controlled system, burdensome political interference, and competition from indigenous practitioners.[5] This has not, however, detracted their dominance over nurses within the hospital; in fact, concern with an authority threatened from many sides may even have increased their preoccupation with protecting professional terrain from nurses. While less autonomous, perhaps, than Western doctors, India's medical profession has exercised a degree of power that has been directly damaging for nurses. Sociologists of nursing often point to the invisibility of the profession, and nowhere is this clearer than in the relative positioning of doctors and nurses in India's health planning. Numbers of doctors, the desirable quantity and quality of medical colleges and the direction of medical research have been regarded as the most important subjects

4 Jeffery, 'Toward a Political Economy of Health Care', p. 279.
5 Jeffery, 'Allopathic Medicine in India', pp. 561–73.

for national health planners and bureaucrats; these are the issues that dominate planning reports and documents. In contrast, nurses have not been viewed as a national concern, instead understood as easily left to the (very unevenly resourced) states. A range of expensive and relatively well-resourced central institutions promoting medical education and research has been maintained, including AIIMS in Delhi and the PGIMER at Chandigarh. In contrast, only a few central nursing schemes have existed, which have struggled continually for adequate funding and resourcing. Typically, the Fifth Five-year Plan, for 1974–79, allocated ₹1,695 lakh to improving undergraduate and postgraduate medical education, while ₹16 lakh was given for nurse education (15 lakh of which was to cover building costs for the college of nursing in Delhi, which, although it had opened in 1946, still did not have a permanent building).[6] Although the alienation of doctors from rural health has been almost as marked as that of nurses, this has not had the same effect in reducing their influence. At least until the 1970s, Jeffery writes, 'the problem of rural medical relief was seen as the absence of doctors'.[7]

The dominance of doctors can be viewed as a consequence of their high status. As a prestigious and publicly well-regarded profession, in comparison to low-status nurses, they have accrued power and influence. Partly, this high status determined the over-direction of resources into medicine, as politicians realised the political capital available through providing medical colleges.[8] At the same time, medical dominance has directly contributed to nursing's ongoing low status. Dignifying nursing required resources and it has been well documented that the successes of the medical profession rested on deflecting resources from nurses and paramedical workers. The phenomenon of 'mushrooming medical colleges' from the mid-1960s, according to Imrana Qadeer, led to a serious under-emphasis and underfunding of the training of all other health workers.[9] This was

---

[6] Planning Commission of India, 'Draft Fifth Five Year Plan 1974–79', p. 247; Anonymous, 'New Building to House College of Nursing', *NJI*, vol. 62, no. 9, 1971, p. 295. A lakh is a unit in the Indian numbering system. One lakh is equal to a hundred thousand.

[7] Jeffery, *The Politics of Health in India*, p. 232.

[8] Ibid., p. 243.

[9] Imrana Qadeer, 'The World Development Report 1993: The Brave New World of Primary Health Care', in Mohan Rao (ed.), *Disinvesting in Health: The World Bank's Prescriptions for Health*, New Delhi: Sage Publications, 1999, p. 52.

directly recognised in the Fifth Five-year Plan, which stated the intention not to expand medical education any further, acknowledging that the education of 'para-medical personnel' was an area of greater need.[10] Despite this, the plan allocated one hundred times the amount of money to improving medical education as it did to nurse education.[11] The inequitable distribution of health resources in favour of doctors was even more strongly recognised in the Sixth Five-year Plan for 1980–85, the first to describe the outcomes of a health planning process that had produced rhetoric emphasising the rural, but which in reality had often served the interests of doctors and of an urban elite. It commented on the overproduction of doctors, the problem of unemployment and the extreme reluctance among the medical profession, even in the face of joblessness, to work in primary health centres and sub-centres.[12] Illustrating the difficulty of putting into practice a policy against the interests of the medical lobby, the Eighth Plan, published in 1992, recognised yet again that the over-resourcing of medical education continued, 'often at the cost of other categories of personnel'.[13]

The problems of the medical profession were thus generally considered a policy issue worth the attention of the centre, while nursing was left to the states. Sunil Amrith writes that independent India, while planning for dramatic improvements in public health, kept 'much of the institutional architecture of its colonial predecessor'.[14] This especially applied to the tendency to leave the majority of responsibility for health to the states, while not allocating them sufficient funding.[15] Nursing has suffered particularly from this trend. The uneven distribution of nurses throughout India and the heavy

---

[10] Planning Commission of India, 'Draft Fifth Five Year Plan 1974–79', p. 237.

[11] Ibid., p. 247.

[12] Planning Commission of India, 'Sixth Five Year Plan', New Delhi: Government of India, c.1980, http://planningcommission.nic.in/plans/planrel/fiveyr/default.html (accessed 24 October 2006).

[13] Planning Commission of India, 'Eighth Five Year Plan', New Delhi: Government of India, 1992, http://planningcommission.nic.in/plans/planrel/fiveyr/default.html (accessed 24 October 2006).

[14] Amrith, 'Political Culture of Health in India', p. 117.

[15] Although, as Jeffery points out, funds allocated by the Central Planning Commission's Five-year Plans have often represented over 50 per cent of all public sector health expenditures, so that the centre has still had considerable influence over the direction of health policy in the states ('Toward a Political Economy of Health Care', pp. 278–79).

national reliance on nurses from Kerala made it quite obvious that building a viable and useful national profession would require the attention of the centre. Figure 5.1 shows the unusual extent of inter-state nurse mobility in India. The picture it gives of nurse movement in 1971 reflects Kerala's status as the producer of nurses for the rest of the nation, and Delhi's position as a magnet for nurses hoping for better work or a path to emigration. States such as Bihar, Rajasthan and Uttar Pradesh have clearly relied extensively on nurses from other states. India has also experienced a chronic imbalance in the state-wise distribution of nurses. In 1974, the nurse to population rate in Delhi was 1:2,856, and 1:4,848 in Maharashtra. In contrast, the ratio in Bihar and Orissa was 1:25,805, in Uttar Pradesh it was 1:23,457.[16] Figures for 2002 reflected similar disparities. For example, Bihar, with 8.1 per cent of India's population, had 1 per cent of GNM nurses. The impoverished newly created state of Jharkand, with 2.6 per cent of the population, had 10 nurses in total. Uttar Pradesh and the new state of Uttarakhand, representing 16.2 per cent of the population, had 2 per cent of nurses. In contrast, Tamil Nadu, with 6.1 per cent of the population, had 18.4 per cent of nurses. Kerala, with 3.1 per cent of the Indian population, had 8.3 per cent.[17] The tendency of the centre to ignore nursing is difficult to comprehend in the face of such extensive evidence of massive inter-state inequalities.

According to Jeffery, the main influence counterbalancing the dominance of the medical profession has been a consistent focus on rural and community health provision, which became markedly more pronounced from the 1970s.[18] This counterbalancing, however, has not benefited nurses, who have been ignored by economist bureaucrats and politicians to the same degree that they have been ignored by doctor administrators, bureaucrats and politicians. As was emphasised in Chapter 4, a strong role for the public health nurse has failed to emerge in India.[19] The consequences for nurses have been grim. Excluded by doctors from authority and influence within the hospital system, they have failed to find an alternative

[16] CAHP, 'Report of a Nursing Survey in India', p. ix.

[17] Central Bureau of Health Intelligence, *Health Information of India 2002*, New Delhi: Central Bureau of Health Intelligence, 2004.

[18] Jeffery, 'Toward a Political Economy of Health Care', p. 279.

[19] Manocha, 'Challenges for Nursing Profession', p. 114.

**Figure 5.1:** Inter-State Mobility of Indian Nurses, 1971

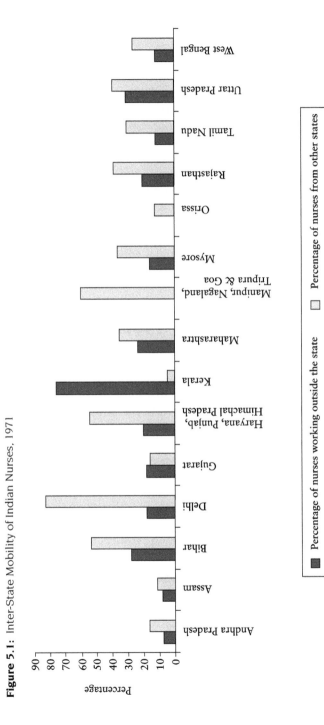

*Source*: CAHP, 'Report of a Nursing Survey in India', 1974.

sphere of authority in the primary health centres and sub-centres, in which nursing roles have frequently remained vacant. The result has been a perception that nursing skill is non-essential in the public health system; that ANMs have worked unsupervised and have been subject to isolation and exploitation; that the public health nurses who do choose to work in the system struggle to have their authority recognised; and that maternal and child health services that ought to have been provided have not been.

This, then, is the background against which the history of nurses' exclusion must be understood. In a health system, dominated on the one hand by the medical profession and on the other by planners attempting to address the massive neglect of rural health, hospital-bound, overworked and under-educated nurses were easily marginalised.

# The Rhetorical Embrace
# of Nursing, 1947–65

The first two decades after Independence saw much enthusiastic rhetoric voiced about the need to develop nursing, but little positive action. Ultimately, this meant that when the politics of health underwent a shift from the late 1960s, the position of nurses was weak. Initially, however, nursing found solid theoretical acceptance among politicians and planners as an essential dimension of modern medicine. It formed a small but significant part of the larger project of the construction of the Nehruvian developmental state, which aimed both to oversee the planning of industrialisation and to intervene so as to bring rapid improvements to the health and education of the population.[20] Amrith describes the general post-Independence feeling among early politicians and health planners that 'a new utopia, a world without disease, seemed within reach'.[21] Nursing, at this early stage, was understood to have a role to play in this envisaged utopia. The eminent Indian doctor and Vice-chancellor of University of Madras, A. L. Mudaliar, even lectured the WHO on the need to

---

[20] For an account of the developmental state, see Partha Chatterjee, 'Development Planning and the Indian State', in *State and Politics in India*, Oxford: Oxford University Press, 1997, pp. 271–98.

[21] Amrith, 'Political Culture of Health in India', p. 114.

expand its horizons to include a stronger role for nurses, declaring that 'no longer can it be said that the health problems of the world can be dealt with by medical personnel alone' and that 'we require the active co-operation of the nursing profession'.[22]

The key health planning document of the early years was the Bhore Report of 1946, which David Arnold describes as 'an epitaph for colonialism's eminent demise'.[23] It revealed a colonial India troubled by an extremely low standard of public health, high levels of preventable mortality and morbidity, the urbanisation of health services and vastly inadequate numbers of doctors, nurses and midwives.[24] The authors ambitiously proposed the establishment of a health system along the lines of the National Health Service proposed for Britain, with universal and high quality health care, accessible to the entire population. As was detailed in Chapter 2, in the case of nursing it endorsed the university-based education of a small elite. It also proposed that an enormous expansion in the number of nurses was necessary and set the target of 740,000 trained nurses by 1971 (by 1972 there were in fact only 82,330).[25]

The ambitious recommendations of the Bhore Report, adopted as the main template of post-Independence planning, provided grounds for considerable optimism. This was reinforced by the favourable orientation of the state towards nursing that developed at the end of the colonial period, as described in Chapter 2. As discussed in Chapter 3, international NGOs and aid organisations also encouraged a focus on the development of nursing, in general heavily emphasising the role of the nurse in a well-functioning national health system. As Rajan emphasises, the Indian state has been keen to maintain its image as modern, liberal, democratic, and motivated by social justice.[26] This has involved a high level of responsiveness to international thinking on development and gender. Thus, the activities of international agencies tended to raise the profile of nursing considerably. Overall,

---

[22] *Collected Speeches of Dr. A. Lakshmanaswami Mudaliar, Vice-Chancellor, University of Madras*, Madras: The Dr A. L. Mudaliar 71st Birthday Celebration Committee, 1957, p. 254.

[23] David Arnold, 'Crisis and Contradiction', p. 351.

[24] Ibid.

[25] Government of India, *India: A Reference Annual 1974*, New Delhi: Ministry of Information and Broadcasting, 1975, p. 82.

[26] Rajan, *The Scandal of the State*, p. 25.

there was thus a significant level of rhetorical support, at least, for the active development of nursing.

At Independence, Adranvala took over from the British nurse, E. E. Hutchings, as nursing advisor to the Government of India and continued as superintendent of nursing at the Directorate General of Health Services (DGHS) until 1966. Adranvala's role in keeping the cause of nursing in the public eye during this period was very significant. As a leader, she was intelligent, diplomatic and productive, and was confident and self-possessed in working with politicians and international agencies. Importantly, and in contrast to the other graduates of overseas education programmes, who usually ended up working in elite educational institutions or in the Christian schools, she was strongly committed to working with governments. Adranvala took on a vital role, as was suggested in Chapter 3, in liaising between state governments and the international agency nurses. She participated in policy forums, and regularly wrote articles and chapters on the nursing profession, advocating the better treatment of students and the development of a stronger nurse role in public health.[27] Although she was a firm supporter of the professionalist cause, in her case this commitment was moderated by a realistic awareness of basic needs at the hospital level. The next generation of nurses produced capable nurses and good leaders, but none who had both her abilities and commitment to work actively with the state and to advocate for nursing in a variety of political and social contexts. As an individual, therefore, Adranvala formed a crucial part of the story of the generally better treatment of nursing during the 1950s and 1960s.

It seemed that, post-Independence, prospects for the development of an overall strong leadership were good, as the infrastructure for nursing authority began to be erected, and gradually to be staffed by capable Indian nursing leaders. The INC was established in 1949 and given responsibility for curriculum, examination, inspection, and the monitoring of registration. Madras was the first to create a post for a nursing superintendent in the office of the surgeon general, but by the end of 1947 five states had such posts.[28] In 1949, India had

---

[27] See, for example, T. K. Adranvala, 'Letter to the Editor', *Indian Journal of Public Health*, vol. 8, no. 2, 1964, pp. 78–79; T. K. Adranvala, 'Nursing Profession in India', p. 173.

[28] T. K. Adranvala, 'Developments in Nursing 1947–57', p. 327.

nine state-level nursing councils regulating registration and train-ing.[29] Strongly encouraged by international agencies that provided 'counterparts' to train nurses in working with the government, the states began to appoint representatives of nursing in their directorates of health services.[30] As detailed earlier, Gool Pestonji Kapadia was appointed as the superintendent of nursing services for Uttar Pradesh in 1957. In 1960, P. V. Prabhu, a male nurse who had specialised in genito-urinary diseases and mental health and had postgraduate qualifications from Columbia University and University of Edinburgh, was appointed as the first superintendent of nursing services in the Government of Mysore.[31] In 1962, Saramma Kunjummen, formerly the superintendent of nursing at the Government General Hospital in Madras, who had studied hospital administration and public health nursing in New Zealand, became the assistant director of health services for nursing in Tamil Nadu.[32] In June 1962, S. Misra, who trained with Jeanette Jackson of USAID, was appointed as the state nursing superintendent for Rajasthan.[33] In 1962, Charlotte Abana,

---

[29] They were: East Punjab Nurses Registration Council, Ludhiana; Assam Nurses, Midwives and Health Visitors Council, Shillong; Madras Nurses and Midwives Council, Madras; Bihar Nurses Registration Council, Patna; Nurses and Midwives Council, United Provinces, Lucknow; Bombay Nurses, Midwives and Health Visitors Council, Bombay; West Bengal Nurses and Midwives Registration Council, Calcutta; Central Provinces Nurses Registration Council, Nagpur; Orissa Nurses Registration Council, Cuttack; and Travancore Nurses, Midwives and Dhais Council, Trivandrum (C. H. Bose to M. Henry, 21 December 1949, UK National Archives, Kew, DT 18/74).

[30] C. I. Abana, 'Report of the Honorary Branch Secretary, Delhi, from August 1945 to June 1946', *NJI*, vol. 38, no. 2, 1947, pp. 82–83; John T. Gentry, Office Memorandum, 11 July 1962, 'Indore College of Nursing Project: Conference with Dr G. L. Sharma, Director of Medical Services, Madhya Pradesh, and Dr B. C. Bose, Principal, Mahatma Gandhi Memorial Medical College, Indore, on July 9, 1962, in Indore', NARA, Box 157, Folder HLS 1–2, Nursing School (College of Nursing — Indore).

[31] Anonymous, 'Personal Notes and News', *NJI*, vol. 51, no. 11, 1960, p. 325; Anonymous, 'Candidates for TNAI Elections October 1972 — Bombay', *NJI*, vol. 63, no. 9, 1972, p. 318.

[32] Anonymous, 'Personal Notes and News', *NJI*, vol. 51, no. 11, 1960, p. 325; Anonymous, 'Candidates for TNAI Elections October 1972 — Bombay', *NJI*, vol. 63, no. 9, 1972, p. 318.

[33] C. C. Brophy, J. S. Jackson, J. B. Sevan, 'Report of Meeting Regarding Creation of College of Nursing', 29 May,1962, NARA, Box 157, Folder HLS 1–2, Nursing Schools (College of Nursing — Jaipur).

in the late 1940s the TNAI branch secretary in Delhi, and who had later taken postgraduate courses in the US and Canada, was working as the special officer for nursing in the Madhya Pradesh Directorate of Health Services and as acting state nursing superintendent. Ms G. Chandramathy, regarded at Columbia University as one of the best international students (described as intelligent, lively and imaginative by the Rockefeller staff in New York), was appointed the first assistant director of nursing for Kerala.[34] The appointment of carefully selected and expensively trained Indian women into these positions was the justifiable cause of considerable excitement and optimism among nursing leaders.

The general sense of optimism during this early period was buoyed by the support of the first health minister of independent India, Rajkumari Amrit Kaur. As was mentioned in Chapter 3, she was an important champion of Indian nurses. A collection of her speeches published by the Lok Sabha Secretariat states that she 'had a deep concern for nurses and nursing services in the country'.[35] One of her major contributions to the profession was swift action to create gazetted rank for matrons, sister tutors and graduate nurses. This meant that senior nursing jobs were regularised in terms of pay and status, and were listed in the Government Gazette alongside other, more prestigious government jobs. Edwina Mountbatten, who as the last Vicereine of colonial India had taken a strong interest in nursing, optimistically commented that in introducing gazetted ranks for nurses, Rajkumari Amrit Kaur had 'brought India to the forefront of those nations who lead in the international field [of nursing]'.[36] Rajkumari Amrit Kaur herself felt this was a major achievement, stating in Parliament that

> the question of status of Nursing profession, the question of giving gazetted status to nurses occupying high offices in the State is

---

[34] 'Memo on Miss Chandramathy', 3 December 1952, RF, Series 2.1 (Post-war Correspondence), R.G. 6.1 (Paris Field Office), Box 44, Folder 403, 'DMPH India, Nursing'; C. P. Thresyamma, *Fundamentals of Nursing: Procedure Manual for General Nursing and Midwifery Course*, New Delhi: Jaypee Brothers, 2002, p. 30.

[35] Rajkumari Amrit Kaur, *Rajkumari Amrit Kaur*, p. 7.

[36] Edwina Mountbatten to Rajkumari Amrit Kaur, 15 August 1948, Nehru Memorial Library, New Delhi, List no. 14, Papers of Rajkumari Amrit Kaur, Correspondence with Edwina Mountbatten, Series M-13.

something for which I worked very hard . . . Maintenance of a high standard of nursing is very necessary.[37]

In 1954, Rajkumari Amrit Kaur supervised the establishment of the Shetty Committee (officially the 'Nursing Committee to Review Conditions of Service, Emoluments, etc. of the Nursing Profession'). The Shetty Committee supported the TNAI's position and that of the international nurse advisors that a stronger institutional relationship was required between profession and state. Among its recommendations, in theory accepted, were the establishment of new nursing schools, the drawing up of a national minimum pay scale for nurses, midwives and ANMs and the appointment of superintendents of nursing to the offices of the directorates of health services in each state.[38] With its emphasis on nurse authority and the dire need for improvements in conditions and education, the Shetty Committee is good evidence for the initially high level of political respect for the concerns of the nursing leadership and the early willingness to endorse their plans for a more organised and professional nursing service.

Valuable evidence of the waxing and waning of state interest in nursing is to be found in India's Five-year Plans. Study of early Plans shows that bureaucrats in the 1950s and 1960s paid a level of attention to the nation's nursing services that has never since been replicated. The First Five-year Plan, for 1951–56, carefully described planned degree programmes, emphasised the need for more sister tutors and outlined a role for the nurse in community health.[39] The Second Five-year Plan, for 1956–61, represented a unique moment in the spotlight of national planning for the profession; it contained a degree of detail and specificity unmatched since. In fact, the thoroughness of the section on nursing seems to suggest that Adranvala wrote it. It advocated better standardisation of training, a large expansion in facilities for the training of GNM nurses, allowing nurses to work part time, and the inclusion of a stronger public health component.

---

[37] Rajkumari Amrit Kaur, *Rajkumari Amrit Kaur*, p. 7.

[38] Government of India, 'Report of the Health Survey and Planning Committee' (Mudaliar Committee), vol. 2, New Delhi: Government of India 1961, Appendix B-29, p. 237; Khaparde, 'Meeting the Needs of the Community', p. 6.

[39] Planning Commission of India, 'First Five Year Plan', New Delhi, 1952, p. 513.

It recommended the expansion of ANM training, to cater for the creation of more rural development programmes, but highlighted the need for avenues for auxiliaries to proceed to full nurse training as their careers progressed, thus supporting the position of the TNAI that the ultimate aim should be for trained nurses to provide the majority of nursing services.[40]

By the Third Five-year Plan, covering 1961–66, the emphasis on nursing had already weakened and less detail was provided. Nonetheless, there is clear evidence that attention was paid to the major needs of the profession as identified by local leaders and foreign experts — better representation and better education. It reflected the ongoing demand (articulated since the mid-1930s), for nurse representation to state government and the profession's emphasis on the great need for more qualified teachers. Lamenting the ongoing shortage of recruits, the Plan reflected the view of professional leaders that a superintendent of nursing for every state would ultimately lead to improved service conditions and thus to more fruitful recruitment efforts.[41]

In June 1959, the Mudaliar Committee (officially the Health Survey and Planning Committee), was appointed by the government to consider developments since the Bhore Report, and to plan for the future of health services. A. L. Mudaliar was a member of the Bhore Committee and showed strong interest in the promotion of nursing; he had even acted as the co-designer of the BSc (nursing) degree at CMC Vellore. The Mudaliar Report reflected the continuing view that nurses had an important role to play in the provision of universal health care and that the question of their professional education was worth consideration. The report made detailed and specific recommendations: nursing teachers and specialists needed more experience prior to promotion; better accommodation must be provided; every school of nursing should have an advisory committee (consisting of the administrative head of the hospital, the nursing superintendent, a senior sister tutor and 'two lady members, one of

---

[40] Planning Commission of India, 'Second Five Year Plan', New Delhi: Government of India, 1956, website of the Planning Commission of India, http://planning commission.nic.in/plans/planrel/fiveyr/default.html (accessed 24 October 2006).

[41] Planning Commission of India, 'Third Five Year Plan', New Delhi: Government of India, 1961, http://planningcommission.nic.in/plans/planrel/fiveyr/default.html (accessed 24 October 2006).

whom should be a non-medical educationist'); schools of nursing should have budgets independent of hospital budgets; and steps should be taken to ensure that the attractions of the nursing profession were equal to or greater than those of the new clerical work opportunities opening up for women at the time.[42] In the context of a larger exercise in health planning, nursing was given considerable attention and the professionalising agenda of nursing leaders was still largely taken for granted as a desirable component of a modern health system.

During this early post-colonial period, there was a strong perception that trained nurses would form an integral dimension of rural public health care. This view was strengthened by the international NGOs working in health that generally promoted the position expressed by a 1951 WHO committee on nursing: 'In countries where medicine is highly developed and nursing is not, the health status of the people does not reflect the advanced stage of medicine. Nursing is essential to the vitalization of the health programme'.[43]

The Bhore Report had advised a central role for the public health nurse. While it suggested that ANMs would play a major role in rural health and recommended that as an 'interim measure' the training of *dai*s should continue, the nurse was to be the supervisor of these less trained carers.[44] The committee advised the creation of a corps of public health nurses, who would be trained nurses with additional qualifications in public health and midwifery. This new type of nurse would be 'able to take part in the extension of preventive health work in all fields of activity in the homes of the people'.[45] The First Five-year Plan, for 1951–56, listed the training of such public health nurses as an important priority.[46] The Plan also advocated a policy that trained nurse leaders had long opposed — expanding the training of auxiliary nurses to provide for rural needs. In contrast to later years, however, the opposition of trained nurses

---

[42] Mudaliar Report, vol. 1, pp. 368–76.

[43] WHO, Technical Report Series 24 cited in Central Treaty Organisation, 'Conference on Nursing Education', Tehran, 14–25 April 1964, p. 132.

[44] Anonymous, 'The Health Survey and Development Committee (Bhore Committee), 1943–46: A Synopsis of the Findings', *Indian Nursing Year Book, 1986–8*, New Delhi: TNAI, 1988, pp. Comm-1–Comm-4.

[45] Bhore Report, p. 170.

[46] Planning Commission of India, 'First Five Year Plan', New Delhi, 1952, p. 513.

was by no means irrelevant; it was not yet the case that plans for constructing a better rural health care system could ignore nurses entirely. The report was careful to spell out that 'it is of the greatest importance that the work of sub-professional personnel should be guided and supervised by qualified persons'.[47] Importantly, the Shetty Committee of 1954 endorsed nurses' demands for a 'single cadre', which would mean that hospital nurses, public health nurses and all junior grades of health workers would be included in the same administrative category, with standardised pay scales and room for nursing leaders to act to make rural work more attractive.[48] Had this suggestion been implemented, the INC and the state nursing councils would have assumed responsibility for a much larger slice of public health work, becoming more involved in the training, regulation and working conditions of ANMs and the many different categories of community-level health worker appointed since Independence.

Throughout the 1950s and 1960s, it was felt to be inevitable that public health nurses would take over from the only existing category of female rural or urban public health worker — the health visitor (ANM training began in earnest only in the later years of the war and was initially designed to staff hospitals rather than primary health centres). Health visitors were matriculates with between six months and a year of training, chiefly in maternal and child welfare. Health visiting was never a successful programme in India. Numbers were always very small, mostly due to the reluctance of women to work in isolated, difficult and often dangerous conditions in rural areas.[49] Adranvala wrote in 1953 that there was a general view that the training given to health visitors was insufficient and that there was 'a trend towards replacing the health visitors by public health nurses'.[50] Hilda Lazarus felt that only highly qualified nurses could do effective community health work, which was beyond the less educated health visitors.[51] By the time the 1961 Mudaliar Report was

---

[47] 'First Five Year Plan', pp. 490–91.

[48] The Mudaliar Report, vol. 2, Appendix B-29, p. 237; Khaparde, 'Meeting the Needs of the Community', p. 6.

[49] According to Lazarus, in 1945 there were only 750 health visitors available in India (Lazarus, *Our Nursing Services*, p. 8). Health visitor training had been available for at least 27 years.

[50] Adranvala, 'Nursing Profession in India', p. 173.

[51] Lazarus, *Our Nursing Services*, p. 8.

published, the health visitor was widely regarded as obsolete, to be replaced with the public health nurse in the imminent future.[52] This has not been the case — a small number of health visitors and large numbers of *dais* and ANMs form the majority of female carers in the public health system. Yet, the confident plans to replace auxiliaries show the strong feeling in these early years that nurses' time would come — with a better public health curriculum and with the expansion of nurse education, public health nurses would begin to take on the central role that had long been predicted for them.

## The consequences of empty promises

The regular attention paid to the needs of nursing during the 1950s and 1960s unfortunately often failed to translate into actual policies or observable improvements in the situation of nurses. In general, there were many promises and little action. When the attention of planners and politicians moved elsewhere in the late 1960s, nurses thus did not prove to have a strong position from which to negotiate.

Such early inaction, of course, was not limited to nurses. The Congress Party Government that took over the reins in 1947 faced a health crisis and minimal resources with which to address it. According to Jeffery, the state's ability to implement new policies to address its 'horrendous health problems' was restricted by the partition of the subcontinent into India and Pakistan, which saw mass killings and created millions of refugees, the demands on bureaucracy caused by the accession of the formerly independent princely states into India, by rebellion in Telengana, and by a 'covert war between India and Pakistan'. This meant minimal time, motivation and resources for the implementation of planned structural changes in India's health services.[53]

Nevertheless, the neglect of nursing was particularly severe. From the beginning the state voiced support for better education and standardisation, while in reality it adopted a pragmatic approach to its urgent need for hospital staff that gave little priority to nurses' desire for more secure and satisfying working lives. Throughout the country, the unregulated training of nursing assistants proceeded with minimal

---

[52] Mudaliar Report, vol. 1, p. 372.
[53] Jeffery, 'Toward a Political Economy of Health Care', p. 277.

222 + Indian Sisters

or no consultation with the nursing leadership. In West Bengal, the government launched programmes for training assistant nurses and 'famine relief aides'.[54] In Mysore, minimally trained women described themselves as 'public health nurses'.[55] Anna Noll, nursing consultant with the Rockefeller Foundation, wrote in 1948 that 'emphasis is on the rapid preparation of some type of nursing personnel for staffing the hospitals, and on doing this as cheaply as possible'.[56] Some nursing leaders reacted to this bitterly. Kumari Lakshmi Devi, secretary of the TNAI and *NJI* editor, wrote in 1950:

> There was a day not long gone when this profession picked and chose those who were privileged to join its ranks, but today we are invaded by many undesirables and thus our cherished name has been tarnished.
>
> We tolerate the employment of 'assistants' and schoolgirls, and knowingly give our sick into their inexperienced hands. We do not protest but seem to encourage the 'training' of these half-educated, immature recruits.
>
> It is quite, quite useless to speak of raising the standard of nursing while we applaud the short-sightedness of those who are lowering the standards by their short-term schemes of 'training'. Have we forgotten those gallant pioneers who courageously fought to raise the standards, and won the battle?[57]

Others more reasonably acknowledged the desperate need for any kind of care, but still expressed the desire that the unregulated, unstandardised training of health assistants should not continue. It was understandable and necessary that large numbers of hospital workers should be prepared, what was unnecessary was the failure to plan organised, regulated programmes for the training of such workers. The predictable consequence of this was a ubiquitous and

---

[54] Anna M. Noll, 'Annual Report on Nursing in India, Pakistan and Ceylon 1949', RF, RG 5.3, Series 464C, Box 204, Folder 2497, p. 8.

[55] Anna M. Noll, 'Semi-Annual Report — Nursing (India and Ceylon), July 1 to December 31, 1948', RF, RG 5.3, Series 464C, Box 204, Folder 2496.

[56] Anna M. Noll, 'Semi-Annual Report — Nursing (India and Ceylon), January 31 to June 30, 1948', RF, RG 5.3, Series 464C, Box 204, Folder 2496, p.5.

[57] Kumari Lakshmi Devi, 'United We Stand', *NJI*, vol. 41, no. 10, October 1950, p. 264.

lasting willingness on the part of many hospitals to economise by employing unqualified or questionably qualified carers in the place of nurses.

Although the INC technically had the authority to register nurses and to monitor educational standards, in practice it did not have the reach or the resources to successfully control the spiralling numbers of unqualified carers, nor did it make much impact on educational practices; as a regulator, it was not given sufficient power. Similarly, the INC was unable to actually enforce government-supported measures to curb the exploitation of student labour. In 1953, Adranvala wrote that in hospitals with nursing schools, the standard of education was low, because 75 per cent of nursing care was given by students and 'the demands of the hospital nearly always have a priority over the need for proper training'. Nursing schools were given until 1960 to meet new requirements for higher standards of classroom teaching, but by 1961, only 97 of the 278 nursing schools in India met the minimum curriculum requirements specified by the INC.[58] The vision of better education and a carefully planned role for trained nurses in public health in practice gave way to the economic imperatives of the hospitals, which were allowed free rein to violate all the regulations and standards set out by nursing leaders.

Not only was the INC given minimal authority, the state also refused a strong official role to any other nurse organisation. The colonial state had never granted the TNAI its desired official government status as the main representative body for Indian nurses, and the independent state continued in this policy. Briefly, from the late 1940s, the West Bengal government required TNAI membership from applicants for government position, but in general there was minimal support for compulsory membership.[59] The TNAI protested this refusal of recognition, arguing that it was the only national, non-religious organisation representing nurses' interests. Throughout the 1950s, Devi lamented the unrecognised status of the TNAI. She wrote in 1958 that:

> With the coming into being of the Indian Nursing Council, the TNAI has been pushed aside until today we are mere observers instead of

---

[58] Julien, 'Case History on Nursing', p. 28.
[59] Anonymous, 'People', *NJI*, vol. 62, no. 3, 1971, p. 96.

active participants in India's nursing education programmes. Granted, the Indian Nursing Council nurses are also members of the TNAI and we have one TNAI representative on the INC but nonetheless, the professional organisation has been overwhelmed by the Statutory Body and I do not like it. I am ambitious for our Association and want to see it in its rightful place and accepted as the voice of India's nurses.[60]

In 1968, Indira Dorabji, general secretary of the TNAI until 1967, grieved that the organisation had still not attained its longstanding goal of official status. This has continued to be viewed as a lost opportunity.[61]

The South African Nursing Association (SANA), similar in origins and orientation to the TNAI, provides an instructive contrast. In 1944 an Act of Parliament established membership of SANA as compulsory for every registered nurse and midwife.[62] This state-supported representative organ's mandate was to 'raise the status, maintain the integrity and promote the interests of the South African Nursing profession' through its 'representations to Government, provincial and local authorities in regard to conditions of employment, salaries, leave and pensions'.[63] Had the TNAI benefited from the financial stability and positive publicity inherent in state-endorsed status and compulsory membership, it may have been stronger and more capable of innovation. Despite oft-voiced rhetoric about concern for the status of Indian women, the state was unwilling to entertain a step that would strengthen the representative organisation of an all-female profession.

Although the state professed support for nurses' professionalising plans, it did not substantially include nurses in planning processes. It was clear that the advice of the TNAI, of Adranvala and of international nurses was heard, but the official inclusion of nurses in the planning process was limited. Committees met to consider health and

---

[60] Kumari Lakshmi Devi to Virginia Arnold, 7 May 1958, RF, RG1.2, Series 464, Box 53, Folder 491, 'India: Trained Nurses' Association, Devi, Kumari Lakshmi, 1958–1960'.

[61] Dorabji, 'Greeting Message', p. 366.

[62] Marks, *Divided Sisterhood*, p. 123.

[63] Charlotte Searle, quoted in Marks, *Divided Sisterhood*, p. 124.

nursing, and although they emphasised the importance of a strong nursing service, they excluded nurses from their ranks. Narender Nagpal, former TNAI president, describes the history of nursing and health committees in India as one of exclusion, in which decisions have been made 'by other people, usually physicians, without the benefit of professional input by Nurses'.[64] The Bhore Committee contained no nurses and appointed no nurse advisors, despite the presence in India of a number of highly trained experts in nursing. Although Mudaliar was a high-profile supporter of nursing and had done collaborative work with nurse leaders before, no nurses were members of his 1959 committee. Officially documented consultation of nurses for the purposes of the Mudaliar Committee was limited to mailing questionnaires to nurse leaders, and holding discussions with local leaders in five of the 15 states that the committee visited.[65] As Devaki Jain comments, gender hierarchy is most obvious and most damaging in this kind of 'failure to take note of, to understand and respect and absorb, women's ideational and intellectual skills'.[66] By denying nurses' capacity to contribute intelligently and to assume leadership, opportunities for them to gain experience and skill in political participation were closed off at this early stage.

Even Rajkumari Amrit Kaur, who took a rare personal interest in the fate of nursing, in practice did not make it a main focus of her work. The Lok Sabha's collection of her speeches shows nursing to be a low priority, mentioned in only a few speeches and discussed only briefly. Rajkumari was preoccupied by such concerns as the education of doctors, their fight to limit the role of traditional medicine in the new health system and the government's campaign against tuberculosis. In 1956 she delivered a 29-page speech on the establishment of AIIMS, which, besides a medical school, dental college and hospital, was to include a nursing college. The role of nursing got a total of six lines.[67] Whilst she recognised that nurses

---

[64] High Power Committee, 'Development of Nursing and Health Care: 1947–2000', in Narender Nagpal (ed.), *History and Trends in Nursing in India*, Delhi: TNAI, 2001, p. 125.

[65] Mudaliar Report, vol. 2, Appendix B-1, pp. 13–25.

[66] Devaki Jain, *Women, development and the UN*, p. 164.

[67] 'All India Institute of Medical Sciences Bill, 1956', in Rajkumari Amrit Kaur, *Rajkumari Amrit Kaur*, p. 166.

were overworked and undertrained,[68] and that the underdevelopment of nursing was a serious problem, it is obvious that there was
an almost complete absence of the kind of strong political pressure
exerted on her by other interest groups such as allopathic doctors,
practitioners of indigenous medicine and homeopaths.

In 1961, the Mudaliar Report confirmed the stagnation of promising early plans for the development of nursing. The Report recognised
the limited extent to which regulations and plans for the development
of nursing had actually been implemented. It pointed out that the
lack of control of nursing schools over their own budget (which in
most cases was managed by hospital administrations) was limiting
the quality of the education delivered. Hospital authorities had been
unwilling to fund the library materials and classroom aids mandated
by the INC as the minimum required for effective teaching.[69] The
Report recognised that progress in the improvement and standardisation of nurse education had been disappointing, suggesting that:

> The present practice of using nurse-pupils for doing all the routine
> duties in a hospital and not concentrating on training and practi-
> cal experience, is not desirable. We agree with the Trained Nurses'
> Association that the duties allotted to the student nurses should be
> specific and that in carrying out these duties emphasis should be given
> to the training programme rather than to the discharge of other inci-
> dental duties in the hospital . . . the tendency in hospitals at present,
> to utilise the services of the probationers for the purpose of reducing
> the number of qualified staff nurses that ought to be available in such
> hospitals, is a retrograde step and is not conducive either to proper
> attention being given to the patients or to the efficient training of the
> probationers.[70]

Post-war, the introduction of nurse representation in government
had been the source of much excitement. Very quickly, however,
it became clear that too much optimism was unwarranted, as in
many cases the working relationship between nurses and government was very difficult. Politicians and bureaucrats often regarded
hard-won institutions for nurse representation in government with
contempt. In 1948 in Madras, where a nursing superintendent had

---

[68] See *Rajkumari Amrit Kaur*, pp. 124, 166, 214–15.
[69] Mudaliar Report, vol. 1, p. 371.
[70] Ibid., pp. 369–70.

been appointed since 1941, the government attempted to appoint a woman doctor. Up until then the English nurse, Dora Chadwick, former TNAI president and co-designer of the BSc course at CMC Vellore, had held the post. Her replacement by a doctor was vigorously protested by international organisations and the TNAI, with the result that the position was just left vacant for several years.[71] In Bombay, Noll wrote in 1949 that the state nursing superintendent, Mehra Doctor, 'is usually not consulted when planning in nursing matters is being done by other officers'.[72] In 1962, Abana reported that the state government of Madhya Pradesh was refusing to make her temporary appointment as state nursing superintendent permanent, which she attributed to 'a continuing failure on the part of the medical authorities to appreciate fully the contributions nurses can make' and the fact that those in government were 'unwilling to have too much authority placed in the hands of a nurse'.[73] Juliette Julien, the leader of USAID's nursing programmes, described the serious problems experienced with a 1950s programme of supplying USAID nurses to state governments in order to train local state nursing advisors. The programme faltered because state directorates of health and health ministries would not give their nurse advisors any responsibility, bureaucrats obstructed nurses or refused any active support and in some cases the local counterparts promised were not even recruited.[74] Ultimately the difficulty of working with state governments led to the termination of the programme (which was replaced by the troubled project of investment in nursing colleges that was discussed in Chapter 3). The INC and its state-level equivalents, the institution of which had been viewed as a great victory for nurses, were subjected to restrictive medical dominance. In 1971, the director general for health services commented on an 'incongruous' history in which the medical profession had headed these councils. The nursing advisor to the government had taken the role of secretary to the INC, but the position of Chair of the INC was reserved for a doctor.[75]

---

[71] Noll, 'Semi-Annual Report July 1 to December 31, 1948'; Adranvala, 'President's Address', pp. 6–8.
[72] Noll, 'Annual Report 1949', p. 8.
[73] Gentry, 'Indore College of Nursing Project'.
[74] Julien, 'Case History on Nursing College Development', p. 10.
[75] Anonymous, 'News', *NJI*, vol. 62, no. 3, 1971, p. 90.

The neglect of nursing was, from the beginning, even more out-standing at state level. Among state governments, even the rhetorical emphasis on the role of nursing evident in central health policy was often less. In Bombay, regarded as a leading state in its encouragement of nurse leadership, the first state Five-year Plan gave minimal space to nursing. One and a half pages are devoted to describing funds for three medical colleges, on which ₹352.71 lakh were being spent; whereas one paragraph describes plans for a new nursing college at Ahmedabad, to cost ₹4 lakh. Typically, considerable detail was given to the expansion of hospital facilities in the state, but none on how best nurses could be trained to staff them.[76]

In Madras during this period, a paradoxical situation developed in which there were both serious nurse shortages and high nurse unemployment, because hospitals saw an opportunity to economise during a period of intense financial strain by replacing nurses with untrained staff. In 1951, Mudaliar commented of Madras that 'even those who have been properly trained are not given opportunities for suitable employment by the State, by philanthropic organizations and by other bodies'. He protested against the short-sightedness of hospital administrations that economised by cutting back on the number of nurses employed, and commented on the general lack of recognition that 'the duties of the doctors can only be performed effectively if there is a proper provision of trained nursing staff to co-operate and collaborate in any scheme of medical relief'.[77] In Andhra Pradesh in 1959, a similar situation was developing. Alice Zachariah, the president of the state TNAI branch, commented:

> The shortage of nurses in this country is not due to lack of applicants to nursing, but is almost entirely due to the fact that funds are not being made available to prepare more nurses, and to create posts for the employment of more graduate nurses.[78]

In the state of Travancore-Cochin (which became Kerala in 1956), whence the majority of India's nurses emerged, the government was actively obstructive to nursing leaders in these early years. The

---

[76] Government of Bombay, 'The Five-Year Plan for Bombay State (1951–52 to 1955–56)', Bombay: Government of Bombay, 1953.

[77] *Collected Speeches of Dr. A. Lakshmanaswami Mudaliar*, p. 238.

[78] Zachariah, 'News from the States', p. 274.

Travancore section of the administration maintained a harsh system of bonding graduates into the mid-1950s, which meant that nurses had to supply five years of service in the state after their training, during which they were not allowed to be married. This meant that most nurses would have had to wait until the age of 25 before marriage, which at the time was considered very late. If they violated these terms, their parents forfeited ₹2,500. In 1948, Noll reported that the school of nursing in Trivandrum was sending out 'distress signals'. It was struggling to attract candidates due to dreadful working conditions and the bonding system, and faced opposition from the government, which had formed a committee opposing nurse leaders' plan to separate the nursing school from the hospital in order to provide better classroom teaching.[79] Mary Elizabeth Tennant, associate director for nursing at Rockefeller's International Health Division (IHD), toured India to report on the general state of nursing in 1952. She reported that the Trivandrum School of Nursing, viewed as one of the most established in the state, had failed an INC inspection because of the poor provision for clinical practice for student nurses, the selection of students for the school without input from any nurse member of staff, the long hours of work required of students, bad conditions on the wards, and the maintenance of the bonding system. Travancore-Cochin, like most states in this early period, generally pursued a policy dictated by the economic advantage of hospitals, rather than seriously addressing itself to improve conditions for nurses.

# The Disappearance of the Nurse from Health Planning, 1965–87

Politicians continued after 1965 to attend nurse graduations regularly, seizing opportunities to lecture their 'noble sisters' on emulating Florence Nightingale. In health planning, however, a new discourse dominated, in which nurses found little room. Rather than being identified as an essential foundation of public health services, they were from this time on often subsumed within a more general category of 'para-professional manpower', their particular role and specific

---

[79] Noll, 'Annual Report 1949', pp. 4–5.

concerns no longer viewed as worthy of separate discussion. While the profession continued expanding and educational facilities grew significantly, little attention was paid to policy and direction.

This was a period of political shift and considerable disillusionment after the first decades of the post-Independence period, which had been characterised by 'a framework of unchallenged unity and integrity of the Indian state', 'political homogeneity' and, to some extent, a national spirit of optimism and excitement.[80] In contrast, from the mid-1960s, there was increased political and social conflict and an end to the stability of the Nehruvian era. In 1964, Nehru's death signalled the impending end of the era of unchallenged Congress Party domination and its accompanying verities. The mid-1960s brought serious food shortages and a foreign exchange crisis caused by massive wartime expenditure on defence. As a result, in 1967, nine states elected non-Congress governments. This brought difficult challenges for a federal system not accustomed to such political variety and indicated, according to T. V. Satyamurthy, 'widespread alienation and disaffection throughout the country'.[81] Indira Gandhi returned as prime minister after the 1967 elections, and a new style of populist politics and the dramatic centralisation of power began. India in the 1970s witnessed new levels of unrest among peasants and industrial workers and the political rise of the 'rural rich', which transformed state politics, especially in north India. In 1975 Gandhi declared a national emergency. She suspended democracy for two years and pursued a range of often oppressive policies presented as 'anti-poverty' initiatives.

All of these events brought profound change to the health system and to health planning. It was increasingly evident that the health of the rural majority had been neglected, and in the 1970s there was a general recognition of this and a reorientation of health planning. Also, the national emphasis on population control and family planning, which had been escalating since the publication of the Third Five-year Plan for 1961–66, reached fever-pitch in the early 1970s. Health resources were overwhelmingly directed into population programmes, at the cost of all other aspects of the health system,

---

[80] T. V. Satyamurthy, 'Impact of Centre-State Relations on Indian Politics: An Interpretative Reckoning 1947–1987', in Partha Chatterjee (ed.), *State and Politics in India*, Oxford: Oxford University Press, 1997, pp. 238, 241.

[81] Satyamurthy, 'Impact of Centre-State Relations', p. 243.

and a violent programme of mass sterilisation was carried out during the years of the Emergency. The short-lived Janata Party government elected in 1977 after the Emergency, according to Partha Chatterjee, represented 'a different developmental strategy, articulated in a Gandhian rhetoric', which was centred on rural areas.[82] Its schemes for the introduction of community-level health workers outlasted it, and proved an important new focus in health planning. On 12 September 1978, the Alma Ata declaration was made at WHO's International Conference on Primary Health Care. Alma Ata proposed a radical, worldwide reorientation of health priorities, emphasising the preventive and promotive, and targeting neglected rural regions. It put forward the influential and oft-cited goal of 'Health for All by 2000', which influenced the health care policy of many developing countries and infused Indian health planning over the subsequent two decades.[83] None of these developments were favourable to nurses, who increasingly found themselves altogether excluded from a planning process in which they were perceived as irrelevant to community health and as a result, to the success of family planning initiatives and rurally-focused schemes.

The attention of planners increasingly focused on schemes for training new types of village-level health workers so as to improve the health access and health outcomes for the rural poor, rather than on nurses. In 1973, the Kartar Singh Committee (officially the Committee on Multipurpose Workers under Health and Family Planning Programme) advocated the introduction of male and female multipurpose workers to boost rural health provision. Under this scheme, workers from the vertical campaigns targeting particular diseases such as malaria and smallpox would be retrained to perform a broader public health role at village level.[84] In 1975, the Srivastava Committee (officially the Government of India Group on Medical Education and Support Manpower) further emphasised

[82] Partha Chatterjee, 'Introduction: A Political History of Independent India', in Partha Chatterjee (ed.), *State and Politics in India*, Oxford: Oxford University Press, 1997, p. 28.

[83] For a discussion of 'Health for All by 2000' in India, see Foundation for Research in Community Health, *Health Status of the Indian People: Supplementary Document to Health for All: An Alternative Strategy*, Foundation for Research in Community Health, 1987.

[84] Ibid., p. 35.

the alienation of the medical profession from rural areas and recommended the training of community health workers.[85] Schemes for new, community-based health workers, according to Jeffery, were not very successful as a variety of factors worked to inhibit their effective recruitment and training.[86] Nonetheless, schemes to promote the training of such personnel have continued. Recent initiatives have included the National Rural Health Mission, which proposed the training of accredited social health activists, female village health workers, who, it was hoped, would have an impact on high infant and maternal mortality rates, particularly in the poorer states.[87]

The new National Health Policy adopted in 1985 is suggestive of the results of these new health planning priorities for nurses. It stated that:

> The existing situation has been largely engendered by the almost wholesale adoption of health manpower development policies and the establishment of curative centres based on the Western models, which are inappropriate and irrelevant to the real needs of our people and the socio-economic conditions obtaining in the country. The hospital-based disease and cure-oriented approach towards the establishment of medical services has provided benefits to the upper crusts of society, specially those residing in the urban areas. The proliferation of this approach has been at the cost of providing comprehensive primary health care services to the entire population, whether residing in the urban or rural areas.[88]

It was clear that nurses were to be regarded as part of a mode of health care 'irrelevant to the real needs of our people' and as personnel working for the benefit of the 'upper crusts of society'. With no clear role to play in the primary health centres and sub-centres, they

---

[85] Report of the Srivastava Committee, in *Health Status of the Indian People*, p. 37.

[86] Jeffery, 'Toward a Political Economy of Health Care', pp. 283–85.

[87] Ministry of Health and Family Welfare, 'National Rural Health Mission', New Delhi, 2005, http://mohfw.nic.in/nrhm.html (accessed 14 November 2006); T. K. Rajalakshmi, 'Birth Control in Disguise', *Frontline*, vol. 22, no. 3, 11 February 2005, pp. 81–82; Anonymous, 'Rural Health Mission Flagged Off', *Deccan Herald*, 13 April 2005; A. K. Shiva Kumar, 'Budgeting for Health: Some Considerations', *Economic and Political Weekly*, vol. 40, no. 14, 2 April 2005, pp. 1391–96.

[88] Lok Sabha Secretariat, 'National Health Policy', New Delhi: Lok Sabha, 1985, p. 35.

struggled unsuccessfully to find relevance in this new health environment. In 1986, a nurse writing in the *NJI* recognised the exclusion of nurses. He described the strong influence of the Alma Ata declaration on health planning and wrote of the urgent need for nurses to find a way into the new community health discourse, stating somewhat tactfully that nurses' 'vital role in influencing healthcare policies and planning nursing component has not yet taken a concrete shape'.[89] Governments at central and state level, caught up in policies for the preparation of vital community health workers, ignored the question of training and employing public health nurses, which had been seen as crucial in the 1950s and early 1960s. A lack of early success in the development of public health nursing had meant the growth of a widely accepted pragmatic view that while no one could really deny the importance of doctors, nurses were ultimately a non-essential in the rural health system.

Planning documents for this period reflect the extent to which nurses vanished from the politics of health. The Fourth Five-year Plan, for 1969–74, abandoned the tendency to comment on the direction of nurse education or on trends in public health nursing. The totality of its comment on nursing was to state the numerical size of the profession.[90] Political upheaval surrounding the Emergency of 1975 meant a much-abridged Fifth Plan, which was only published in 1976, well into the plan period of 1974–79 — it did not mention nursing.[91] The Ministry of Health's annual report for 1976–77 also contained no information about national policy or priorities in nursing, merely a description of the centrally administered Rajkumari Amrit Kaur College of Nursing.[92] The Sixth Plan gave up the use of the term 'nurse' entirely, choosing to treat the various grades of health care workers, including the minimally trained community health volunteers and multipurpose workers employed at village level,

---

[89] C. P. B. Kurup, 'Nurses' Role in Health Care Policies', *NJI*, vol. 77, no. 11, 1986, p. 284.

[90] Planning Commission of India, 'Fourth Five Year Plan', New Delhi: Government of India, 1969, http://planningcommission.nic.in/plans/planrel/fiveyr/default.html (accessed 24 October 2006).

[91] Planning Commission of India, 'Fifth Five Year Plan', New Delhi: Government of India, 1976, http://planningcommission.nic.in/plans/planrel/fiveyr/default.html (accessed 24 October 2006).

[92] Ministry of Health and Family Welfare, 'Annual Report 1976–77', New Delhi: Government of India, 1977.

ANMs, technicians, radiographers, and nurses as one group of 'public health and paramedical workers'.[93] In 1980, the Ministry of Health and Family Welfare's annual report gave half a page to the nursing profession.[94] During the 1980s, the tendency to eschew the use of the term 'nurse' continued; in 1983 Nagpal reported that a Central Council of Health conference on leprosy had included nurses in the ranks of 'non-medical technical personnel'.[95] The Seventh Plan, for 1985–90, again made next to no direct mention of trained nurses, although it did advocate training more ANMs and *dais*.[96] The trained nurse seemed to have faded into non-existence, denied a meaningful role by new health terminology that was used to eliminate awareness of her specific function in the health system.

At state level, policy on nursing was similarly contemptuous. This was particularly clear in the states where, during the 1970s, nurse unemployment emerged as a major problem. As the joint survey of the profession conducted by the Coordinating Agency for Health Planning (CAHP) and TNAI in 1974 observed, 'this was rather obviously due to lack of budget to pay them than to any surplus of nurses'.[97] In some states, there were finally enough nurses to satisfy officially mandated nurse–patient ratios, but officials were unwilling to sanction the funds needed to appoint them. This resulted in the parallel existence of shortage and surplus in some states during the early 1970s. A. Cherian, the nursing advisor to the Indian government, commented in 1972 on 'the acute shortage of trained nurses and the unwillingness of the authorities to appoint more staff nurses to maintain the nurse–patient ratio'.[98] In the early 1970s unemployment was an increasingly pressing problem, particularly in the following states: in Andhra Pradesh it was 15.6 per cent, in Delhi 13 per cent, in Kerala 23.3 per cent, and in Maharashtra 12.8 per cent.[99] This heightened nurses' resentment of the widespread

---

[93] 'Sixth Five Year Plan'.

[94] Ministry of Health and Family Welfare, 'Annual Report 1979–80', New Delhi: Government of India, 1980, p. 64.

[95] Narender Nagpal, 'The Joint Conference', *NJI*, vol. 73, no. 9, 1982, p. 229.

[96] Planning Commission of India, 'Seventh Five Year Plan', New Delhi: Government of India, 1985, http://planningcommission.nic.in/plans/planrel/fiveyr/default.html (accessed 24 October 2006).

[97] CAHP, 'Report of a Nursing Survey in India', Preface.

[98] Anonymous, 'Realities of Nursing', *NJI*, vol. 63, no. 12, 1972, p. 418.

[99] CAHP, 'Report of a Nursing Survey in India', p. x.

employment of untrained women instead of nurses. Accordingly the TNAI requested national implementation of INC ratios and better regulation of private hospitals, the chief culprits in the employment of untrained women. Neither demand was acted on. It also protested against the problematic policy in some states of forcing recent graduates to remain in their home state under systems of bonding, despite the fact that there were no jobs available at home, and many vacant elsewhere.[100] In Rajasthan, for example, in a context of widespread unemployment, nurses were forced to observe a five-year bond period. Rajasthani nurse unemployment existed in spite of the fact that the nurse–patient ratio observed on a 1971 TNAI tour was typically one nurse to 50 or more patients.[101] Nurses in Bihar, who at that stage still had no official presence in the state health ministry, were required to complete a three-year bond in the early 1970s.[102]

In Orissa, the draft Fifth-five Year Plan reported in 1973 that the general dilapidation of the public health infrastructure was such that a significant proportion of nurses graduating in the state could not be employed.[103] In Orissa in 1975, according to Jeffery, the government sanctioned only two posts for public health nurses, although 50 qualified applicants were available.[104] Moreover, while a national shortage of nurses that was described by the chief minister of Maharashtra in 1972 as 'nothing short of a scandal' continued, eager candidates were increasingly turned away from nursing schools.[105] Despite the fact that, as the deputy union minister for health, A. K. Kisku, reported, there had been 35,000 applications for 7,000 seats in nursing in 1971, the nursing education system expanded only very slowly.[106] At state level, therefore, the willingness to simultaneously accept nurse shortages in hospitals and nurse unemployment illustrated the complete lack of political and bureaucratic interest in nursing.

---

[100] Anonymous, 'Abortion Act: Nurses' Rights on Moral Grounds Defended', *NJI*, vol. 62, no. 11, 1971, p. 352.

[101] Anonymous, 'Problems of Nurses in Rajasthan: Memorandum Submitted', *NJI*, vol. 62, no. 3, 1971, pp. 75–76.

[102] Anonymous, 'News', *NJI*, vol. 62, no. 3, 1971, p. 90.

[103] Planning and Coordination Department of the Government of Orissa, 'Fifth Five Year Plan of Orissa (Draft)', Bhubaneswar: Government of Orissa, 1973.

[104] Jeffery, *The Politics of Health in India*, p. 241.

[105] George Mathew, 'Fair Deal to Nurses', *NJI*, vol. 63, no. 12, 1972, p. 401.

[106] Kisku, 'Nursing Education Needs Change', p. 409.

The career and pay structures for nurses established by state governments also reflected their continuing marginalisation. In Kerala, for example, a 1978 revision of pay scales provided for the assistant director of health services for nursing to be paid on the scale of ₹800–1,550 per month, whereas the non-nursing assistant directors were placed on a scale of ₹1,125–1,725.[107] The report on the revision of pay scales noted that in general it took Kerala staff nurses 14 years to be promoted to head nurse, and allotted a pay rise for this promotion of about '40 per month. In Rajasthan, the principal of the state's college of nursing was paid on the scale of ₹930–1,500, less than the general rate for principals of degree colleges, which was ₹1,150–1,650 and less than principals of higher secondary schools, who got ₹1,000–1,600.[108]

# The Recognition of Neglect, 1987–2006

Recent decades have seen a political climate more favourable to nurses. More powerful imperatives for politicians to pay attention to nursing have developed. At the same time, the pattern witnessed in earlier years has again applied. The theoretical recognition of nurses' concerns has not translated into substantive action.

This recent reorientation of the state towards nursing was in part caused by a new political and social context that was more woman-focused. As was discussed in Chapter 4, politics and planning were increasingly characterised by awareness of the state's developmental failures in regard to women, recognition of the need for a gendered approach in future development projects and by the accompanying growth of a new wave of Indian feminism. The rapid development of high-end private hospital facilities, a growing medical tourism industry and lucrative opportunities for Indian nurses to migrate abroad have also directed more state attention to the profession. Since the mid-1990s, India has seen fast growth in high quality, expensive private hospitals, such as the Apollo Group, whose network spans India and the Gulf states, the Escorts Heart Institute and Research Centre and the Amrita Institute of Medical Sciences. These provide

---

[107] Government of Kerala, 'Report of the Third Pay Commission', p. 160.

[108] 'Report of the Rajasthan Pay Commission', Jaipur: Government Central Press, 1981, pp. 248, 685.

high-tech medical care in five-star-hotel style surroundings to wealthy Indians, as well as to a growing clientele of expatriates from the Gulf states, Asia, the US, and Britain. A recent *Business India* special issue on medical and health tourism pointed out, however, that the continuing growth of this lucrative industry depends on high quality nursing care.[109] At the same time, nursing has been galvanised by opportunities to migrate (discussed in the next chapter) and there has been state recognition of the potential for India to develop a Philippines-style role as supplier of nurses to the world. Health planners have recognised that this will require the maintenance and improvement of standards in nurse education.[110]

The first marker of renewed interest in nursing was the appointment in 1987 of the High Power Committee on Nursing. The late 1980s brought a long-delayed state recognition of the dangerous, unsatisfying conditions in which nurses continued to work. Escalating nurse activism in the capital led to the appointment of the Committee to consider the problems of Indian nurses in general. Nurses had lobbied for the appointment of such a committee since 1977. Consistent with the usual approach to nursing issues, this demand was not accepted until 1984, when Mrs Gandhi approved the proposal, while the committee was not actually appointed until 1987. When it was finally appointed, its chairperson was a doctor, Jyoti Trivedi, former Vice-chancellor of SNDT University, Bombay. The committee was composed of 12 members, of whom only five were nurses.[111] Nonetheless, this state attention was welcome and the committee was given a wide brief, charged to consider:

> Conditions and status of Nurses, staffing norms, problems of training all categories of Nurses and Midwifery Personnel, study and clarification of the role for Nursing personnel in the health care delivery system, [and] the need for organisation of Nursing personnel at the national and state levels.[112]

---

[109] Radha Venkataachalam and Krishna G. Seshadri, 'Think Health, Think India: A Few Fast Measures will see the Corporate Indian Healthcare Industry Continue to Rise', *Business India*, 12–25 April 2004, Health Supplement, pp. 93–94.

[110] Satish Chawla, 'Address to XX TNAI Biennial Conference', *NJI*, vol. 95, no. 1, 2004.

[111] Narender Nagpal, 'The High Power Committee', *NJI*, vol. 78, no. 10, October 1987, p. 253.

[112] Nagpal, 'The High Power Committee', p. 253.

The findings of this High Power Committee on Nursing highlighted in strong terms the exploitation of nurses and the lethargy with which state governments had approached nursing reform. The Committee's section on the issue of minimum staffing levels, an issue with enormous implications for patient and nurse welfare, recorded that 'no State has implemented even the norms set out 35 years back'.[113] The Committee saw a pressing need for: reform of the rules and procedures for the recruitment of senior nurses; a reduction in working hours to 40 hours per week; a guarantee of adequate promotional avenues for nurses; a provision for access to higher education after five years of service; and for improvements in accommodation and transport.

In 1987–88, in response to the High Power Committee, as well as to the INC's ongoing attempts to develop better continuing education for nurses, the central government launched the 'Development of Nursing Services' scheme, which is still in progress. It has four pillars — the opening of new schools of nursing to alleviate nurse shortages (to be focused on areas where there were large Scheduled Caste [SC] and Scheduled Tribe [ST] populations);[114] the strengthening of existing schools of nursing; the provision of accommodation for nurses in Delhi; and a continuing education programme.[115] This scheme has resulted in some substantive action. Between 1992 and 1999, 19 new nursing schools were opened.[116] Investment in the continuing education scheme has been consistent. In 2001, ₹100 lakh was allocated for short continuing education courses, which were to focus on management techniques for administrators, educational technology for teachers and clinical specialisations for staff

---

[113] Quoted in Manocha, 'Challenges for Nursing Profession', p. 115.

[114] Scheduled Castes and Scheduled Tribes are sections of the community given special status by the Indian Constitution, due to the severe historical discrimination they had experienced and their relative disadvantage. Under a national affirmative action policy, there is a quota reserved for them in government universities and employment services.

[115] Ministry of Health and Family Welfare, 'Annual Report 1998–99', New Delhi: Government of India, 2000, http://mohfw.nic.in/reports/1998-99Er/enpart2_Chapter%206.pdf (accessed 16 November 2006).

[116] Ministry of Health and Family Welfare, 'Annual Report 1999–2000', New Delhi: Government of India, c. 2000, http://mohfw.nic.in/reports/1999-20Er/Contents.pdf (accessed 16 November 2006).

nurses.[117] The 'strengthening of existing schools' component of the programme was designed to remedy the serious shortage of educational resources in most schools. Grants of ₹10 lakh were given to individual schools to fund audiovisual aids, furniture, books, transport, and improvements to often dilapidated buildings. In 2005–6, ₹14.24 crore (or 142.4 million) was allocated for this purpose. In 2004–5, 60 schools of nursing were 'strengthened', in 2005–6, 41.[118] The Development of Nursing Services scheme, therefore, has been a relatively solid and practical means of addressing some of the most serious problems identified by the profession, as well as enhancing numbers of nurses trained (although from 2002 the opening of new schools was discontinued as the private sector expanded).

The Eighth Five-year Plan, for 1992–97, marked a higher level of attention to the state of the profession than had been seen for many years. It directly acknowledged the neglect of nursing in health planning since at least the 1960s, although the states were blamed for it.[119] The Plan recorded:

> While the States have been more than anxious to start new medical colleges, their efforts to develop institutions for training of para medical staff have been entirely sub-optimal. This has resulted in a considerable mismatch between the requirement and availability of health personnel of different categories. Ideally, the doctor-nurse ratio should be 1:3 but currently there are less than 300,000 registered nurses against 400,000 registered medical graduates.[120]

The Ninth Plan, covering 1997–2002, restated the negative consequences of the longstanding neglect of the education of 'para-professional manpower'. It added a proposal, first mooted by the Bajaj Committee of 1986, to set up an Education Commission of Health Sciences, the responsibilities of which included establishing several universities of health sciences (four of which were already operating), which would create academic environments in which all the faculties

[117] Ministry of Health and Family Welfare, 'Annual Report 2000–2001', New Delhi: Government of India, c. 2001, http://mohfw.nic.in/reports/Annual%20Report%20 2000-01.pdf/Part%20-I-6.pdf (accessed 16 November 2006).

[118] Ministry of Health and Family Welfare, 'Annual Report 2005–2006', p. 169.

[119] There was no Plan for 1989–91 due to political and economic instability. Only Annual Plans were published between 1990 and 1992.

[120] 'Eighth Five Year Plan'.

of the health sciences might interact, providing models for successful health teams. This proposal held out potential for improvements in the problematic doctor–nurse relationship in India. At the same time, the Ninth Plan, although it clearly referred to some of the pressing issues in nurse education and practice, managed to entirely omit direct reference to nurses or their specific concerns. Rather, trained nurses were again subsumed within the non-specific categories employed by the report, such as 'para-professional manpower', 'health care professionals' and 'health manpower'.[121] This was also a feature of the Tenth Plan, which speaks of 'improving the content and quality of education of health professionals and para professionals', of ensuring that all 'health personnel' are attuned to national health needs and of the 'skill upgradation of all health care providers'.[122] The distinctions between the needs and functions of ANMs, trained nurses, multipurpose workers, and health visitors are again ignored. There are doctors, and there are 'health care providers'.

The ministry of health's 2000–2001 annual report, responding to the increasing demand for Indian nurses abroad and the growth of specialised, expensive private hospitals at home, specified the importance of introducing a higher level of scientific and technological expertise into nurse training.[123] This was not discussed in any detail, but there was some desire evident to increase the skills of the women who will staff well-resourced, technologically sophisticated urban institutions at home and abroad. Recent years have witnessed Indian nursing leaders' concerns for educational improvement finally tying in with major state priorities — the desire to encourage the profitable health services sector and the will to profit from a potentially very lucrative additional source of overseas remittances, as nurse migrants come to match the numbers of engineer, doctor and IT worker migrants. There has thus been something of a state reorientation towards nurses, motivated both by more restive and less easily

---

[121] Planning Commission of India, 'Ninth Five Year Plan', New Delhi: Government of India, 1997, http://planningcommission.nic.in/plans/planrel/fiveyr/default.html (accessed 25 October 2006).

[122] Planning Commission of India, 'Tenth Five Year Plan' New Delhi: Government of India, c. 2002, p. 83, http://planningcommission.nic.in/plans/planrel/fiveyr/default. html (accessed 25 October 2006).

[123] Ministry of Health and Family Welfare, 'Annual Report 2000–2001', New Delhi: Government of India.

ignored nursing organisations and new developments in health that have made good quality nursing education a higher priority.

## 'Gathering dust in the Government archives': Rhetoric without action, again

Nagpal wrote in 2001 that 'the retarded development of Nursing and the Nursing profession seems to be mainly due to the fact that no serious thought has been given to this discipline by the Government over the years'.[124] As Nagpal's words indicate, the recent refocusing of state attention on nursing described earlier did not ultimately involve 'serious thought' or 'timely action'. Action to remedy neglect of nurses has been partial and unsatisfactory; in general, reform and improvements have focused more on education and less on working conditions.

Despite the High Power Committee of 1987's strong recommendations for the implementation of better promotional structures, the average nurse's career has remained stagnant, with minimal prospects of advancement, increased responsibility or pay rises. The Academy for Nursing Studies in Hyderabad's comprehensive 2005 report on the state of nursing recorded: 'there are very few higher-level posts for nurses who complete higher education. The career ladder is poorly constructed'. This, they felt, had caused 'stagnation, decline and decay'.[125] In 2000, the All India Government Nurses' Federation (AIGNF, the national wing of the DGNU) stated that the High Power Committee's report was with its predecessors, 'gathering dust in the Government archives', and re-listed the criticisms of working conditions made by the report, which remained equally pertinent 13 years later.[126] They pointed out that most nurses in India still stayed at the lowest pay bracket for 15–20 years. The majority retired having received only two pay increases during their careers.[127] This represents little change from 1952, when a USAID report recorded that it took

[124] Nagpal, 'Development of Nursing', p. 125.

[125] Academy for Nursing Studies, 'Situational Analysis', p. 37.

[126] AIGNF, 'Representation to Honourable Prime Minister, Government of India, in respect of Nursing Profession, on behalf of Fourth National Convention on 26th–27th , 2000, at New Delhi', New Delhi: 2000, pp. 1–5.

[127] Ibid., p. 1.

an average of 12–15 years before the average nurse received her first promotion.[128] According to the AIGNF's analysis, there was only one nursing superintendent for every thousand Indian nurses. Moreover, the starting pay for a nursing superintendent in 1997 was ₹8,000, compared to ₹9,400 for a junior resident doctor.[129] The High Power Committee also highlighted the false economy of leaving senior nurse roles unfilled or underpaid, a practice that has continued apace in most states.[130] The Committee was thus another chapter in the sorry history of committee reports that were not implemented.[131]

The Hyderabad Academy of Nursing Studies also recorded that nurses' demand for a single cadre (meaning that public health nurses and health workers would be united and administered by the INC and state councils), had still not been implemented, despite the fact that in theory this recommendation was accepted by the state in 1954.[132] Public health continued to be another field in which the administrative and authoritative capability of nurses was denied, and the chance to develop such capability refused.

It has also been the case that the most basic foundation of institutionalised trained nursing — the regulation of lower nursing grades and the protection of trained nurses from cheaper, less educated competitors — is yet to be firmly established. In 1998, the TNAI was still lobbying for proper attention to this issue, requesting the appointment of full-time nurse registrars in all the states and for a majority of nurses on state registration boards.[133] Although registration has long been in place in all the Indian states, in most parts of the country the employment of semi-trained or untrained staff is common practice. In 2004, the TNAI branch secretary for Goa,

[128] Julien, 'Case History on Nursing College Development', p. 2.

[129] AIGNF, 'Representation to Honourable Prime Minister', p. 1.

[130] The Maharashtra state government typifies the approach: in 2003 it directed the LT College of Nursing, at SNDT University in Mumbai, 'to fill 2 thirds of the vacancies on basic pay scale not on complete scale', effectively requiring the majority of new appointees to accept less than the salary government pay scales allotted to them. The principal asked, 'with this restriction, who will come?' (Falaknaaz, 'India Faces Acute Shortage of Teaching Staff').

[131] Nagpal, 'Development of Nursing', p. 125.

[132] Academy for Nursing Studies, 'Situational Analysis', p. 17.

[133] Anonymous, 'The Trained Nurses' Association of India: An Introduction', *Indian Nursing Year Book 1996–97*, New Delhi: TNAI, 1997, p. 11.

Patsy Joseph, lamented the recent growth of private institutions there that trained nurses for six months and then gave them certificates in 'basic nursing', unendorsed by any recognised nursing or health authority.[134] In 1987, Jaiwanti P. Dhaulta described the frequent employment by private hospitals of community health workers, trained for basic rural health work in villages, instead of nurses.[135] Manocha comments on the alarmingly high presence of totally unqualified 'nurses' in personnel-starved rural areas.[136] In Thiruvananthapuram, the nurse principals I interviewed stated that the employment of untrained carers was rife in the private hospital system, which appointed 'trainees', who retained this status indefinitely and were paid a low wage to provide nursing care. This widespread disregard for the INC and the state-level councils as regulators has been enabled by the fact that they have not had sufficient funding to take meaningful action and have frequently been headed and staffed by non-nurses. A key recommendation of the Hyderabad report was that nursing councils should be strengthened and better structured. The report recorded that:

> Nursing Councils were poorly structured and administered. They did not enjoy professional autonomy to undertake measures of quality of education and maintain standards. Most were headed by non-nursing persons, they were housed in poorly equipped offices and many posts were vacant . . . The nursing profession was found to be weak at the top administrative level at state and district level. Most of the key administrative positions were vacant or were occupied by lower cadres or were being officiated by non-nursing persons.[137]

The longstanding issue of violence against nurses seems, if anything, to have worsened, and no agency of the state has proved willing to take meaningful action to address it. Indeed, in its inaction to either punish offenders or compensate victims, the state has seemed increasingly complicit in anti-nurse violence. One of the most recent cases to gain public attention was the rape of a Delhi nurse by a ward

---

[134] Anonymous, 'International Nurses' Day: Celebrations throughout the Country', *NJI*, vol. 95, no. 11, November 2004, pp. 246–50.

[135] Dhaulta, 'A Report on the Community Nurses' Meet', p. 17.

[136] Manocha, 'Challenges for Nursing Profession', p. 114.

[137] Academy for Nursing Studies, *Situational Analysis*.

attendant in the Shanti Mukund Hospital in 2005.[138] In a difficult to comprehend act of state-endorsed violence, the nurse concerned was requested by the judge in the case to consider an offer of marriage made by the 'remorseful' defendant.[139] Pledges made by committees such as the High Power Committee to improve workplace safety have not been enforced. Whereas some of the wealthy private hospitals, such as the Indraprastha Apollo in Delhi, have introduced CCTV and metal detectors and employed women security guards on the wards, in the government sector measures long ago approved for the improvement of security have not been implemented.[140] Agnes writes of the legislative victories won by women activists in the 1980s that the progressive intent of the new laws was destroyed by the manner in which they were interpreted and implemented, which was 'totally contradictory to the spirit of the enactments'.[141] Similarly, the continuing tolerance of violence against nurses suggests the weak and partial commitment of a male-dominated state to safety for working women.

Fortuitously, the interests of the state now seem to be in fostering better nurse education, given the potential this holds out of profit and business development. To some extent, a more gender-sensitive political environment has made nurses more difficult to ignore. As in the 1950s and 1960s, nursing initiatives can again be proclaimed as evidence of the state's commitment to international developmentalist orthodoxies. As before, however, the extent to which rhetoric has become practice has clearly been limited.

---

[138] It was reported that Shanti Mukund initially refused treatment to the victim, denied all responsibility for the case and, following protests from the victim's family and neighbours, admitted her but attempted to charge ₹7000 for treatment (Anonymous, 'Delhi Rape Case', 2003).

[139] Anonymous, 'On Rape Judgment Day, Court to Victim: He wants to Marry you', *Express India*, 3 May 2005, http://cities.expressindia.com/fullstory.php?newsid=127644 (accessed 6 May 2005); Anonymous, 'Shanti Mukund Rape Victim declines Convict's Marriage Proposal', *Hindustan Times*, 4 May 2005, http://www.hindustantimes.com/news/181_1347603,000600010001.htm (accessed 12 May 2005); Anonymous, 'Delhi Hospital Ward Boy gets Life Sentence for Rape', *Outlook India*, 4 May 2005, http://www.outlookindia.com/pti_news.asp?id=295969 (accessed 6 May 2005); Anonymous, 'Judge asks Victim to Consider Marrying Rapist', *The Age*, Melbourne, 5 May 2005, p. 11.

[140] Dogra, 'Delhi has a Long way to go'.

[141] Agnes, 'Protecting Women against Violence?', p. 522.

# Conclusions

The relationship between state and profession has been characterised by contempt and exclusion, confirming Rajan's analysis that 'the denial of women's work and of women's identity and productivity as workers predominates in state law and policy as common sense'.[142] Neither planners nor politicians have seen any incentive to construct a positive, ongoing relationship with the nursing profession. The early years of health planning promised much, but delivered little. Governments paid lip service to the importance of good nursing but, in reality, it was a distant last in health priorities. In later years, even the rhetorical emphasis on nursing vanished. The profession remained underdeveloped and from the mid-1960s became easier and easier to ignore, until in some cases it even disappeared altogether from government plans and reports. The late 1980s, however, saw the beginnings of an improvement. The historical neglect of the profession was recognised and some policies for professional development were implemented. At the same time, nurses have continued to struggle. As always, victories won on paper have proved difficult to win in practice and the issues identified by the High Power Committee persist.

The marginalisation of nurses illustrates some brutal truths about the state and the sincerity of its regularly reiterated commitment to improving women's lives in India. Its inaction has institutionalised the contempt that has long been expressed for nurses as women who work, as women who work with bodies, as women who tend to men, as women who are mobile and independent, and as non-elite women. It has maintained a one-sided, disempowering relationship with nurses (although periodically castigating itself for doing so via committees that result in no action). The history of nurses' interaction with governments suggests that the state has largely been impervious to nurses' problems, but at the same time it highlights the extent to which improving things for nurses depends on forcing the state and its agencies into action. Even though it replicates and reinforces the brutal patriarchy of the hospital workplace, the state must be confronted somehow. It is to be hoped that the signs of rejuvenation in nursing organisation identified in the previous chapter will ultimately

---

[142] Rajan, *The Scandal of the State*, p. 27.

produce a more balanced and productive relationship, where past approaches have failed.

In recent years, nursing has been transformed by expanding opportunities to emigrate to the West. Chapter 6 questions the prevailing orthodoxy that this has represented a status revolution for nurses, suggesting that some of the less publicised results of emigration in fact confirm the problematic relationship of the state with its nurses that have been identified in this chapter.

# The Dean
## C. Chandrakanthi

Had she been born a generation earlier, C. CHANDRAKANTHI might have finished her career as an august TNAI leader or a respected advisor to local nursing schools. Instead, in the days of expanding nursing emigration, her career as a nursing leader is culminating in the transition into a successful businesswoman.[1] It took me at least 10 telephone calls to set up an interview with the impressively busy Chandrakanthi, who is the Dean of the College of Nursing at the privately-run Amrita Institute of Medical Sciences and Research Centre in Kochi, as well as the Chairman of the Board of Studies in Nursing at the (also privately-run) Mahatma Gandhi University.

Her evident enjoyment of her power and influence was in dramatic contrast to the more sedate, polite atmosphere of the TNAI headquarters in Delhi. In many ways, she seemed the private sector equivalent of Mrs Khurana — pioneer of nursing unionism in Delhi — another forceful woman who has also found professional fulfilment by forging new paths of leadership.

Chandrakanthi is unusual in that she has also had a political career outside nursing. In 2000 she was elected to the local council as the member for the Medical College district of Trivandrum, winning the election by a large majority.

Like Mr Khurana, Chandrakanthi's husband too was quietly supportive of her work. My interview took place in the family home, a house called 'Rajakanthi', a combination of her name and that of her husband, which strongly suggested that theirs was, at the very least, a partnership of equals.

---

[1] This profile is based on my interview with C. Chandrakanthi, Thiruvananthapuram (Trivandrum), 4 December 2005.

As a young woman, Chandrakanthi took up her nursing career against the wishes of her family. Her father, who worked for the Indian Railways, was strongly opposed to the idea. Fortunately, the family was connected by marriage to G. Chandramathy, one of the earliest Malayali nurses who had been sponsored by Rockefeller to study nursing at Columbia University in New York, and who returned to become an influential leader of nursing in Kerala. Chandramathy begged Chandrakanthi's father to reconsider, and permission was granted.

Chandrakanthi, after taking two years of a pre-university course, enrolled at the newly established School of Nursing in Trivandrum, and was a member of the first batch of students to study with Lucy Peters (a student of Aleyamma Kuruvilla and the first principal of the Trivandrum school). Peters identified her as a capable and well-educated student with potential for leadership, and gave her extra responsibilities. Chandrakanthi then went on to take Peters' pioneering post-basic BSc programme, the first of its kind in South and South-east Asia.

She studied for her Master's degree at CMC Vellore, after which she returned to Trivandrum to work as a teacher at the local College of Nursing. From there she was selected by WHO for a fellowship in medical-surgical nursing, to be taken up at the Frances Payne Bolton School of Nursing at Case Western Reserve University in Cleveland, Ohio. She very fondly remembered her time there, particularly her close relationship with her supervisor, Ruth M. Anderson. She felt that the specialised knowledge gained through the programme greatly enhanced her teaching skills upon her return to India.

Chandrakanthi became the Director of the Trivandrum College of Nursing, a post she occupied for 12 years. In 1982 she was deputed to launch the new government nursing college in Kottayam. Despite some opposition, she successfully argued for the admission of male students into the new college. In 1987, she superintended the launching of Trivandrum College's Masters degree. She is former Vice-President of the Kerala Nurses and Midwives Council and former President of the INC.

After her retirement, she was able to take advantage of expanding opportunities in the private sector, particularly after 2002–3, when the Kerala Government removed a prohibition on private sector colleges of nursing. This brought the prospect of rich profits, as hitherto those girls who did not qualify for admission to one of Kerala's three government colleges had enrolled in large numbers in the colleges of Tamil Nadu and Karnataka. The change in the rules led to the opening of a number of new private colleges, many under the advice of Chandrakanthi. She headed the launch of five new nursing colleges associated with the privately-run Mahatma Gandhi University and assisted in establishing a nursing college at the Amrita Institute. She very strongly feels that part of the solution to the national shortage of teachers lies in permitting and encouraging the private sector to expand, particularly in allowing it to teach more postgraduate courses.

The Amrita College claims on its website that it 'will always be in the forefront in moulding intellectually creative, morally responsible, spiritually enlightened, emotionally mature and socially committed nurses'. It also provides an English language training course geared to pass the Commission on Graduates of Foreign Nursing Schools (CGFNS) test for entrance to the US and the International English Language Testing System (IELTS) examination, essential for work in a number of Western countries.[2]

The rapid opening of new nursing schools and colleges is providing opportunities for retired nurses such as Chandrakanthi to take up creative and profitable new positions of authority. It is unsurprising, therefore, that she is wholly in favour of an expanding role for Kerala as a supplier of nurses to the hospitals of the world.

◘

---

[2] Amrita Institute of Medical Sciences School of Nursing, http://www.aims.amrita.edu/school-of-nursing/nursing-home.php (accessed 12 March 2013).

# 6

# 'Nurses Anytime'

## Emigration and
## the Status Question

◘

A career in Indian nursing has, since the 1990s, been reshaped into a lucrative route to work overseas. A multi-faceted industry has sprung up around emigration, with agencies, supported by an eager state, promising 'nurses anytime' to the hospitals of the West.[1] The phenomenon has drawn unprecedented public attention to nursing and has largely been celebrated in India. This chapter draws on interviews with nursing school and college principals and other nursing leaders (conducted in New Delhi and Thiruvananthapuram in 2005 and 2006), as well as on the growing literature on the global trade in nurses, to direct attention to domestic ramifications of large-scale migration. It suggests that frequent claims that emigration has revolutionised the status of nursing must be carefully qualified. While it is fair to argue that emigration has radically improved individual nurses' social status, the status of the profession in general and of nurses in the workplace continues to be low, and may even be reduced by the strains emigration is placing on the national health system.

This chapter suggests that the position of the central government on the issue of nurse emigration reveals its continuing contempt

---

[1] The phrase is borrowed from a Bangalore agency, Nurses Anytime, which gives training to nurses in computer literacy and 'cross-culture etiquette, accent orientation, intonation and smart grooming' (Habib Beary, 'Indian Nurses' American Dream', BBC News Online: International Version, 1 September 2003, http://news.bbc.co.uk/2/hi/health/3191525.stm [accessed 15 December 2005]).

for the profession. The state has chosen to focus on the rewards of positioning itself as a Philippines-style global exporter of nurses, while ignoring the costs of such a role. Already, these costs include escalating rates of staff turnover, severe understaffing in some areas, a critical shortage of nursing teachers, and an enormous, rapid, under-regulated, and geographically imbalanced expansion in private nursing education. Nursing organisations have largely been excluded from discussion and action on the issue. The emigration debate, it is argued, thus reflects the fact that nursing has still not found acceptance with the state as an integral dimension of a functioning health system.

In recent years, the literature on the gendered dimensions of international migration from Asia has expanded greatly. This literature draws attention to what Oishi describes as 'the feminisation of migratory populations around the world'.[2] Accounts of gender in migration explore both the agency and potential empowerment of women who migrate alone, and their vulnerability to exploitation in a global, under-regulated trade in services.[3] This literature also provides some relevant insights into the role of the state in international migration. Young, for example, contests the suggestion that international migration is an example of globalisation threatening sovereignty. He writes that states 'continue to play a critical role, not in opposing globalisation, but as facilitators of globalisation', an analysis borne out in the dynamics of nursing emigration in India.[4]

On the issue of nurse migration in particular, Mireille Kingma's study identifies the ethical dilemmas the contemporary global trade in nurses creates. Her suggestion that migration may delay effective solutions to personnel problems in both host and source countries, leading to a 'strange version of musical chairs where there are always more empty seats than players', underpins much of my analysis.[5] Catherine Ceniza Choy's account of nursing migration from the

---

[2] Oishi, *Women in Motion*, p. 2.

[3] See, for example, Gulati, 'Asian Women Workers', pp. 46–72; Ehrenreich and Hochschild, *Global Women*; Jolly, et al., *Gender and Migration in Asia*; Roy and Arya, 'When Poor Women Migrate', pp. 19–48.

[4] Young, 'Globalization and the Changing Management of Migrating Service Workers in the Asia-Pacific', p. 16.

[5] Mireille Kingma, *Nurses on the Move: Migration and the Global Health Economy*, New York: Cornell University Press, 2005.

Philippines also has resonance for the student of India. Ceniza Choy describes the way in which a nursing system developed by the colonial power, according to the North American ethos of professionalism, has provided the perfect solution to contemporary US nursing shortages.[6] There is also a small but fascinating literature on the experience of Indian nurse migrants. Sheba George, studying Kerala nurses in the US, describes the complex negotiations of traditional gender roles involved in nurse-led migration.[7] Marie Percot's research highlights the emergence of nursing work in the Middle East as a 'stepping-stone' strategy in nurses' plans for permanent emigration to the West.[8] In this chapter, however, I emphasise the fact that nurses are not only skilled individuals in demand on an international labour market, but also a crucial dimension of the national health system. Rather than focusing substantially on the experiences of nurses as migrants, I highlight the effects of migration on the status of the profession at home.

## The First Wave of Nursing Emigration from India, 1940–95

The family of Thankamma Cherian, the principal of the private Cosmopolitan School of Nursing in Thiruvananthapuram, is illustrative of the long history of nurse migration in India. Cherian comes from a family of six daughters, of whom five are nurses. Two of her sisters now live in Canada, and another spent decades in the Gulf. As this family history indicates, the prospect of work abroad has long shaped the culture of Indian nursing. Although the percentage of nurses who emigrated permanently was small in the early years, most nurses were aware of the possibility and many knew or knew of colleagues reputed to have found higher salaries and more respect

---

[6] Ceniza Choy, *Empire of Care*. For the Philippines, see also R. Ball, 'Divergent Development, Racialised Rights: Globalized Labour Markets and the Trade of Nurses: the Case of the Philippines', *Women's Studies International Forum*, vol. 27, no. 2, 2004, pp. 119–33.

[7] George, *When Women Come First*.

[8] Percot, 'Indian Nurses in the Gulf: Two Generations of Female Migration', pp. 41–62; Percot, 'Indian Nurses in the Gulf: From Job Opportunity to Life Strategy', pp. 155–76.

abroad. Given the international orientation of nursing culture developed by Western leaders and a programme of overseas scholarships in place since the 1930s, this was not at all surprising. In many ways, the emergence of India as a source of nursing labour for the West is a logical outcome of the process of professional development, which was overseen by British and American nurses and which valorised the West as the source of nursing culture and the highest standards of practice. Ceniza Choy writes that

> the desire of Filipino nurses to migrate abroad cannot be reduced to an economic logic, but rather reflects individual and collective desire for a unique form of social, cultural and economic success obtainable only outside the national borders of the Philippines.[9]

Similarly, the culture and history of Indian nursing has always oriented its nurses outward.

A steady trickle of Indian nurses has thus travelled abroad to work in the hospitals of the West since Independence, although their numbers and experiences have remained largely undocumented. In Britain, nurses formed a small group in a much larger wave of post-Independence migration from South Asia. Shakuntala Bhansali, the Punjabi nurse emigrant talked about in Chapter 1, came to Britain in 1957. She told me that at that stage most of the Indian nurse arrivals in England drew on their contacts with missionaries.[10] Although the numbers arriving were small, by the late 1960s there was awareness in the British government of growing enthusiasm among Indian nurses for work in Britain. During 1967, problems arose at the ministry of labour over a scheme for granting Category B work vouchers, which allowed Commonwealth nurses to enter the country without having the sponsorship of an employer. The scheme was designed to attract white nurses, but instead drew large numbers of Indian nurses. From January to November 1967, 172 Indian nurses had been granted Category B vouchers, compared to only 24 Australians, 16 Canadians and six New Zealanders.[11] In September 1967, the ministries of

---

[9] Ceniza Choy, *Empire of Care*, pp. 6–7.

[10] Author interview with Shakuntala Bhansali, London, 8 August 2005.

[11] R. B. Mayoh to B. H. Heddy, 18 December 1967, Commonwealth Office (General and Migration Department), UK National Archives, Kew, (henceforth UKNA), FCO 50/84, 'Immigration/UK/: Trained Nurses: Difficulties Of'.

labour and health were corresponding with the Commonwealth office about the handling of the issue, emphasising that the government was 'not anxious to stimulate a flow of nurses from India or Pakistan'. An official of the ministry wrote that 'many Indian girls are coming to this country as nurses without an adequate knowledge of English ... they are quite inadequate to undertake staff nurse duties because they cannot understand the instructions given by the doctors and senior nurses'.[12] Later in the year, the two offices debated measures that might be taken to ensure that nurses from Australia and New Zealand were more easily able to work in Britain. It was clearly the case, officials felt, that Antipodean nurses could 'be expected, both clinically and socially, to be well up to the standards we expect of our own British girls' in comparison to Indian nurses, whom they felt to be dubiously qualified and in general less desirable.[13] This wave of nurse migration to some extent was stemmed by raising the standard of qualification asked of professional migrants, leading to the cutting from the waiting list of large numbers of 'Indian and Pakistani teachers and other (allegedly) professionally trained people'.[14] Debate over desirable sources of foreign nurses reflected a considerable race-based anxiety to stem the flow of South Asian nurses into Britain. It also, however, showed that there was a very early awareness among Indian nurses of the possibilities for work abroad, as well as a high level of sensitivity to adjustments in British immigration policy.

India's nurses continued throughout the 1960s and 1970s to seek work in the West. George writes that nurse shortages in the US during the 1960s prompted the extensive recruitment of Asian nurses, including nurses from Kerala, of whom there has been a continuing flow ever since.[15] Mejia's early study of physician and nurse emigration from India gives some figures for the late 1960s and 1970s,

---

[12] D. C. Anderson to P. Gill, 20 September 1967, Commonwealth Office (General and Migration Department), UKNA, FCO 50/84, 'Immigration/UK/: Trained Nurses: Difficulties Of'.

[13] B. H. Heddy to R. B. Mayoh, 11 December 1967, Commonwealth Office (General and Migration Department), UKNA, FCO 50/84, 'Immigration/UK/: Trained Nurses: Difficulties Of'.

[14] Note for the Secretary of State's talk with Lord Robens, 1967, UKNA, FCO 50/84, 'Immigration/UK/: Trained Nurses: Difficulties Of'.

[15] George, *When Women Come First*, p. 19.

although he is likely to have underestimated the number leaving.[16] He found that each year between 1969 and 1974, on average 84 Indian nurses were licensed in the US, 160 in Canada and about 80 in the UK. During this period, therefore, on average 324 Indian nurses left per year for the three countries. In 1972, out of India's 82,300 nurses, 250 went abroad.[17] Including those who were working in the Gulf, in 1972 there were about 4,000 Indian nurses in work abroad, or about 5 per cent of the domestic nurse workforce. The TNAI president for 1976, A. Cherian, was concerned about the numbers leaving and felt that this could potentially undermine efforts to improve conditions at home:

> Similar to other professional personnel, there is brain drain among nurses. The better-qualified nurses seek employment abroad for recognition and improved remuneration. It is natural that everyone desires to better oneself but our country needs these valuable members to work for our people and the profession. The desired situation can be achieved through hard work and not by running away . . . It would seem that this is the best time to pull ourselves together and help in nation-building.[18]

Throughout the 1970s and 1980s, although migration was predominantly to the Gulf, there was also a pervasive professional awareness of the possibility of new lives for nurses in the West. George records the extensive professional and personal networks that facilitated the early flow of Kerala nurses to the US.[19] Ramanamma's 1984 survey of 254 nurses found a strong general awareness that conditions were better overseas and that generally there was a very common desire to emigrate.[20] Although, as is the case today, the *NJI*

---

[16] There are many factors that affect the accuracy of statistics on the migration of Indian nurses. Many went to the Gulf before continuing to the West and were thus not counted as emigrants to the West, better records were kept of nurses emigrating from the government than from the private sector, and some nurses took further qualifications in their host country and thus were not necessarily registered there as overseas trained nurses.

[17] A. Mejia, H. Pizurki and E. Royston, *Physician and Nurse Migration: Analysis and Policy Implications*, Geneva: WHO, 1979, p. 73.

[18] A. Cherian, 'Role of Nursing in India Today', *NJI*, vol. 67, no. 11, 1976, p. 259.

[19] George, *When Women Come First*, p. 199.

[20] A. Ramanamma and Usha Bambawale, 'Occupational Attitudes of Nurses: A Sociological Study', *The Journal of Sociological Studies*, January 1984, p. 88.

seems to have largely ignored the controversial issue of emigration, to some extent its pages also reflected the international mobility of some of its readers. Throughout the 1970s, it carried an advertisement for Swissair's 'Special Service Department for Nurses', catering for those flying to Canada and the US.[21] In 1970, a long article by an Indian nurse documented the far greater state and public support for the public health nurse she had witnessed in the US.[22] Fairly low numbers actually left India, but the culture of emigration and an awareness of opportunities in the West thus pervaded the profession.

## Migration to the Gulf, 1940–95

A crucial part of the emigration story is the longstanding presence of Indian nurses in the Gulf states. As Percot observes, nurse migration to the Middle East was mostly an 'economic strategy' designed to create a better life at home, compared to the permanent migration of many nurses to Western countries.[23] Thankamma Cherian told me that by going to work in the Gulf, 'we can collect some money and come back to our Kerala, and make a house and stay here'. In comparison, leaving for the US brought the prospect that 'the children are taking their culture', daughters would go 'running with the boys' and Kerala families would turn into American ones.[24] The Gulf, therefore, has chiefly functioned as an opportunity to earn an enormous salary in comparison to Indian rates. These salaries have then been used to ensure the social mobility of nurses' families through the purchase of better education and housing back home.

A small number of Indian nurses worked in the Gulf from as early as the 1940s and 1950s, when Indians were first recruited by newly established oil companies.[25] In 1941, the *NJI* reported the formation

---

[21] See for example, *NJI*, vol. 67, no. 7, 1976, inside back cover.

[22] Bachu, 'Public Health Nursing', pp. 361, 373.

[23] Percot, 'Two Generations of Female Migration', p. 42.

[24] Author interview with Thankamma Cherian, Thiruvananthapuram, 22 November 2005.

[25] For a description of this early recruitment of migrants from Kerala to the Gulf, see K. C. Zachariah, E. T. Mathew and S. Irudaya Rajan, *Dynamics of Migration in Kerala: Dimensions, Differentials and Consequences*, Hyderabad: Orient Longman, 2003, pp. 65–67. Prema Kurien reports that nurses from the predominantly Christian Kerala village of Kembu had migrated to the Gulf since the 'post-Second World War period' (Kurien, *Kaleidoscopic Ethnicity*, p. 136).

of a new district branch of the TNAI in Bahrain, with a Mr Daniel as the honorary provincial secretary.[26] Nurse migrants of the 1940s and 1950s worked in austere and lonely conditions; during the 1950s it was reported that they were housed in mud huts without electricity.[27] The face of nurse migration to the Gulf changed dramatically, however, with the oil price rises of the early 1970s and the new wealth that this brought to the states of the Gulf region. Rapidly expanding health systems needed large numbers of new nurses, and so Indian nurses began to be recruited in much greater numbers. From then on, many of these nations have relied on them.

Nurse migration to the Gulf was dominated by nurses from Kerala, who had a long-established tradition of high domestic mobility. Difficult conditions in their home state and more lucrative work elsewhere had motivated them to train and work in other Indian states since the 1930s, as was discussed in earlier chapters. From the 1950s, they were a ubiquitous presence in Indian hospitals from Bihar to the Andamans. This pre-existing tradition of domestic mobility allowed a rapid response to the opportunities that arose to work in the Gulf.

Their response must also be understood in the context of the extensive general participation of Malayalis in Gulf migration. Kerala has a longstanding tradition of mass migration, upon which the economy of the state relies. The presence of Kerala migrants in the Gulf began from the late 1940s and sharply escalated from the early 1970s.[28] Percot writes that by current estimates, there are over 4 million Indian migrants working in the Gulf, of which almost half are from Kerala (although the state of Kerala contains just 3.1 per cent of the population of India).[29] Forced by high unemployment and economic stagnation to leave home, most Malayalis can claim a high level of cultural familiarity with the Gulf.

---

[26] Anonymous, 'Extracts from the Minutes of the Conference of the TNAI, Delhi, 1941', *NJI*, vol. 32, no. 4, April 1941, p. 111. The same edition of the *NJI* carried an advertisement for a nursing sister to run the Men's Block in a Persian Gulf hospital.

[27] Narender Nagpal, 'It's not all Green on the Other Side of the Hedge', *NJI*, vol. 67, no. 7, 1976, p. 160.

[28] See, for example, Zachariah et al., *Dynamics of Migration in Kerala*, pp. 66–67.

[29] Percot, 'Indian Nurses in the Gulf: Two Generations of Female Migration', pp. 42–43.

The documentation of nurse migration during this period was limited, but the presence of Indian nurses in the Gulf was certainly significant. Mejia and his co-authors found that in 1971, at the beginning of large-scale nurse migration to the Middle East, there were 416 Indian nurses working in Bahrain and 269 in Oman.[30] Bahrain had a total foreign nurse workforce of 566 at that stage, meaning that Indian nurses in that year were 73 per cent of the overseas nurse workforce there.[31] In 1976, Narender Nagpal wrote that official statistics had been impossible for her to find due to the variety of channels nurses used to find work in the Gulf, some through the government, some through travel agents and some through friends already in the Gulf. She felt that a conservative estimate of numbers in the Gulf was that 3,000 Indian nurses were working in Oman, the United Arab Emirates, Qatar, Kuwait, Iraq, Jordan, and Iran. In 'Saudi Arabia, Bahrain and other Arab-African republics' there were approximately 5,000.[32]

Nurse migrants to the Gulf faced considerable hardships, including restrictions on their mobility in conservative Muslim states and isolation from their families and children. They were also frustrated by workplace discrimination that meant Arab and Western nurses were paid more and preferred for promotions, whilst they were stereotyped as submissive and lacking in initiative.[33] On the other hand, salaries comparatively were far higher than at home, and working conditions were excellent.[34] In the late 1970s, the average staff nurse in the Gulf was paid a starting salary of between ₹2,000 and

---

[30] Mejia et al., *Physician and Nurse Migration*, p. 279.

[31] Ibid., p. 44.

[32] Nagpal, 'It's not all Green', p. 160. Documentation and commentary on the role of Indian nurses in Africa is even more rare than that on the Gulf during this period, but the joint survey of the Coordinating Agency for Health Planning (CAHP) and the TNAI in 1974 mentioned Africa as an important destination for the increasing numbers of migrating nurses. Many nurses in Kerala mention colleagues or relatives who worked in Zambia, Uganda and Zimbabwe (CAHP, 'Report of a Nursing Survey in India', Preface).

[33] Nagpal, 'It's not all Green', pp. 160–62.

[34] Although Nagpal reported that nurses employed in the private sector rather than by government hospitals struggled with high costs of living, as they had to rent their own accommodation and cover living expenses, these nurses also lacked job security and some were pressured to sign unfavourable contracts (Nagpal, 'It's not all Green', p. 161).

₹3,000 per month.[35] An advertisement carried in the *NJI* in 1976 for
a senior sister tutor to work in Bihar offered ₹550.[36] Kurien writes
that by the late 1980s an Indian nurse in the Gulf received between
₹10,000 and ₹30,000 per month, whereas in Kerala nurses were paid
between ₹800 and ₹1,500.[37]

## The consequences of first wave migration for the status of nursing

Nurse migration to the West and to the Middle East from the 1940s
through to the 1990s had a strong effect on professional status in
India, and gives some indication of what to expect from the recent
escalation in migration. The growing profile of nurses as professionals in demand overseas reduced the stigma historically attached
to nursing, and the social experience of the nurse improved. Early
Malayali migrants to the Gulf were paid very high wages and forged
a tradition of international nurse mobility, in the process revising
prospective nurses' expectations of what a nursing career would
provide. In most Kerala towns, local residents are able to point out
the grand residences of 'Gulf-returned' nurses. It became clear that
nursing abroad was a successful strategy of social mobility and,
according to Kurien, this was widely recognised. The continuing
high demand for nurses in the Gulf and in the US from the 1960s
meant that the numbers of nursing students in Kerala grew steadily,
despite the cessation of the payment of a stipend to student nurses
from the mid-1960s.[38]

Work in the Gulf often paid for the crippling dowry expenses of
nurses and their relatives and the experience of migration was both
planned and circumscribed by the families of nurses, so migration
cannot be straightforwardly represented as a source of empowerment. At the same time, it is also usually agreed that nurses' status
as high-earning professionals in demand in an international market
brought new levels of personal autonomy and social respect. George's
account of Malayali nurses in the US shows the effect of migration

---

[35] Nagpal, 'It's not all Green', p. 160.
[36] Advertisement for staff at Magadh Medical College, Gaya, *NJI*, vol. 67, no. 7,
1976, p. 162.
[37] Kurien, *Kaleidoscopic Ethnicity*, p. 141.
[38] Kurien, *Kaleidoscopic Ethnicity*, p. 152.

on nurses' status in the private sphere.[39] Nurses in the US continued to negotiate and live within a Kerala culture of 'connectivity', in which individual experience is determined, restricted and enriched by extended family structures. Migration brought with it difficult and stressful marital conflict and even domestic violence. Nurses' husbands often had limited work opportunities, and nurses were required to balance their status as breadwinners with cultural expectations of them as wives, mothers and daughters. Nonetheless, many found professional stimulation and satisfaction at work and also new levels of influence within the family. George concludes that, to some extent, nurses in the US were able to negotiate a reconfiguration of the structures of patriarchy.[40]

The popularity of Malayali nurses abroad and their capacity to command high wages, however, did little for the status of the profession at home in Kerala. The state was winning a reputation worldwide for its remarkable achievements in social development, but conditions for nurses were among the worst in India, and professional organisation, in a context of exceptionally strong general labour activism, was at its weakest. Malayali nurses, focused on work abroad, were not easily mobilised around local issues. It is also true that although the stigmatisation of nurses decreased somewhat as their opportunities abroad grew, much of this stigma remained. Kurien, in a study of Kerala migrants in three villages, found that nursing was regarded as an effective strategy for social mobility, but that it had not come to be seen as a desirable career:

Among the second-generation migrants, young women (even daughters of nurses) were almost never sent for nurse training. Of the more than dozen cases that I was acquainted with directly or indirectly, I did not come across a single instance where the daughter of a nurse became a nurse herself. This was due to the stigma that was still (though to a lesser degree) attached to nursing. Thus the profession continued to be perceived as one entered into by poorer women unable to afford a college education (which was considered far more prestigious).[41]

---

[39] George, *When Women Come First*.
[40] Ibid., p. 204.
[41] Kurien, *Kaleidoscopic Ethnicity*, p. 156.

Recognition of nurses' earning potential abroad thus by no means entirely removed the stigma attached to nursing in Kerala, and in fact high mobility could even contribute to the stereotyping of nurses as morally suspect. As George writes, nurses' freedom of movement was often viewed as indecorous and the many nurses who travelled outside of Kerala for their training were particularly stigmatised.[42]

Generally, the high status of nurses abroad and the value placed on them in overseas labour markets contrasted glaringly with the low esteem held for their services in India. Nagpal wrote of the intense frustration she felt at the frequency with which nurses were blamed for the poor condition of India's hospitals. It was clear, she felt, that nurses were not in fact to be blamed. In the hospitals of the Gulf states, many staffed mainly by Indian nurses, conditions were clean and pleasant, and hospitals ran efficiently. At home, nurses were the scapegoats in a malfunctioning and under-resourced system; abroad, they were highly sought-after professionals.[43] Nurses as individuals were better-regarded, less stigmatised and more empowered, and were increasingly sought-after in the marriage market. Individual status, however, could be separated from professional status. Emigration, even though it attracted more and better candidates into nursing and brought a more positive public profile for nurses, was not a source of empowerment for nurses working in the hospitals of India. This earlier history thus casts doubt on contemporary claims that new opportunities for emigration will result in better conditions for nurses at home.

## Mapping the Second Wave of Emigration, 1995–2006

Twenty-first century emigration involves much larger numbers, and holds the prospect of a far-reaching transformation of the nursing profession, as India comes to play a new role in an increasingly permanent global market. This market has been created by 'crisis-level' nurse shortages in the West (although invariably nurse–patient ratios in host countries are far higher than in the nurse-sending countries of Asia and Africa) and by hospitals' new, institutionalised practice

---

[42] George, *When Women Come First*, p. 46.
[43] Narender Nagpal, 'Why Blame the Nurse?', *NJI*, vol. 67, no. 7, 1976, p. 153.

of recruiting nurses directly from developing countries. It is widely recognised that these serious nurse shortages in developed nations are likely to continue for at least 10 to 20 years.[44] Already, Western health systems have become dependent on International Registered Nurses (IRNs). Australia experienced a 'dramatic ethnic diversification' in nursing between 1995 and 2000.[45] Britain in 1999 was said to be experiencing the 'worst nursing shortage crisis in 25 years' and recent expansion of the NHS has made it a major employer of overseas-trained nurses.[46] The number of IRNs working in Britain doubled between 1999 and 2002 to 42,000.[47] In Ireland in 2002, two-thirds of new entrants to the register were IRNs from India, Europe, Australia, and South Africa.[48] In May 2006, the US Senate approved immigration reforms removing restrictions on the number of foreign nurses entering the country, suggesting that the role of IRNs in the American system will expand.[49] Linda Aiken and her co-authors comment that the projected requirements of the UK, Canada, Ireland, Australia, and New Zealand alone are 'large enough to deplete the supply of qualified nurses throughout the developing world'.[50]

Nurses have always been a mobile group. The current situation, however, is something radically different from the smaller streams of migrant and traveller nurses that existed until around the early 1990s. Now, overseas recruitment is a large-scale, state-endorsed strategy to resolve shortages in Western hospitals. Brush and Vasupuram write

---

[44] Kingma, *Nurses on the Move*, p. 8.

[45] Lesleyanne Hawthorne, 'The Globalisation of the Nursing Workforce: Barriers Confronting Overseas Qualified Nurses in Australia', *Nursing Inquiry*, vol. 8, no. 4, 2001.

[46] The Baroness Gardner of Parkes, quoted in Sandra Meadows, Ros Levenson and Juan Baeza, *The Last Straw: Explaining the NHS Nursing Shortage*, London: King's Fund, 2000, p. 3.

[47] Linda H. Aiken, James Buchan, Julie Sochalski, Barbara Nichols and Mary Powell, 'Trends in International Nurse Migration', *Health Affairs*, vol. 23, no. 3, 2004, pp. 69–77.

[48] Kingma, *Nurses on the Move*, p. 3. After recent years of economic expansion, Ireland has moved from being a well-regarded exporter of nurses to suffering considerable shortages and is emerging as a newly popular destination for developing world nurses (Aiken et al., 'Trends in International Nurse Migration', pp. 69–77.)

[49] Rana Rosen, 'From East to West', *Outlook*, 24 July 2006, YaleGlobal Online, website of the Yale Center for the Study of Globalization, http://yaleglobal.yale.edu./index.jsp (accessed 27 July 2006).

[50] Aiken et al., 'Trends in International Nurse Migration', pp. 69–77.

of the US that 'hiring foreign nurses is no longer a short-term solution to the nursing shortage problem'.[51] In 2002, the RCN in Britain wrote: 'Nursing is a global profession and the international mobility of nurses is nothing new. What is new, however, is increasing large-scale, targeted, international recruitment by developed countries to address domestic shortages'.[52]

In recent years, India has emerged as the largest supplier to the UK and Ireland. In the UK, the number of Indian nurses, as shown in Table 6.1, has grown rapidly. In 1998–99 there were 30 applications from Indian nurses for UK registration, by 2003–4 there were 3,073.[53] An RCN project development officer told me that the numbers of Indian nurses working in the private sector was increasing particularly quickly.[54] The presence of Indian nurses is also notable in Ireland, which has recently increased its direct recruitment efforts (see Table 6.2). Australia poses a somewhat more difficult market for

**Table 6.1:** Number of New Indian Registrants in Britain, 1998–2006

| 1998–99 | 2001–2 | 2002–3 | 2003–4 | 2005–6 |
|---------|--------|--------|--------|--------|
| 30 | 994 | 1833 | 3073 (compared to 5594 from Philippines) | 3551 (compared to 1541 from Philippines, 751 from Australia, 378 from South Africa, 200 from Pakistan). Indians were 41 per cent of the total of new IRNs; nurses from Africa were 14 per cent. |

*Source:* James Buchan and Delanyo Dovlo, 'International Recruitment of Health Workers to the UK: A Report for DFID'; World Health Organization, 'Efforts Under Way to Stem "Brain Drain of Doctors and Nurses"'; James Buchan and Ian Seccombe, 'Worlds Apart? The UK and International Nurses'.

---

[51] Barbara Brush and Rukmini Vasupuram, 'Nurses, Nannies and Caring Work: Importation, Visibility and Marketability', *Nursing Inquiry*, no. 13, 2006.

[52] Royal College of Nurses UK (RCN), 'Working Well Initiative: Internationally Recruited Nurses: Good Practice Guidance for Health Care Employers and RCN Negotiators', London, July 2002, p. 5, http://www.rcn.org.uk/publications/pdf/irn-insides-001-788.pdf (accessed 20 July 2006).

[53] World Health Organization, 'Efforts Under Way to Stem "Brain Drain of Doctors and Nurses"', *Bulletin of the World Health Organization*, vol. 83, no. 2, 2005, p. 85.

[54] Author interview with Jennifer Doohan, RCN Project Development Officer, London, 11 August 2006. Since July 2006, however, the direct recruitment of staff nurses to Britain from abroad by NHS trusts was prohibited, although some grades

**Table 6.2:**  Applications for New Registration in Ireland,
1 January 2005–8 May 2005

| Country of Origin | Number |
|---|---|
| India | 874 |
| Philippines | 208 |
| Ireland | 153 |
| United Kingdom | 66 |
| Nigeria | 61 |
| China | 1 |

*Source:* 'Applications for Registration', *An Bord Altranais News*, 2005.

Indian nurses to enter, given that there is no direct recruitment and most must undertake an expensive and time-consuming process of Competency-Based Assessment (CBA) and verification of language skills upon arrival in Australia. Nonetheless, in 2005–6, India was the third biggest supplier of IRNs in the state of Victoria, after Britain and Ireland, with an 80 per cent increase from the previous year. The CGFNS, which runs examinations for nurses wishing to immigrate to the US, now has four centres in India — at Kochi, Bangalore, Mumbai, and New Delhi — more than in any other country.[55] Khadria found that during 2004–5, approximately 10,000 nurses in Delhi alone had entered the CGFNS application process required to work in the US.[56]

As Percot documents, new global opportunities for Indian nurses have transformed the nature and purpose of their migration to

---

of specialised and highly experienced nurses were exempt from this ('Supporting UK nurses — band 5 nurses to be taken off the Home Office shortage occupation list', UK Department of Health Press Release, 3 July 2006, http://www.gnn.gov.uk/environment/fullDetail.asp?ReleaseID=211686&NewsAreaID=2&NavigatedFromDepartment=False [accessed 24 July 2006]). This does not mean greater legal restriction on foreign nurses entering Britain, but limits the much more accessible emigration route provided by direct recruitment drives in India. This will probably mean that the highly mobile nurse migrants will turn to Ireland and the US, where entry is becoming less rather than more restricted.

[55] Commission on Graduates of Foreign Nursing Schools (CGFNS) web site, http://www.cgfns.org (accessed 7 August 2006).

[56] Binod Khadria, 'International Nurse Recruitment in India', *Health Services Research*, vol. 42, no. 3, part II, 2007, p. 6, http://www.blackwell-synergy.com/doi/abs/10.1111/j.1475-6773.2007.00718.x (accessed 14 April 2012).

the Gulf.[57] There are still 40–50 thousand Indian nurses employed there, and as before the Gulf continues to function as a temporary rather than a permanent destination for nurse migrants.[58] Now, however, work in the Middle East functions as a stopover for Indian nurses in a long-term and carefully planned 'stepping-stone' process of migration to Western countries. High salaries and the absence of language and skill-testing mean Gulf work is now a way of saving for the educational and travel costs of migration to the West. Thus, new patterns of migration have incorporated and refashioned the old. A long tradition of Indian nurse migration to the Gulf has enabled the rapid uptake of opportunities in the West, both in terms of the creation of a professional culture of international mobility and in practical terms.

## Emigration and the Individual Status of Nurses

At the personal and individual level, this second wave of emigration has brought enormous change to the lives of nurses in India. The 'marriage market' provides some indication of women's status, and nurses, previously relatively unpopular as brides, are now in great demand. It is widely known that nurses who make it to the US can access salaries of US$50,000 and higher, frequently augmented by bonuses, incentive payments and additional benefits including cars, assistance with purchasing houses, educational funding, and holidays.[59] As a result, families seeking wives for their sons now often specify nursing qualifications, and those who have already passed the CGFNS are particularly sought after.

The experience of A. Nirmal Jose, a nurse I interviewed in Kochi, demonstrates the extent to which the social position of the nurse has changed in India over a relatively brief period. Jose told me that when she embarked on nursing training in 1988, 'we had some stigma at that time'. She met with considerable opposition from her family, who were 'dead against' the idea of a nursing career, feeling it would not bring 'respect and dignity'. A doctor aunt advised her not to

---

[57] Percot, 'Two Generations of Female Migration', pp. 41–62.
[58] Percot, 'From Job Opportunity to Life Strategy', p. 155.
[59] Kingma, *Nurses on the Move*, p. 45.

take up nursing, because it was too difficult, but Jose persisted. By the time she had graduated in 1992, family attitudes had changed, with an uncle in the US encouraging her to sit for the CGFNS, and good marriage proposals were flooding in. She comments that 'at that time, I thought, I had selected [a] good profession'. Things had changed a great deal for nurses over the course of her career and she felt that 'I don't have that stigma now', and in contrast to the past, 'everywhere I'll go I'll say I'm a nurse, I won't say I'm a professor or teacher. I'll say I'm a nurse'.[60]

Nurses' new status is frequently seen to have brought increased autonomy in the private sphere. Percot writes that emigration has 'changed the status of nurses in India, which used to be rather low'.[61] The young nurses in her study were motivated not just by money, but by the prospect life abroad offered of enhanced autonomy and the opportunity to concentrate on the nuclear family, free from the pressures of the Kerala joint family. They carefully planned life-strategies designed to 'secure more autonomy or agency, as women, than they can get in their own country'.[62] At the same time, the old prejudices have not completely disappeared. To some extent societal contempt for nursing work remains a problem. A Kerala doctor told me:

> What I feel is that there are still status problems. Educated classes find it a rather low occupation . . . and even if they have a lot of money, more than any doctor . . . whether they have emigrated or not, the money and dollars and all, they are still a nurse. Nobody considers them equal, say, to a doctor who has emigrated, or an engineer who has come back, or a teacher who came back.

She went on to comment of the rising numbers of male nurses drawn to the profession by chances to work abroad, that they were merely 'taking a simple degree and wandering abroad'.[63] Stereotypes of nurses as unintelligent and morally questionable still persist in India, and to a degree are reinforced by increased international mobility. George found that, despite the recent new attractiveness of nurses

---

[60] Author interview with Nirmal Jose, Lisie Hospital College of Nursing, Ernakulam, 5 December 2005.

[61] Percot, 'Two Generations of Female Migration', pp. 41–42.

[62] Ibid., p. 42.

[63] Author interview with Dr Sreelatha, Mental Hospital, Thiruvananthapuram, 11 November 2005.

on the marriage market, a deep ambivalence about the profession remained.[64] Sreelekha Nair found in her interviewing with Delhi nurses in 2004 that there was defensiveness among nurses stemming from frequent questioning of their respectability and morality. She also felt that nurses differentiated between their economic status, which had improved dramatically in recent years, and their social status, which they felt was still a major problem. Nair's conclusion was that the high levels of mobility and independence among Malayali nurses, in particular, continued to contribute to their low status within Kerala society.[65] It is thus clear that nurses do continue to encounter stereotypes of nursing as undemanding work pursued by 'loose women'. In general, however, these stereotypes have been challenged and destabilised as never before, and the social status of the nurse seems rapidly on the rise.

## The Status of the Profession

Mrs Vasantha, a middle-aged nurse who is the superintendent of nursing at the short-staffed Thiruvananthapuram Mental Hospital, told me that emigration has had a 'personal impact', rather than a professional one.[66] Status gains have accrued to individual nurses, but the workplace experience of nurses as a group may even have worsened. In comparison to the issue of individual nurses' societal status, this question of the status of the profession, as a whole, is less straightforward.

One important aspect of the question lies in the fact that the profession is poised at the beginning of a profound demographic transition, the consequences of which are difficult to predict. A casual visit to almost any nursing school in India, but especially one in Kerala or Karnataka, makes this obvious. In 2005, I chatted in the forecourt of the Thiruvananthapuram College of Nursing with Jinu, a male nursing student about to enrol for a PhD in nursing at the college. Around us, female students were talking and laughing in

---

[64] George, *When Women Come First*, p. 175.

[65] Sreelekha Nair, Paper on 'Nurses, Status and Stigma', Centre for Women in Developing Societies, New Delhi, 6 February 2006.

[66] Author interview with Mrs Vasantha, Mental Hospital, Thiruvananthapuram, 11 November 2005.

groups on the veranda. The large square of garden around which the college was built, however, had been colonised by numerous rowdy men students playing soccer, with errant kicks flying hazardously. Jinu told me that he had entered nursing because of the chance to emigrate to the West. His career plans centred on becoming a nursing lecturer, because he could not bring himself to actually practise nursing. Emigrating as a teacher, however, was much more difficult than emigrating as a practitioner, and he had thus been forced down a frustrating, expensive and seemingly quite unstimulating path of further education, taking a BSc, then an MSc, and next, a PhD. He was now, it seemed, quite desperate in his search for a route to the West which did not involve working in the career for which he had undertaken three degree courses.

Jinu's experience and the ambience of his college point to an interesting reworking of Indian nursing's status as exclusively a women's profession. It has been credibly claimed that the number of male nurses is rising by 10 per cent annually, which my interviewing in Kerala seemed to confirm.[67] Chandrakanthi told me that a quarter of her student body at the Amrita College was now male, and that 'they are very much interested in nursing because they can get jobs abroad'.[68] Sulochana Bai, the principal of the school of nursing at SUT hospital in Thiruvananthapuram, reported that 20 per cent of her students were male, a figure which she said would be larger except that they were limited by the difficulty of arranging accommodation for men students.[69] At the KIMS school of nursing in Thiruvananthapuram, 10 out 60 students were male.[70]

The Government of Andhra Pradesh until very recently maintained a ban on male nurses, who were not admitted to nursing courses in the state.[71] In 2005, however, a quota of 5 per cent was allocated to

---

[67] C. Chandrakanthi, quoted in Center for Nursing Advocacy, 'Could Shortage-driven Migration Change Nursing's Gender Gap?, http://www.nursingadvocacy.org/news/2005aug/23_new_kerala.html (accessed 5 June 2006).

[68] Author interview.

[69] Author interview with Sulochana Bai, Thiruvananthapuram, 3 December 2005.

[70] Author interview with Rachel Mathew, principal, KIMS School of Nursing, Thiruvananthapuram, 23 November 2005.

[71] Joy Das and Moumita Ghosh, 'The Main Attraction: Hefty Salaries', *The Hindu*, 22 November 2004, Education Plus, Karnataka, http://www.hinduonnet.com/edu/2004/11/22/stories/2004112200250400.htm (accessed 19 January 2006).

male nursing students. An eager group of male applicants protested that this was unjustly low, given that in other courses women were given 33 per cent of seats.[72] In Rajasthan, a state which has historically been unable to create a sustainable recruitment base of educated, willing women to train as nurses, instead relying heavily on Malayali women, nursing is now gaining popularity as a career for men.[73]

It also seems likely that the class profile of nursing students is shifting, given its newfound status as a guaranteed route to the West. Several of the principals I interviewed felt that students from 'better families' were now drawn to nursing, which had previously predominantly attracted poorer Kerala families. Thankamma Cherian, the principal of the private Cosmopolitan School of Nursing, for example, observed that 'now from higher families, very educated parents are sending daughters for nursing'.[74]

The consequences of such changes in the long-term are difficult to predict. It is possible that the gender transformation may, as the Center for Nursing Advocacy postulates, be empowering, creating a vast new recruitment pool, ending the stigma of 'women's work', and changing the social profile of the profession.[75] On the other hand, the all-female environment of the nursing school is being radically and quickly transformed, and this may have its costs. Throughout November and December 2005, the Kerala newspapers reported on the drugging and gang rape of a *Dalit* BSc nursing student, the daughter of a tea-stall owner, by men students on her course, suggesting a potential dark side to this gender transformation of nursing education.[76] Reportage on the issue frequently suggested that

---

[72] Anonymous, 'Nursing Admissions: Male Aspirants' Quota "Meagre"', *The Hindu*, 18 August 2005, http://www.hindu.com/2005/08/18/stories/2005081821070300.htm (accessed 30 January 2006).

[73] Rana Rosen, 'Male Nurses from Rajasthan', Medill News Service, posted on Immigration Here & There Project website, http://www.immigrationhereandthere.org/2006/06/male_nurses_from_rajasthan.php (accessed 12 December 2006).

[74] Author interview.

[75] Center for Nursing Advocacy, 'Shortage-driven Migration'.

[76] See, for example, Anonymous, 'Sexual Assault Reports False, Fabricated, say Students', *Indian Express*, Thiruvananthapuram, 19 November 2005; Anonymous, 'KGMCTA Condemns Ongoing Campaign and HC Dismisses Students' Plea', *The Indian Express*, Thiruvananthapuram, 19 November 2005; Anonymous, 'Directive to Complete Probe in Rape Case', *The Hindu*, Kochi, 10 January 2006, http://www.thehindu.com/2006/01/10/stories/2006011007090500.htm (accessed 12 January 2006). The term *Dalit* was adopted by the community formerly described as 'untouchable' under the Indian caste system.

sexual harassment was endemic in many Kerala universities, and it now seems that nursing classrooms will not be immune to this. The effects of a class and gender transition in nursing are thus various and difficult to predict at this stage, but the current pace of change suggests that they will be profound.

## Emigration and state contempt

An easier question to address is the significance of central and state governments' approach to the nursing trade. The political positioning of India as a nation with nurses to spare reveals the continuing low esteem the state places on the services of its nurses. In effect, it reinforces a longstanding disengagement from the problem of dangerous, unstimulating working conditions for nurses at home. State policies on nurse emigration have placed value on nurses as the earners of remittances and as workers in demand in the West, but not as crucial deliverers of care in the national health system. Whereas some developing nations have adopted policies to retain health professionals, such as increased salaries, compulsory service requirements and educational benefits, the Indian state has only encouraged emigration.[77] The state has sought to foster the growth of India into a Philippines-style provider of nurses to the global market, allowing overseas health care systems to effectively outsource education to India. In accordance with this policy, the Indian government allowed the development of a formal NHS programme, run from the British High Commission in New Delhi, for the supply of nurses to Britain.[78] The programme for several years conducted marketing, screened applications, provided information, and arranged interviews in person and by video conferencing. As of December 2005, around 1,000 Indian nurses had come to Britain through this channel (although it is now suspended due to funding shortfalls in the NHS).[79] The Indian government also signed an agreement with

---

[77] Commonwealth Secretariat, 'Companion Document to the Commonwealth Code of Practice for the International Recruitment of Health Workers'. London, 2003, p. 9, http://www.thecommonwealth.org/Internal/34044/codes_of_practice/ (accessed 26 July 2006).

[78] NHS Employers, 'International Nursing Recruitment', http://www.nhsemployers. org/workforce/workforce-527.cfm (accessed 24 July 2006).

[79] NHS Employers, 'Indian Nurses Programme: Guidance for Trusts', http://www. nhsemployers.org/workforce/workforce-540.cfm (accessed 24 July 2006).

Britain in 2001, listing India as an ethical nurse provider, with the restriction that recruitment must not occur in Andhra Pradesh, Madhya Pradesh, Orissa, and West Bengal.[80] This was an important step, as it allowed British hospitals to recruit from India directly, a practice forbidden in most African countries. Some state governments have also promoted migration, with Tamil Nadu, for example, establishing a government-run agency to place Tamil nurses overseas. After operating for six months, this agency had 3,000 nurses in its database, had reportedly placed 500 nurses and had received 1,800 expressions of interest from Ireland alone.[81]

The argument for policies to promote nurse migration has some strength. India's nurses possess highly transferable skills and have historically displayed high mobility and adaptability. India has an extensive, longstanding and organised culture of migration and its economy benefits greatly from remittances. The importance of these remittances is not to be underestimated; Non-Resident Indians (NRIs) send home the largest flow of remittances in the world, seven times the size of that sent by Chinese diaspora.[82] The former UN Secretary-General Kofi Annan has pointed to the fact that in most countries remittances significantly exceed both foreign direct investment and international aid flows.[83] The central government has a ministry specifically to administer NRI affairs, which provides support and attempts to systematically harness the earning potential of the diaspora.[84] Goa, Rajasthan, Tamil Nadu, Andhra Pradesh, Uttar Pradesh, Karnataka, Gujarat, and Kerala all have NRI departments.[85] In terms of its nursing personnel, India does not face the crisis-level situation of many African countries, such as Zimbabwe, where in

---

[80] NHS Employers, 'Indian Nurses Programme'.

[81] Vani Doraisamy, 'Global Demand for Trained Indian Nurses Skyrocketing', *The Hindu*, Chennai, 20 September 2005, http://www.hindu.com/2005/09/20/stories/2005092015530500.htm (accessed 10 August 2006).

[82] Naeem Mohaimen, 'The Other NRIs Come to India', *The Subcontinental*, 22 January 2004, available at the India Resource Center website, http://www.indiaresource.org/news/2004/1005.html (accessed 22 August 2006).

[83] Kofi Annan, 'Managing Migration Better', *The Hindu*, 29 January 2004, p. 10.

[84] Website of the Ministry of Overseas Indian Affairs, http://moia.gov.in (accessed 3 August 2006).

[85] 'State Nodal Officers for Matter Related to Overseas Indians', website of the Ministry of Overseas Indian Affairs, http://moia.gov.in/showinfo1.asp?linkid=315 (accessed 3 August 2006).

2001 the number of nurses who registered in the UK was larger than the number that graduated from the country's nursing schools that year, or Ghana, where in 2000 twice as many nurses left the country as had graduated.[86]

At the same time, the position promoted by the government that India has nurses to spare is problematic.[87] The astute observer may immediately question this, given the somewhat ridiculous terms of agreement struck between the Indian government and the British NHS. This agreement is oxymoronic, stipulating that India has a surplus of nurses, except for the four large populous states of Andhra Pradesh, Madhya Pradesh, Odisha, and West Bengal, where there is a shortage. These states together hold over a quarter of India's population, casting doubt on the idea that India can possibly have a 'surplus' of nurses while they suffer shortages. Moreover, the agreement to recruit only from some states seems impossible to enforce. It pretends ignorance of the widely recognised interdependency of national and transnational migration.[88] In the case of nursing, a venture abroad is usually preceded by a stint of work in a major city, often in a different state. Under the agreement, it seems uncertain whether, say, a Bengali nurse in Delhi could be recruited, or a Malayali nurse in Odisha.

The notion of a surplus also contradicts the evidence of nurses on the ground. In New Delhi, an urban centre relatively better supplied with nurses, government hospitals routinely function with nurse–patient ratios of one to 50 or 60, rising to 80 or 90 for the night shift.[89] At Chandigarh's elite PGIMER hospital, considered a prestigious posting by nurses, there was severe understaffing in 2002,

---

[86] Kingma, *Nurses on the Move*, pp. 2, 12–13.

[87] 'India Exporting Nurses to UK and US', *The Guardian*, 23 September 2004, available at the India Resource Center website, http://www.indiaresource.org/news/2004/1037.html (accessed 1 September 2006).

[88] Roy and Arya write that 'transnational and internal migrations cannot be studied independently of one another since both unfold within the larger framework of development practices and economic policies, structures of inequality, and the social and cultural practices that inform them' (Roy and Arya, 'When Poor Women Migrate', p. 27).

[89] Author interview with Mrs G. K. Khurana, AIGNF, 6 February 2006; Author interview with Evelyn Khannan, assistant secretary at the TNAI, 27 January 2006; Author interview with Nanthini Subbiah, deputy secretary general at the TNAI, 27 January 2006.

with a shortage of 140 nurses.[90] Interestingly, a recent article about Kenya described a national health crisis resulting from the exodus of nurses to the West. Hospital wards there were being run on ratios of one nurse to between 40 and 70 patients, slightly higher than the ratio apparently accepted as a sign of surplus in New Delhi.[91]

'Unemployment' of Indian nurses also often stems from state and central governments' failure to fund sufficient nursing positions to staff the nation's hospitals and clinics properly.[92] In some areas, there may indeed be more nurses than there are jobs sanctioned for them, but it is universally acknowledged that not enough jobs are authorised. Kilgour, in his analysis of medical migration, comments that in developing countries the need for doctors is usually far greater than that of developed nations on all measures except for 'effective demand'.[93] That is, although patients urgently need doctors and nurses, faulty planning or scarce resources mean that jobs are not available for them. The willingness of the Indian government to promote the idea that India is a country with too many nurses is thus questionable on many levels, and places profit before the objective of ensuring that the nation's hospitals are functional.

State policies towards nurse migration have also been characterised by a degree of practical disengagement that further reinforces the seeming invisibility of nurses. As Thapan writes of Asian female migrants in general, nurses are 'still not perceived as equal actors worthy of being accounted for'.[94] While willing to sign agreements allowing nurses to leave India, governments at the centre have paid

---

[90] Anonymous, 'Nurses, Technicians join Anti-OPD Chorus', *Chandigarh Tribune Online Edition*, 28 November 2002, http://www.tribuneindia.com/2002/20021129/cth3.htm (accessed 26 July 2006).

[91] Tracy McVeigh, 'Nurse Exodus leaves Kenya in Crisis', *The Observer*, 21 May 2006, http://observer.guardian.co.uk/world/story/0,,1779773,00.html (accessed 15 August 2006).

[92] As John L. Kilgour pointed out in 1971, the absence of 'effective demand' does not mean that demand does not exist, but rather that serious inefficiencies exist in health planning (John L. Kilgour, 'Foreign Medical Graduates in the United Kingdom', in John Z. Bowers and Professor Lord Rosenheim (eds), *Migration of Medical Manpower: Papers from an International Macy Conference*, New York: The Josiah Macy, Jr. Foundation, 1971, p. 7).

[93] Kilgour, 'Foreign Medical Graduates in the United Kingdom', p. 7.

[94] Meenakshi Thapan, 'Series Introduction', in A. Agrawal (ed.), *Migrant Women and Work*, New Delhi/Thousand Oaks/London: Sage Publications, 2006, p. 9.

the most minimal practical attention to emigration. In general, support for it has been a casual and non-specific policy. The 2006 Annual Report of the Ministry of Overseas Indian Affairs, for example, makes one mention of nurses throughout its entire report. Table F in the Annexure section, point 11, lists nurses as among the categories of workers who do not need an emigration check. The remainder of the report, which concerns itself with gender in migration, the exploitation of migrants and trends in migration makes not a single mention of the exodus of nurses.[95] In general, there is a complete absence of data on the numbers of nurses leaving to work abroad, illustrating a lack of serious engagement with its consequences.

In contrast, the extensive migration of doctors since Independence caused ongoing national concern.[96] In 1971, the Indian government, according to P. N. Chhuttani, had an explicit policy of trying to retain its doctors and to encourage the return of those who were abroad. The Council of Scientific and Industrial Research even financed returning doctors' expenses until they found employment and offered loans on attractive terms to assist them in establishing private practices. Chhuttani, who as an experienced leader in the medical profession had participated in various government forums, stated that 'our government's policy is to try its best to remove the causes that generate emigration'.[97] The debate over nurse migration reveals the strange gender blindness of the Indian state, which, in opposition to received wisdom on the subject, saw the mass departure of doctors as a more serious problem than that of nurses. The discourse of

[95] Ministry of Overseas Indian Affairs, 'Annual Report 2006', New Delhi: Government of India, 2006, http://moia.gov.in/showsublinklevel2.asp?sublink2id=187 (accessed 3 August 2006).

[96] The Indian state has dealt with the mass emigration of its doctors virtually since Independence. A conservative estimate in 1971 was that 10,000 out of a stock of just over 100,000 doctors had emigrated. The most highly qualified graduates of the most prestigious schools were the fastest to leave. From the 1960s to the present, approximately half of all graduates of the All India Institute of Medical Sciences (AIIMS), the most prestigious medical school in India, have emigrated (P. N. Chhuttani, 'India', in John Z. Bowers and Professor Lord Rosenheim (eds), *Migration of Medical Manpower: Papers from an International Macy Conference*, New York: The Josiah Macy Jr. Foundation, 1971, p. 17; Phillip L. Martin, *Highly Skilled Labor Migration: Sharing the Benefits*, Geneva: International Institute for Labour Studies, 2003, p. 18, http://www.ilo.org/public/english/bureau/inst/download/migration2.pdf [accessed 3 August 2006]).

[97] Chhuttani, 'India', pp. 18–19.

nursing emigration thus powerfully reveals, as Davies puts it, the devaluation of nursing as gendered labour and the clear difference between 'valued manpower' and 'devalued womanpower'.[98]

Like their colleagues in the central government, Kerala politicians have encouraged migration while showing little concern for the fate of hospitals at home. Government hospitals maintain polices wherein staff nurses are given leave periods of up to five or six years to pursue work abroad. During this time, they are allowed to retain their government job (jobs that, in comparison to private work, are highly sought after). Unfortunately, no one is employed in their place. The result of this is that large numbers of coveted government positions are vacant, waiting for their occupants to return from overseas. At the Thiruvananthapuram Mental Hospital, five staff nurses out of 65 were on long leave in the Gulf, positions which would remain unfilled until they returned or resigned.[99]

The desire of the Indian government to follow the example of the Philippines is itself questionable. The Philippines has a long record of nursing emigration and maintains a worldwide reputation for the education and ability of its nurses, who have found work in numerous Western countries. Ceniza Choy writes that between 1966 and 1985, 25,000 Filipino nurses went to work in the US alone. She recorded in 2003 that Filipino women made up 18 per cent of all nurses in New York City.[100] The Filipino experience, however, emphasises the complex consequences of becoming caught up in the 'global structure of power' and the 'empire of care' that defines the exchange of nurses between the developing and developed world.[101] Understanding nurse emigrants as skilled women taking advantage of their training to find high salaries and good conditions abroad does not capture the whole picture, which also needs to include the cost to the home country of nurse emigration. In recent years, it has seemed the case that the Philippines has been overwhelmed by global demand. Aiken et al. reported in 2004 that 85 per cent of Filipino nurses were working abroad. In 2001, a quarter of all nurses working in Filipino hospitals left the country. As a result, there were 30,000

[98] Davies, *Gender and the Professional Predicament*, p. 79.
[99] Author interview with Mrs Vasantha.
[100] Ceniza Choy, *Empire of Care*, p. 1.
[101] Ibid., p. 2.

vacant nursing positions.[102] The Philippines has found itself in the situation of having an efficient, high quality nurse education system that produces large numbers of nurses, but at the same time is suffering severe nursing shortages and worsening hospital conditions. The Indian government's explicit pursuit of a model based on the Philippines casts further doubt on its regard for nursing.

## The big business of nurse emigration and its consequences

The transformation of nursing has brought with it the growth of a nexus of business interests capitalising on both Western hospitals' need for staff and the new enthusiasm of Indian students for nursing careers. The unrestrained and under-regulated rush to profit from this new trade in nurses has had a profound impact on the quality of nurse education and casts further doubt on emigration as the source of better professional status.

The recruitment of Indian nurses is an increasingly profitable venture. Small agencies, minor private hospitals, Christian hospitals, large agencies, and governments all make money from sending nurses out of the country. Across India, young women and increasingly also men, visit agencies that improve their English, help them to cram on aspects of American nursing and adjust their accents, bearing and dress along Western lines.[103] As Brush and Vasupuram comment: 'Women are increasingly produced as export products and, with the help of recruitment agencies, processed as products that meet the cultural expectations of competing market buyers'.[104]

In Kerala, a college lecturer informed me, every coconut palm boasts an advertisement for CGFNS coaching. Manjoorams, a coaching college for prospective nurse emigrants with 10 branches in Kerala and Karnataka, is typical of such businesses. It charges ₹6,000 for a two-month preparation course for the CGFNS and ₹5,000 to prepare for the less difficult IELTS. The company has expanded rapidly and frequently conducts business with agents from the UK and US. It has recently established a long-distance arm that

[102] Aiken et al., 'Trends in International Nurse Migration', pp. 69–77.
[103] Beary, 'Indian Nurses' American Dream'.
[104] Brush and Vasupuram, 'Nurses, Nannies and Caring Work'.

allows nurses to take its courses while working in the Gulf.[105] New Delhi, Bangalore, Mumbai, and Chennai and the towns of Kerala host hundreds of similar coaching colleges and nurse recruitment agencies, as well as frequent visiting contingents of overseas recruiters. Dr Mark McKenney of Nurses for International Cooperative Exchange (NICE), a US-based recruitment organisation, stated that in January 2005, his organisation was placing 200 nurses in the US, and anticipated an escalation in business as shortages became more severe.[106] Some Western companies have gone further than merely recruiting already trained nurses. Blue Cross Healthcare UK has set up a programme to train specialist mental health nurses for work in the UK. Sponsoring hospitals pay for all training costs in return for a three-year commitment from candidates.[107]

Indian hospitals also negotiate deals with Western employment agencies and hospitals to host their recruitment drives, allowing agents to conduct seminars and information sessions and then fund the chosen candidates' CGFNS or IELTS examination costs. In 2003, for example, Narayana Hrudayalaya, a specialist heart care hospital in Bangalore, was negotiating with British Columbia Institute of Technology in Canada to train Indian nurses for work in Canada.[108] The well-known Indian private health care business, Apollo Health Resources, advertises the provision of free board and lodging at its Kottayam training centre for prospective migrants, which also supplies free training, funds the exam fee for the CGFNS and teaches 'soft skills' in American culture.[109] In his analysis of nurse migration, Binod Khadria describes these entrepreneurial hospitals and agencies as engaging in 'business process outsourcing' (BPO). He found that an Indian hospital investing between US$4,700–7,000 into the training of a nurse could expect a profit of up to US$47,000 once she or he was placed abroad through one of these international

---

[105] Author interview with Ms Bella Mary Jacob, 30 November 2005, Manjooram's Group of Institutes, Thiruvananthapuram office.

[106] Nurses go West', *Times of India*, 19 January 2005, City Supplement, Bombay, http://timesofindia.indiatimes.com/articleshow/995616.cms (accessed 15 January 2005).

[107] Helene Mulholland, 'Plan to Train Indian Nurses as RMNs then bring them to UK', *Nursing Times*, vol. 99, no. 25, p. 4.

[108] Beary, 'Indian Nurses' American Dream'.

[109] Advertisement on the Kerala Nurse website, http://www.keralanurse.com/modules/news/article.php?.storyid=38 (accessed 13 December 2006).

partnerships.[110] Hospitals thus facilitate and profit from the exodus of their own nursing staff. The growth of this large and complex business, unaccompanied by effective policy measures to guard the nation's stock of nurses, seems nothing less than the reckless commodification of care. Short-term profits are pursued vigorously while long-term consequences are rarely considered.

Sizeable profits have also gone to investors in nursing education, who have capitalised on the enormous rush of enthusiastic potential emigrants into nursing. As occurred in the Philippines, nursing schools have become a fail-safe means for hospital owners to make large profits, by charging very high fees to students.[111] Almost all of the private nursing schools in Kerala have opened in the last four to five years, as hospitals have rushed to take advantage of the low level of investment and high returns available in nurse education. For many of the large number of new private hospitals in Kerala, the nursing school in fact provides the major source of income.

These fast profits stem from the enormous and rising enthusiasm of Kerala students for nursing as a route to emigration. In Kerala, the private nursing school principals I interviewed all estimated that between 80 and 100 per cent of their students plan to emigrate. Thankamma Cherian, for example, told me that 95 per cent of her students plan to leave India. She qualified this, however:

> The thing is, family planning, is very forcefully conducted in Kerala. So we have only two children, or one. So we are not ready for them to go abroad, because [there would be] nobody to look after us . . . otherwise a hundred percent would like to!'.[112]

A. Joykutty, the principal of the prestigious LT School of Nursing at SNDT University in Mumbai, stated in a 2005 interview for *The Times of India* that there was an 'exodus of nurses' to foreign countries and that on average over 80 per cent of her student body applied for visas to work abroad.[113]

---

[110] Khadria, 'International Nurse Recruitment', pp. 5–6.
[111] Kingma, *Nurses on the Move*, pp. 84–85.
[112] Author interview.
[113] 'Nurses go West', *Times of India*, 19 January 2005, City Supplement, Bombay, http://timesofindia.indiatimes.com/articleshow/995616.cms (accessed 15 January 2005).

This new enthusiasm for nursing education has put flashing dollar signs into the eyes of politicians, doctors and businessmen, and India has consequently witnessed the fast and uncontrolled growth of nursing education and a fall in standards. Figure 6.1 illustrates the rapid expansion in numbers of schools and colleges of nursing, and Figure 6.2 shows the very fast move to private sector provision. Statistics on the relative role of the state, the Christian churches and the private sector in 2005 are an approximation, but the picture of a uniquely fast expansion in private sector education is accurate.[114] As opportunities for nurse emigration have risen, the private sector

**Figure 6.1:** Growth of Nursing Schools and Colleges, 1970–2005

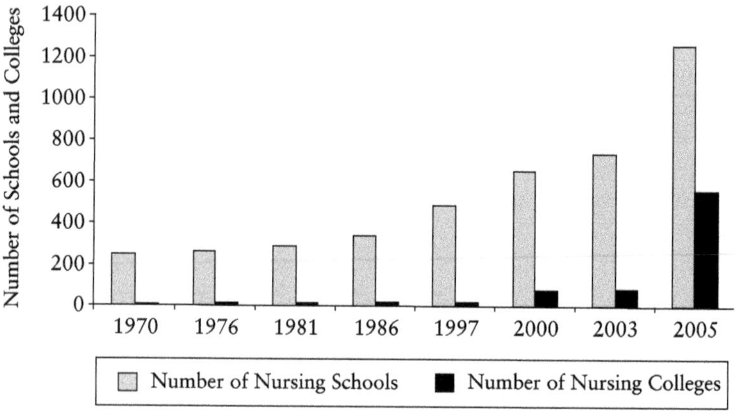

*Source:* Indian Nursing Council, 'List of Schools of Nursing Recognised and Permitted to Admit Students for the Academic Year 2005–2006'; Indian Nursing Council, 'List of Colleges of Nursing for Basic B.Sc (N) Programme who are Permitted to Admit Students for the Academic Year 2005–2006'; CAHP, 'Report of a Nursing Survey in India', 1974.

---

[114] I have based figures for 2005 on the INC's lists of its schools and colleges in 2005, which required judging which sector the institution belonged to purely using its name. It is likely that this will have underestimated the number of church- or government-run institutions. I think the extent of the error is likely to be fairly small, however, as the names are in general quite clear (government schools usually include this status in their name and Christian schools very often take the name of a saint, the word Christian, or have missionary origins that are easily recognised), and the figures tend to tally with observers' comments on the very fast expansion of the private sector in relation to the state sector (Indian Nursing Council, 'List of Schools of Nursing Recognised and Permitted to Admit Students for the Academic

**Figure 6.2:** Sectoral Share of Nursing School Education, 1970 and 2005

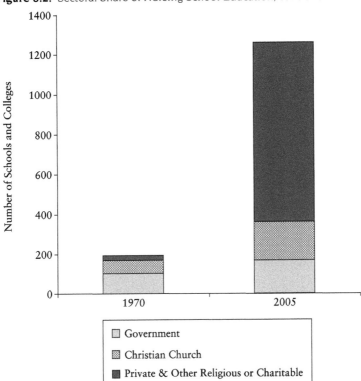

*Source:* Indian Nursing Council, 'List of Schools of Nursing Recognised and Permitted to Admit Students for the Academic Year 2005–2006'; Indian Nursing Council, 'List of Colleges of Nursing for Basic B.Sc (N) Programme who are Permitted to Admit Students for the Academic Year 2005–2006'; CAHP, 'Report of a Nursing Survey in India', 1974.

in nursing education has expanded incredibly quickly and the result has been a total transformation in the pattern of nurse education provision.

A 2003 report for the International Labour Organization (ILO) lauded the fact that 'the private sector in India and the Philippines

---

Year 2005–2006', New Delhi, 2005; Indian Nursing Council, 'List of Colleges of Nursing for Basic B.Sc (N) Programme who are Permitted to Admit Students for the Academic Year 2005–2006', New Delhi, 2005.

**Table 6.3:** State-wise Distribution of Nursing Schools and Colleges in India (by Share of Nursing Schools in Descending Order)

| State | Population (Percentage of Indian Population) | Number and Percentage of Nursing Schools | Number and Percentage of Nursing Colleges |
|---|---|---|---|
| Karnataka | 5.1 | 381 (30.3) | 233 (41.8) |
| Andhra Pradesh | 7.4 | 177 (14.1) | 108 (19.4) |
| Kerala | 3.1 | 128 (10.2) | 59 (10.6) |
| Tamil Nadu | 6.1 | 97 (7.7) | 49 (8.8) |
| Punjab | 2.4 | 89 (7.1) | 18 (3.2) |
| Maharashtra | 9.4 | 67 (5.3) | 22 (3.9) |
| Rajasthan | 5.5 | 64 (5.0) | 4 (0.7) |
| Uttar Pradesh | 16.2 | 45 (3.6) | 6 (1.1) |
| West Bengal | 7.8 | 37 (2.9) | 5 (0.9) |
| Madhya Pradesh | 5.9 | 23 (1.8) | 22 (3.9) |
| Odisha | 3.6 | 20 (1.6) | 8 (1.4) |
| Bihar | 8.1 | 10 (0.8) | 0 |
| Himachal Pradesh | <1 | 5 (0.4) | 0 |
| Jammu & Kashmir | <1 | 2 (0.2) | 0 |
| Chandigarh | <1 | 0 | 1 (0.2) |
| Uttarakhand | <1 | 0 | 2 (0.4) |
| Haryana | 2.1 | 24 (4.3) | 2 (0.4) |
| North-eastern states (except for Assam)* | 1.2 | 21 (1.7) | 3 (0.5) |
| Delhi | 1.3 | 17 (1.4) | 5 (0.9) |
| Assam | 2.6 | 11 (0.9) | 1 (0.2) |
| Jharkhand | 2.6 | 7 (0.6) | 0 |
| Chhattisgarh | 2 | 2 (0.2) | 9 (1.6) |
| Andaman & Nicobar Islands | <1 | 1 (0.8) | 0 |

*Source:* Census of India 2001; Indian Nursing Council, *List of Schools of Nursing Recognised and Permitted to Admit Students for the Academic Year 2005–2006*; Indian Nursing Council, *List of Colleges of Nursing for Basic B.Sc (N) programme who are Permitted to Admit Students for the Academic Year 2005–2006.*

*Note:* The figures in parentheses indicate the percentage of nursing schools.

*Sikkim, Arunachal Pradesh, Nagaland, Manipur, Mizoram, Tripura, and Meghalaya.

has quickly added the capacity to train IT workers and nurses for jobs abroad, including developing the financial infrastructure that can assess potential returns and make loans to students'.[115] This is a rosy view of the situation in India, which is belied by an increasingly troubling reality. Aiken et al. provide a more nuanced analysis of the challenge of expanding nurse education to meet the needs of a Western market:

> A number of less developed countries, such as India, China and some of the Newly Independent States of the former Soviet Union (NIS) aspire to train nurses for export following the Philippine example. That model is based mainly on the provision of private-sector education. Countries considering the development of nurses for export face challenges because of limited access to capital to build an appropriate nursing education infrastructure that meets Western standards and by the emigration of nurse faculty and leaders to developed countries.[116]

As this analysis suggests, the expansion in educational facilities has been at the expense of good quality education, and it has occurred at the same time as the number of teaching staff has drastically declined. As Table 6.3 shows, the increase in nursing schools and colleges is concentrated in Kerala, Karnataka and Andhra Pradesh, while the poorest states, such as Bihar, Odisha and Uttar Pradesh, have profited little. This table shows only the schools approved by the INC. In reality the state of Karnataka, in particular, has hosted hundreds of more new schools than these statistics show. In August 2006, a government taskforce reported that Karnataka had an astonishing 843 nursing schools or colleges operating, some with INC approval but many without. It was found that 63 per cent of these lacked appropriate resources, such as teachers and classroom equipment.[117] The development journalist, P. Sainath, found that numerous colleges in Kerala and Karnataka provide a substandard nursing education. Many, he discovered, are not attached to teaching hospitals and

---

[115] Martin, 'Highly Skilled Labor Migration', p. 28 (footnotes).

[116] Aiken et al., 'Trends in International Nurse Migration', pp. 69–77.

[117] 'Steps to Close Down Unapproved Nursing Institutes in Karnataka', *Kerala Kaumudi*, 2 August 2006, p. 7.

charge extortionate tuition fees.[118] Satish Chawla, former TNAI president, commented that the 'mushrooming of nursing colleges is harming the nursing profession' and that it was sad to note that as a result of rapid expansion, 'hundreds of students who did not even know how to pick a vein, had been certified as qualified to take up the profession'.[119] According to Bella Mary Jacob, who works as a head tutor at Manjoorams, the most common cause of failure in the CGFNS examination for the US is not poor English, but poor clinical knowledge. Manjoorams did not just hothouse its students on grammar and spoken English, it also helped them to cram the nursing knowledge that their schools had not provided.[120]

Politicians, businessmen and hospital administrators have in many cases made shady profits from the expansion of nursing education, which has brought with it increasing levels of corruption. Efforts to close down the hundreds of substandard nursing schools in Karnataka stumbled against the obstacle that a large proportion were owned by powerful politicians, including the state's deputy chief minister B. S. Yadiyoorappa.[121] The school principals I interviewed all referred to the common practice of auctioning nursing school places in government-aided private schools to the highest bidder, under the government-sanctioned 'management quota' (which allows a percentage of each intake to be admitted other than by merit). 'Donations' and influential connections guaranteed places for students, who could then be continually asked for further fees throughout their schooling.

The increasing fees charged to students, as well as confidence in the large salaries available abroad, has meant that students now take big loans to fund their nursing education. A post-state-election debate screened in May 2006 on Doordarshan, Thiruvananthapuram, the Indian government's television station, raised the issue of loans to

---

[118] P. Sainath, 'Commerce and Crisis hit Wayanad Students', *The Hindu*, 30 January 2005, India Together website, http://www.indiatogether.org/2005/jan/psa-student. htm (accessed 4 June 2005).

[119] Anonymous, 'Nurses who don't even know how to Pick a Vein', *The Hindu*, 15 October 2004, http://www.hindu.com/2004/10/15/stories/2004101514410300. htm (accessed 3 August 2006).

[120] Author interview with Bella Mary Jacob.

[121] Anonymous, 'Steps to Close Down Unapproved Nursing Institutes in Karnataka', p. 7.

nursing students, who in Kerala often come from lower-income families. It suggested that it is now common for nurses to take out loans requiring repayments of ₹20,000 per month, which will only be possible on an overseas salary. A farmer interviewed predicted that, if assistance is not provided in the next few years, there would be a spate of nurse suicides similar to the mass farmer suicides in Karnataka and Kerala that have attracted worldwide attention. In the three weeks leading up to the debate, two Malayali nursing students had already committed suicide, both motivated by financial difficulties.[122]

When asked whether she encouraged or discouraged her students to leave India for work, one Thiruvananthapuram principal of a private school of nursing told me, 'I don't tell them anything. Because, even if they think it is bad, they have no option because their life situation requires this'.[123] For many of the new brand of nursing students, their 'life situation' includes a large-scale, stressful financial investment entirely dependent on them finding a means to leave India. Intensive Western recruitment can bring with it an accompanying set of pressures, such as these higher debt levels for students, meaning nurses end up with no option other than entering the global market.[124] Kingma asks:

> Is migration a matter of choice or is it imposed on nurses as an obligation or a constraint? For many nurses, migration may seem to be a matter of free will. Yet, when we delve deeply, we see that social and economic conditions in their homelands may practically oblige them to abandon their homes and families to find employment abroad.[125]

Meanwhile, even in the best schools and colleges of nursing, students' educational experience is declining in quality due to the rush of qualified teachers abroad. The 2002 introduction to the INC's *Guide for Schools of Nursing in India* acknowledges that 'due to shortage of trained nursing faculty and other reasons, nurses may enter

---

[122] Post-election Debate, screened on Doordarshan Thiruvananthapuram, 11 May 2006.
[123] Author interview with Sister Sylvia, principal of the Little Flower School of Nursing, Jubilee Hospital, Thiruvananthapuram, 25 November 2005.
[124] Kingma, *Nurses on the Move*, p. 3.
[125] Ibid., p. 5.

teaching careers without attaining the laid down requirements'.[126] In Kerala, the centre of nurse emigration in India, Chandrakanthi told me that the nurse education system faced 'acute shortages of postgraduate qualified nurses' and that as a result there was a severe lack of qualified faculty throughout the state.[127]

In a group interview, students of the Thiruvananthapuram College of Nursing's MSc course told me that they had taught themselves the entire syllabus of their course, each student preparing handouts and a presentation for a given topic.[128] At the end of the course, they hired and paid their own examiner. Sister Sylvia, principal of the Little Flower School of Nursing in Trivandrum, had recently had four of her teachers depart simultaneously to work abroad, leaving her and her vice-principal to teach all four batches of 20 students. This meant that until final examinations finished at the local college of nursing and new graduates could be recruited as teachers, the students spent much of their day 'simply sitting'.[129]

Increasingly, recruitment efforts from countries such as Ireland target nurses with specialist skills and postgraduate qualifications in maternity nursing, paediatric nursing and psychiatric nursing, which means that important expertise is lost from the education system.[130] At Jose's college, only 5 out of 19 teachers had the qualifications mandated by the INC for teaching BSc (nursing). Jose commented that 'as seniors, we are dealing with important subjects, and we are delegating the other subjects to junior teachers. We are not happy about that. Still we can't help it'. As well as draining away current nurses with qualifications adequate for teaching, mass emigration opportunities are also jeopardising the future supply. Jose finds little interest in her students for the postgraduate qualifications that she herself pursued with enthusiasm. Instead, most of the students 'just want to finish their course and go abroad and earn money'.[131]

---

[126] S. A. Samuel, 'Introduction', in *Guide for School of Nursing in India*, New Delhi: Indian Nursing Council, 2002.

[127] Author interview with C. Chandrakanthi.

[128] Author interview with MSc (nursing) students at the college of nursing, Medical College Hospital, Thiruvananthapuram, January 2005.

[129] Author interview with Sr Sylvia.

[130] Author interview, Ernakulam, 5 December 2005.

[131] Author interview with A. Nirmal Jose.

Principals in Kerala were anxious about the quality and motivation of students entering nursing in the current climate, expressing a concern that many students now had little real interest in nursing. Sulochana Bai, principal of the Sree Uthradom Thirunal Hospital School of Nursing in Thiruvananthapuram, felt that among her generation of nurses there had been 'a 100 per cent service mentality', whereas now nursing was 'just like another job opening' and 'service mentality is only 50 per cent'.[132] Similarly, Jolly Jacob, the principal of Lords School of Nursing, said of her students that 'to mould them is really quite difficult nowadays', and that the commitment to care had declined considerably. She felt that nowadays 'I, my, myself, that is the attitude'.[133] Sister Sylvia, struggling with heavily indebted students and a critical lack of staff, was also somewhat despondent over the changing orientation of those entering nursing:

> The difference is, in the past, students used to join mostly motivated by service mentality, service. Dedication, commitment. And they used to be very dedicated also. Hardworking. More study. They would study spontaneously, not need of much pushing. But now, totally different. Now they join, not with much dedication, service mentality, but [only wishing that] they should leave to get a job and to go abroad. Secondly, regarding their training, they are not interested to study much. They want to get a degree, but their study is the difference. They don't like to study.[134]

Jose (a much younger woman than the others and therefore without the same generational distance from her students) similarly felt that contemporary nursing students, stimulated by opportunities abroad, rushed into the course 'without knowing the cause or the difficulties they face' and were too often pushed by their families. Her students, she felt, were largely motivated by job opportunities; an interest in caring work had not usually figured in their decision to become nurses. These new students often did well with classroom work, but when it came to clinical practice, she had noticed that 'some irritation is there, hesitation is there'. On average, she felt that only 5 out of the 50 students in each batch had come with a genuine interest in nursing and without family pressure to take nursing as a route out

---

[132] Author interview with Sulochana Bai.
[133] Author interview with Jolly Jacob, Thiruvananthapuram, 1 December 2005.
[134] Author interview with Sr Sylvia.

of India.[135] Sulochana Bai told me that sought-after places at government schools and colleges attracted students with science scores of around 80 per cent, but her private school accepted students with scores of around 50 to 53 per cent. Out of an average batch of 40 students, she felt that 10 were good students, 10 were average, and 20 were not good at all. In government schools, she felt, students were 'able to catch the subject', whereas in her school, 'we have to teach them, force them, help them, encourage them, generally they will be able to complete the course'.[136]

It was clear that all the nursing principals with whom I spoke, with the exception of the entrepreneurial Chandrakanthi, felt some ambivalence about the overwhelming desire among their students to emigrate, an unsurprising fact given the stretched, strained context in which they had to work. They had no option but to watch their students participate in coaching for visa examinations, and were not in any position to influence the links that hospital management established with agencies and overseas partners. They did, however, deny encouraging their students to leave. As Sulochana Bai succinctly told me when I asked her what the school's attitude to emigration was, 'I am not putting any interest and we are not taking any interest. They make their own interest'.[137]

The effects of the emigration business are not limited to education. The increasing mobility of nurses means an increasingly transitory workforce. In Kerala, hospitals have adapted to a mode of functioning in which the great majority of nursing staff are transitory. Nurses work one or two years in order to get the necessary experience and then apply to go abroad, meaning a constant staff turnover. At Lisie Hospital, Jose commented that apart from a small number of religious sisters and some specialist nurses on the cardio-thoracic ward and in the dialysis unit, 'they don't have permanent nurses', as most nurses 'stay for one, or two, maximum two years, and by that time they'll get one opportunity in Gulf country or any other country and they'll go'. Local hospitals come to function merely as the source of clinical experience needed to get work abroad. As Kingma points out, 'continuity of care, a needed dimension of health services to the population, is put at risk when a critical mass of personnel is

---

[135] Author interview with A. Nirmal Jose.
[136] Author interview with Sulochana Bai.
[137] Author interview with Sulochana Bai.

undergoing constant turnover'. Lesley Mackay describes the constant reliance on a staff composed almost entirely of young graduates as 'the disposable workforce ethos — use once and throw away'.[138] The new reliance on a transient workforce may thus reinforce the existing tendency of the state to devalue the work of nurses, as well as reducing the standard of care received by patients.

Under such conditions — with increasingly poorly educated graduates, students taking on burdensome loans that remove the element of choice from migration, a crisis-level teaching shortage and a very high staff turnover in Indian hospitals — the claim that emigration is raising nursing's status must be qualified. In fact, the unregulated and unchecked expansion of nursing schools and the failure to devote policy attention to the educational crisis suggests the continuing low status of the nursing profession in health politics. The state is willing to allow numerous interests to profit from nurses' popularity abroad, but unwilling to address the growing strain on its hospitals.

## The absence of a professional voice

It is perhaps the case that in the long-term the profession will be empowered by emigration, as levels of confidence rise and the social experience of nurses improves. Evelyn Khannan, for example, felt that Indian nurses were already less submissive and more willing 'to raise their voices and fight' due to the new opportunities to emigrate.[139] Several of the principals I interviewed said that students were becoming more assertive and demanding. At the same time, the voicelessness and marginalisation of organised nursing in the emigration debate is pronounced. The INC and the state nursing councils have always been relatively weak regulatory bodies, with little support from the state in their attempts to standardise education and to enforce minimum standards for new schools to meet. In the face of the profiteering hospitals and business interests that have accompanied the new opportunities for emigration, they have been sidelined as never before. In Karnataka, for example, despite appointing a taskforce to report on uncontrolled expansion in nursing schools, the government declared its intention to continue the

---

[138] Quoted in Davies, *Gender and the Professional Predicament*, p. 81.
[139] Author interview with Evelyn Khannan.

practice of allowing them to disregard INC minimum standards.[140] It is quite clear that, as occurred with the enormous expansion of medical colleges during the 1970s, the state is pursuing the political and financial advantages of unregulated expansion, and ignoring the professional regulator.[141]

Professional organisations have made only the most minimal contribution to the public debate on nurse emigration. The TNAI has preserved an almost complete silence on the issue, with not a single article in its journal addressing migration until 2006. In July 2006, an article was published by Simmy M. Varkey, a lecturer from Kottayam, a large Kerala town whence many emigrants have come. Varkey pointed out some of the negative experiences of Indian nurses abroad, but her general point was that the government was doing too little 'to raise the standard of nursing to international levels'. She urged the immediate implementation of policies to 'raise the competitive edge of our nurses' and advised the restructuring of education 'to cater to the needs of receiving society (for example, more geriatric hours in syllabus)'.[142] This seemed an interesting starting point for a broader debate, but as yet the TNAI has not promoted any extensive debate on emigration and its consequences for local nurses. International meetings on the issue of migration have not included Indian nursing representation and researchers writing on this issue have rarely been able to find a professional voice from India.

The TNAI officials I interviewed recognised that there would be negative consequences for Indian health and that the state was not adequately addressing these, but seemed to feel paralysed by the enthusiasm of nurses for opportunities abroad. With the competing imperatives of a strong organisational narrative of national service and a constituency clamouring to work abroad, the preservation of a dignified silence had emerged as the preferred option. The one

---

[140] 'Steps to Close Down Unapproved Nursing Institutes in Karnataka', p. 7.

[141] Jeffery describes the unchecked growth of medical colleges during the 1970s and the protests voiced by the Indian Medical Council (IMC) and the Indian Medical Association (IMA). Declining standards in Indian medical schools was the official explanation for controversial de-recognition of Indian medical degrees in Britain in 1975 (Jeffery, 'Allopathic Medicine in India', p. 569).

[142] Simmy M. Varkey, 'Immigration of Nurses: Problems, Prospects and Challenges', *NJI*, vol. 97, no. 7, 2006, p. 258.

active step taken by the organisation was the removal in 2005 of a ban on emigration-related advertising in the *NJI*. Leaders explained to me that there was no point in keeping up the ban, when it was manifestly clear that the government was going to take no action to address the 'push factors' underlying migration.[143] Yet this was not a position that was publicised, and in general, nursing organisations are not advocating the protection of nurses and nursing in the context of rapidly increasing migration.

In comparison, professional bodies elsewhere have been vocal on the issue and have expressed a range of positions on nurse migration. For example, the Democratic Nursing Organization of South Africa in 1997 publicly criticised Nelson Mandela for his successful advocacy of a ban in the UK on the direct recruitment of South African nurses, pointing to the hypocrisy of a ban that restricted the opportunities of nurses while the free migration of doctors was allowed and South Africa itself continued to recruit doctors and nurses from its poorer neighbours.[144] In host countries, the exploitation of IRNs has been an ongoing concern. The RCN in Britain has produced a series of publications strongly geared towards protecting the rights of the IRNs, especially their right to equal treatment and access to professional development.[145] British nursing organisations have condemned the unethical practices of migration agencies. In both Australia and Ireland, nursing unions have vocally defended the rights of IRNs.[146] The comparative voicelessness of organised nursing in India suggests the lower status of nurses there. In India, those in power who have debated the desirability of nurse emigration have generally done so without input from the nursing leadership.

---

[143] Author interviews, TNAI, New Delhi, 27 January 2006.

[144] Kingma, *Nurses on the Move*, p.127.

[145] See for example, RCN, 'Internationally Recruited Nurses: Good practice Guidance'; RCN, 'Success with Internationally Recruited Nurses', p. 7; J. Buchan, 'International Recruitment of Nurses: United Kingdom Case Study', London: RCN, 2002, http://www.rcn.org.uk/publications/pdf/irn-case-study-booklet.pdf (accessed 22 May 2006); J. Buchan, 'Here to Stay? International Nurses in the UK', London: RCN, 2003, http://www.rcn.org.uk/publications/pdf/heretostay-irns.pdf (accessed 20 July 2006); Beverly Malone, 'Government Targeting of Overseas Nurses Beggars Belief, says RCN', 3 July 2006, http://www.rcn.org.uk/news/mediadisplay.php?ID=2067&area=Press (accessed 20 July 2006).

[146] Julia Limb, 'Foreign Nurses Exploited, Union says', 19 October 2005, The World Today, ABC Radio, http://www.abc.net.au/worldtoday/content/2005/s1485986.htm

# Emigration and the Media

Emigration has brought nurses into the public eye to an unprecedented extent. 'Rags to riches' narratives of nurses seeking their fortunes abroad have proved popular with journalists, and so, for the first time in history, India has seen regular and positive reporting of nursing. Media coverage, however, often reinforces and uncritically accepts the dichotomy between individual nurse status and the troubled position of the profession as a whole. Most media reports celebrate the achievements of nurses in winning visas to emigrate, but fail to consider their importance to the national health system. Coverage of nurse emigration has an overwhelmingly individualised focus, with rosy accounts of determined and courageous individual nurses with the gumption and skill to escape the trials of the Indian health system. A 2004 article in *The Hindu*, 'The Main Attraction: Hefty Salaries', typifies this. For the article, Joy Das and Moumita Ghosh interviewed a group of nurses extensively about their motivations for leaving India. They documented their enthusiasm for high salaries and excellent conditions and their frustration with the Indian system, but drew no conclusions from this about the importance of nurse departures for Indian health.[147] Another article from *The Hindu* in 2003 described a typical émigré in similarly enthusiastic and optimistic terms:

> Cynthia Kennedy is a nurse who has 'always loved challenges in life'. 'Before I went to Saudi Arabia, there were many people who asked me not to go there'. And she ignored them . . . Cynthia is not alone. Many more like her are queuing up at Bangalore's agencies that have begun recruiting nurses for the West. They are encouraged by fat pay packets there and discouraged, among other things, by a lack of respect for the profession here.[148]

---

(accessed 26 July 2006); Mary Henry, quoted in Anthony Garvey, 'Counting the Costs: The Irish Government is under Fire after a Recent Tragedy Revealed the Extent of the Funding Crisis in the Country's Nursing Services', *Nursing Standard*, vol. 17, no. 46, 2003, p. 12.

[147] Das and Ghosh, 'The Main Attraction: Hefty Salaries'.

[148] D. Dasgupta, 'Nursing High Hopes', *The Hindu*, 31 July 2003, http://www.thehindu.com/thehindu/mp/2003/07/31/stories/2003073100250100.htm (accessed 15 November 2004).

News coverage often points to some of the issues that make nursing in India an unrewarding career, which may be of value in drawing public attention to the profession's problems, but at the same time exhibits a fatalistic acceptance of the status quo. Many journalists dwell on the good luck of nurses in getting a chance to escape mistreatment at home; only a few argue for reform or suggest that individual good fortune might, in the bigger picture, translate into patient suffering. The position adopted by *The Times of India* article is typical: 'often treated shabbily by both patients and employers, the nursing community could not have hoped for a better bonanza . . . Nursing aspirants should grab the carrot being offered by the US with both hands'.[149] The US-based Center for Nursing Advocacy, which was established to monitor the world media's representation of nurses and nursing, comments on a *The Times of India* article typical of journalists' heady, unqualified enthusiasm for nurse migration:

> It fails to address the likely effects of this trend on Indian health, instead comparing it to the superficially similar trend in the migration of IT professionals — a trend that we do not believe is the result of a life-threatening shortage in developed nations, nor a cause of such a shortage in the developing nations from which they recruit.[150]

The tendency of the media to ignore the ramifications of nurse migration is lamentable and also rather hypocritical, given that these same newspapers also publish critical accounts of a hospital system troubled by understaffing and poor quality nursing that is certainly related to migration.[151] The claim that emigration has caused a major shift in the status of nursing in the public eye therefore requires qualification. The media presents feel-good stories about migrants, but at the same time replicates and reinforces the general lack of comprehension of the importance of nursing in the health system.

---

[149] Anonymous, 'Nursing Dreams: Medical Caregivers to get U.S. Green Card within one Year', *Times of India*, 19 July 2005, p. 24.

[150] The Center for Nursing Advocacy, 'Go West, Young Nurse?', http://www.nursing advocacy.org/news/2005jan/19_times_india.html (accessed 26 July 2006).

[151] See, for example, Rai, 'Forging a Bond in a Government Hospital'; and Purba Kalita, 'Nursing System in Poor Health', *Times of India*, 9 September 2003, http://timesofindia.indiatimes.com/cms.dll/html/uncomp/articleshow?msid=174084 (accessed 3 March 2004).

# Conclusions

Nurse emigration has captured the imagination of Indian media and society. It has done great things for the social experience of the average nurse, who is now popular on the marriage market and recognised as a professional in global demand. In many ways, however, hailing migration as a historic victory in the battle to improve nursing's status in India is problematic. It may now be far less embarrassing for nurses to inform a group of in-laws or strangers of their occupation, but they must continue to turn up for work in an underpaid job in dangerous conditions. Media coverage of migrants lauds the courage of individuals embarking on new lives abroad and sometimes even recognises the dire conditions for nurses at home, but rarely draws attention to the domestic consequences of India becoming a nurse exporter or advocates reform in the local health system. Meanwhile, at home, a crisis in education continues to unfold, with the large-scale production of heavily indebted, under-skilled nurses. India's development as a nurse exporter has also been peculiarly noteworthy for the absence of a professional voice in debates over the issue.

Restricting the freedom of nurses to emigrate does not seem a desirable solution. As Thapan writes, state efforts to restrict women's migration tend to 'strengthen and perpetuate the exploitation and abuse of women', rendering them more vulnerable to agencies and middlemen.[152] Nor is it even the case that, were emigration halted tomorrow, India's public health problems would be solved. It is unlikely that the droves of new nurses attracted to the profession by emigration would, in this scenario, flock to work in the rural primary health centres where shortages are most pressing. At the same time, the contours of the issue as described in this book show that it is complex, and that the ramifications of becoming a large-scale supplier of nurses to the West are unpredictable. Already, standards of care in many hospitals are likely to be slipping, as poorly prepared nurses graduate from under-resourced schools, and staff turnover rises in many parts of the country. A transient, highly mobile, increasingly urbanised nursing workforce brings many problems. There is a need to search for policy solutions to address the mounting crisis in nursing education and somehow to address the consequences of emigration

---

[152] Thapan, 'Series Introduction', p. 16.

for staffing patterns. It is, of course, no surprise that this has not occurred. This reflects the contention throughout this book that the state has failed thus far to recognise the need for women's caring work in its health system. The modern, globalising Indian state sees nurses as remitters, society is starting to see them as high-earners with access to the West, but none of this is sufficiently informed by their status as essential carers, whose loss will cause pain and suffering in the nation's hospitals.

# Conclusion
## The Four Feet upon
## which a Cure must Rest

◘

A major fault line that runs through narrations of history and their
knowledge base — whether it is political, economic or social history
. . . is the failure to take note of, to understand and respect and absorb
women's ideational and intellectual skills and outputs in the area of
theoretical and analytical knowledge . . . recognition of the intellectual
and leadership powers of woman has remained in the ghettos. The
minds of men have not changed.

— Devaki Jain, 2005[1]

For over a century, nurses in India have been viewed as incapable
and unworthy of authority and responsibility by those in power,
reflecting Devaki Jain's contention that 'the minds of men have not
changed'. A patriarchal state has consistently refused the possibility
and desirability of a strong nursing leadership and in doing so, it has
rendered nursing an often unstimulating and dangerous occupation.
This book contends that the state has never shown any practical
understanding of the role of the nurse in modern medicine. The place
of the nurse as the custodian of the hospital ward, the administrator
of medication, the leader in patient care, and the public health supervisor has been enshrined in words, but stymied in practice. This has
created a destructive cycle. Nurses have not wielded authority, have
not had opportunities to prove themselves worthy or to develop bases
of strength, and so policymakers' assumption that they are irrelevant
to health planning has emerged as the depressing reality. The system
limps along with a scarce, a disempowered and an oppressed nursing

---

[1] Jain, *Women, Development and the UN*, pp. 164–65.

staff, or in the case of public health, almost without any nursing staff at all, and this is accepted as the status quo.

The roots of this situation were in the orientation of the colonial state towards nursing. As distinct from the Philippines and Japan during this period, the Indian state was content to leave the development of nursing to the missions.[2] By and large it fatalistically accepted that Indian society could not come to terms with nursing as an occupation for its women, and throughout the period relied on the easy but unsustainable policy of recruiting Anglo-Indian and domiciled European women, as well as a large corps of untrained or minimally trained male servants. The lack of involvement of the state meant that, in contrast to Britain, the US, Japan, and Philippines, nursing was never reshaped as a patriotic career which middle and lower middle class girls might proudly enter.

Without the missions, there would have been even fewer Indian nurses in 1947. It is indisputable that, as Rosemary Fitzgerald's work has highlighted, this was one of the most important legacies of Christian work in India.[3] Western mission nurses forged close working relationships with Indian nurses and often spent three or four decades of their lives training nurses and caring for local communities. In the end, however, the effects of mission monopoly were problematic. The missions often served the very poorest people, and created communities of formerly 'untouchable' converts to Christianity. The ranks of their nursing staff were filled by women from the worst-off stratum of this already socially stigmatised group, often destitute widows or orphans. Nursing, which, given the nature of the work it required, was already liable to be viewed as too close to the work of sweeper castes, became identified with Christianity, poverty, desperation, and untouchability.

Independent India inherited much of the colonial state's health infrastructure, and its approach to nursing was heavily determined by this infrastructure, as well as by the colonial orientation to the profession. In some ways, this legacy benefited nursing. The dying years of colonialism saw a rush to reform the profession, as the inability to provide for wounded soldiers became embarrassingly

---

[2] Takahashi, *The Development of the Japanese Nursing Profession*, p. 31.

[3] Fitzgerald, 'Making and Moulding the Nursing of the Indian Empire'; Fitzgerald, 'Rescue and Redemption, pp. 64–79; Fitzgerald, 'A "Peculiar and Exceptional Measure"', pp. 174–96.

apparent. In 1946, the publication of the Bhore Report, which was taken as the template for post-Independence health planning, saw the adoption of the professionalising plans of the colonial leadership. These plans were viewed as synchronous with a health planning agenda that focused on all that was progressive and modern. The goal of a well-educated corps of nurses, with a role to play in public health, headed by a group of degree-educated leaders was accepted in post-colonial India as the non-negotiable basis for planning for nursing services.

Unfortunately, a pattern of ignoring the need for nursing, refusing engagement with nursing leaders and excluding the profession from health planning at the centre was also part of the legacy. As the rosy optimism of the early 1950s faded, it became clear that nurses would continue to experience an obdurate state deaf to the voices of their leaders. The refusal to fund positions of authority for nurses was one of the most serious failures. At the centre as well as state level, the nursing councils have been weak, dominated by non-nurses, under-funded, and often barely functional throughout the post-Independence period. In hospitals, positions for superintendents and charge nurses have been left vacant as a mode of economising and those who have occupied these positions have had their authority heavily restricted. Most nurses, even today, will be promoted only once or twice during 30- or 40-year careers, with minimal salary increases. The failure to fulfil promises to enhance and respect nurse authority has made nursing a stagnant career, and the profession has unsurprisingly struggled to produce strong and effective leaders, or to contribute to national health policy.

In 1971, a Malayali nurse named Saramma K. U. wrote to the *NJI* to describe the financial ruin and physical injury she had experienced as a result of the failure of her employer, the district hospital at Amaravati, to provide liveable accommodation. Sleeping in her room, the roof had collapsed on her, breaking her spine and both her legs. She took five months to recover, which the hospital insisted should be taken as leave without pay, and she paid all her medical expenses on her own. Concluding her letter, she wrote, 'I realise that I am a nurse and for poor nurses there are no facilities in this world but of course they will be rewarded in heaven'.[4] This experience was extreme, but by no means without precedent, and

---

[4] Saramma K. U., 'The Sad Plight of Nurses', *NJI*, vol. 62, no. 1, 1971, p. 29.

it suggests another of the key state failures during this period. The problem of unsuitable accommodation was a serious issue at the start of the century and it continues to be so today. In general, the state has failed to address even the simplest and cheapest of nurses' problems with working and living conditions. They continue to be regularly attacked on unsafe wards, on the way home at night on unsafe transport or while walking to unsafe living quarters. The failure to improve conditions has had an effect on the fortunes of nursing which is enormous, although difficult to measure. It is certain that, at least, it has ensured that many talented women took up other occupations wherever possible, and that the image problems of the profession have persisted.

Another outstanding feature of nursing's history during this period has been nurses' pronounced invisibility to the eyes of politicians and planners. Studying planning documents, it seems remarkable at times that there are any nurses at all, given the frequency with which nursing seems not to merit consideration. The proliferation of the dangerously untrained on the hospital wards of India, and their ubiquitous presence as 'nurses' in the wards of private hospitals and nursing homes, must be seen at least partly as the result of the absence of nursing and auxiliary nursing from the work of health planners. Given a free rein, hospital administrators have unsurprisingly pursued the cheapest option.

Nurses' invisibility has been a particularly remarkable feature of the politics of the centre. Whereas the problems of the medical profession have preoccupied central planners at some length, nursing has been left to the unevenly resourced states. This, again, is a direct legacy of an unreformed colonial system that substantially delegated health responsibilities away from the federal government. The most cursory look at the nursing profession in India reveals nursing to be manifestly deserving of attention at the federal government level. One state, Kerala, has supplied a large number of other states with significant proportions of their workforces, while others, mainly the big, populous and poor states of north India, have failed to develop much educational capacity at all, and attract an extremely small number of nurses. Yet, the mid-1960s ushered in what could be seen as a 'planning holiday' for nurses, during which their particular concerns were ignored, and they were subsumed within under-defined categories such as 'paramedical personnel'. It was only from the 1980s that this neglect at the centre began to be addressed.

The experience of nurses has thus dramatically reinforced the contentions of feminist scholars of the Indian state that it is characterised by duality towards women.[5] On the one hand, influenced by a founding national rhetoric of social justice, the state has committed itself to the creation of a strong and empowered nursing profession, convening a series of sympathetic committees that have promised the world. On the other, little has been done in practice to address the dangers and frustrations of nurses, and the state can even be viewed as complicit in anti-nurse violence — refusing to assist victims, facilitating attacks by accepting under-staffing and accepting a situation in which rapists and attackers are often its own agents, including the contractors and security guards hired by the government.

Through most of this period, nurses have also been limited by a problematic organisational culture. Leaders have struggled effectively to organise nurses and to represent their concerns. Professional organisation was moulded by the Western nurses who set up organisations such as the TNAI and the CNL. It has focused on education, the search for professional status and emphasised the international nature of nursing, but it has proved unable to achieve a great deal regarding the most serious concerns of nurses, which centred on poor working conditions. This pattern of organisation, which reflected the concerns of a small, often degree-educated elite, while neglecting the majority, was also the legacy of international nursing programmes in the 1950s. North American nursing advisors, although they perceived themselves as pursuing an entirely different project to that of their colonial predecessors (whom they often regarded as hopelessly old-fashioned), in truth reinforced the existing professionalist, elitist and internationalist orientation of nursing organisations.

Nursing organisations found little voice in health planning and were easily marginalised. Combined with the tendency of the state to disregard the role of nursing, a situation evolved in which nursing was seen as tangential to policymaking and to the attempts to improve poor national health outcomes. This was self-reinforcing: the more nursing was shoved to one side, the weaker it became. A strain of thinking emerged which postulated the irrelevance of nurses to health outside the cities. As James S. Tong, the executive secretary of

---

[5] Rajan, *The Scandal of the State*, p. 25; Rai, 'Women and the State in the Third World', p. 15; Agnes, 'Protecting Women against Violence', p. 522.

the Coordinating Agency for Health Planning (CAHP) group, wrote, 'by increasing the number of starched angels in the city hospitals, we do not meet the health needs of the 300 million neglected people mostly in the rural areas'. [6] This kind of thinking increasingly justified ignoring the role of the nurse in the public health system. Yet, although it is undoubtedly true that the villages were neglected and that trained carers at the local level were urgently needed, it was at the same time strange to contend that this could be addressed while ignoring nurses. The structure of India's primary health care system was designed around a rung of public health nurses, who would supervise the work of ANMs. At the very least, if nothing was to be done about encouraging the nurse to work in the country, the system needed restructuring. Instead, the structure remained in place, but with a major section entirely absent.

The nurse, moreover, is able to perform important functions such as overseeing the effective administration of drugs and vaccines (tasks which ANMs have reportedly struggled to perform unsupervised). Minimally educated village carers or even ANMs, who have suffered greatly from lack of supervision, cannot provide the same care as a trained nurse. Doctors, who have been almost as urbanised as nurses, have never suffered from the same suggestion that they are not really worth paying for in the primary health care system. The choice to ignore the role of nurses has been a choice to ignore the many policy options that might have encouraged them into public health work, such as strengthening nurses' public health education by providing real, practical and financial support; or creating statewide nursing services with authority to transfer nurses; or setting up incentive schemes for nurses to work in the country; or seriously investigating male nursing. Nor has the state ever substantially addressed the profession's own well-justified contention that the role of the public health nurse was even worse paid than that of the hospital nurse, and even less likely to lead to any sort of promotion or rise in salary.

Aside from the low participation of nurses in rural health, it must also be suggested that the skills of hospital nurses are important. The 'starched angels' mockingly mentioned by Tong are usually, in fact, overworked and under-recognised providers of health care to enormous numbers of people. Many patients not provided for

---

[6] CAHP, 'Report of a Nursing Survey in India', Preface.

in the country come to city hospitals, which often cater to a very large catchment area. The exclusion of nurses from planning that this book identifies cannot only be explained by the urbanisation of the profession. The acceptance at state level of nurses' absence from public health has in reality represented an outstanding instance of state contempt for the work and skills of women.

The future holds some hope for redressing the neglect of nursing and for the creation of more respect for the skills of nurses. Recent large scale increases in numbers of nurses, attracted by opportunities to emigrate, might mean that it will be more politically difficult to ride roughshod over the profession's concerns. At the individual level, nurses are experiencing higher social status as their diplomas and degrees are increasingly regarded as passports to prosperity in the West. Most promisingly, recent years have seen the emergence of confident and assertive nurse-led unions, with activism entirely focused on improvements to working conditions. Defined against colonial traditions of frocks and deference, these organisations are perhaps finally proving the farsightedness of a 1957 ICN report, which suggested that:

> Nurses in each country have to fight their own battle for recognition even if they get moral and sometimes financial support from other countries. The solution to the problem of strained relationships lies in the life and soul of each individual country, her customs and beliefs.[7]

Yet, the astonishing pace at which Indian nurses have experienced the globalisation of health also suggests discouraging continuities in the orientation of the state to the profession. The state has expressed its willingness to participate in the shaping of nursing education into an export industry, but has proved unwilling to consider the serious domestic ramifications of creating such an industry. The refusal to consider the value of nurses, or to investigate how best the state might work with the profession to create a nursing service better shaped by India's health needs, is thus as obvious as ever.

---

[7] Yvonne Schroeder, 'Post-Basic Nursing Education: Principles of Administration as Applied to Advanced Programmes in Nursing Education, Volume I', London: ICN, 1957, pp. 26–27.

# Further Research

The undervaluation of India's nursing profession is indicated by the scarcity of information about its various important aspects. These await future research. This book, for example, turned up little information on any role played by nurses in India's struggle for Independence. The papers of Rajkumari Amrit Kaur, independent India's first health minister and an important participant in the Independence movement, seemed a likely source, especially as she regarded herself as nurses' greatest champion, but they did not address this. It is possible that nurses at that time were a lower middle class group of relatively disempowered women who were unlikely to have had the financial or social freedom to have participated in significant numbers in this movement. Given their long history of invisibility to policymakers, historians and the media, it is also possible, however, that nurses' role was overlooked. It is certain that some individual nurses, nevertheless, made a contribution. A 1972 article in the *NJI*, for example, mentions a woman called Pramila Shantaram, who had been a successful nurse and activist working with rural women in Maharashtra, and adds as an afterthought that she had been jailed for six months for her role in the Independence movement.[8] The nationalist sentiment that swept India in the 1930s and 1940s certainly enthused numerous nursing students: it is mentioned a number of times in the *NJI* as a concern for British teachers keen to maintain order and discipline. Chapter 1 considered the role the ethos of nurse internationalism played in suppressing this tension between British nursing lecturers and their Indian students: as members of a universal sisterhood, notions of colonial oppression and the joys of national freedom supposedly became irrelevant. Overall, however, the involvement of nurses in the struggle for freedom is an area that may reward further, deeper historical investigation.

Nurses working in the Indian Army have a different status than civilian nurses, and have generally been better regarded. The pages of the *NJI*, however, do occasionally record discontents over low salary and a slow rate of promotion compared to the rest of the army. Military nursing also seems to have been strongly shaped by its colonial roots. For many years after Independence, army nurses

---

[8] Anonymous, 'Nursing world', *NJI*, vol. 66, no. 4, 1975, p. 81.

were forbidden to marry. Male nurses are still not allowed to join the army. This is a regulation that is surely grounded in the struggle for professional control experienced by British military nurses over the much larger numbers of male Indian orderlies and 'ward boys' who worked alongside them in the first half of the 20th century, often undertaking quite sophisticated medical tasks. The army, however, is not easy to penetrate. There is little published information about the experience of the army nurse and I found obtaining interviews was extremely difficult. This, again, remains an area that should be a rewarding site for future research.

The role of general paramedical and government worker unions also requires further investigation. Particularly in the northern states such as Rajasthan and Punjab, these broader unions attracted numerous nurses into their ranks, but ultimately seem to have disappointed them. It is likely that the wider societal prejudices against nurses and the tendency to ignore their concerns were a factor in this; with union leaders probably no less likely than politicians and health planners to minimise the concerns of nurses. This is another nursing story that remains to be told.

The phenomenon of nurse emigration has transformed the profession with astonishing speed, and the effects of this have by no means been comprehensively covered here. It remains to be seen how emigration will affect nurses' status in the long term in northern states such as Rajasthan and Uttar Pradesh, where it has in the past been most difficult for women to become nurses. Recent years have also seen a surge in the numbers of nurses produced in India's north-east: this may be linked to emigration and is certainly a trend worthy of further investigation. At a global level, it also remains to be seen how unpredictable and sweeping changes in the international economy and the resulting swingeing cuts to Western health budgets will touch the lives of potential Indian nurse migrants.

## In Conclusion

In the context of persistent state neglect and contempt, it can be suggested that the story of nursing's low status, of its battle with moral disapprobation, of the notion of nurse work as polluting, is ultimately stale. After all, if the rise of emigration has done nothing else, it has shown the power of the prospect of material reward, plain and simple, to transform the profession. The future rests on the further development of a grounded and enthusiastically supported nursing leadership strong enough to tackle head on the task of placing nursing on the centre stage of policymaking. In doing this, what Celia Davies describes as the 'masculine vision that is built into our organizational life' must be recognised, and the deep-seated reluctance within this framework to take women's work seriously must be confronted courageously.[9] The end result of this, it might be suggested, is contained within the writings of the Susruta Samhita, the most ancient account of caring roles in Indian society. Susruta described nurses not as handmaidens or as ministering angels. Rather, together with the doctor, medicines and the patient, the nurse is simply one of the 'four feet upon which a cure must rest'.[10]

---

[9] Davies, *Gender and the Professional Predicament*, p. x.
[10] Kisku, 'Nursing Education Needs Change', p. 409.

# Bibliography

◘

## Archival Sources

*The Burke Library of the Union Theological Seminary in the City of New York*

Rh. India A — American Baptist Mission, Hospital for Women and Children and School of Nursing.
Rh India C — Clough Memorial Hospital.
Rh India N — Nowrosjee Wadia Maternity Hospital.
Florence Harriette Martyn, 'A Bibliography: Plan of Organization and Administration Provincial Division of Nursing, Pakistan and India, 1950', Masters of Science in Nursing Education, Dissertation, Catholic University of America, 1950. Record number AuM358.

*Cambridge University Library*

Royal Commonwealth Society Library, Indian Nursing Collection of Diana Hartley, RCMS 77.

*Christian Medical College Vellore Archives*

'Nursing staff (Foreign) 1950–1958', D/41/50, C/120, Box 6.
'Director's Office File, Nursing Staff, Correspondence, 1958–1965', D/24/58, Box 18.
'Director's Office File, Dean, School of Nursing 1958–1969', D/47/58, Box 19.

*Imperial War Museum, London, Department of Documents*

Papers of Miss E. Campbell (88/5/1).
Papers of Miss E. D. C. Palmer (Conservation Shelf).
Marian Carswell. 'The Chota Sister Sahibs'. Enclosed with Miss M. Robertson, '14th Army Nurse' (83/27/1).
Mrs C. Hutchinson. 'My War, and Welcome to it' (02/36/1).
Hilda Nield. 'A Short History of the V. A. D. Unit, India, 1944 to 1946' (Misc 183 [2751]).

Mrs E. Stevenson. 'The Last Lap: Autobiography 1912–1986' (86/29/1).
Mrs Margery A. A. Thomas. 'My Life in the Army during the Great War 1914–1918' (85/39/1).

*Nehru Memorial Library, New Delhi*

Papers of the All India Women's Conference, Institutional List No. 38.
Papers of Rajkumari Amrit Kaur, Institutional List No. 14.

*Oriental and India Office Collections, British Library, London*

L/WS/1/876, 'Nurses and V. A. Ds. India'.
L/MIL/9/430, 'Indian Nursing Service, January 1903–August 1916'.
L/WS/1/888, 'Distribution of Doctors and Nurses in first six months of 1945'.
L/WS/2/72, 'Working Party on Nurses 1946'.
V/24/694, 'Papers of Lady Ampthill's Nurses Institute and South India Nursing Service'.
MSS Eur E316, Alice Edith Isaacs, 'Lady Reading Collection'.
MSS Eur D1182, 'Eileen Palmer Collection'.
MSS Eur C251, Constance A. Wilson, 'Never in Poona'.
MSS Eur C812, 'Diary of Miss Partington, Sister at Military Hospitals in Delhi and elsewhere'.
MSS Eur Photo Eur 263, 'Diaries of Pauline Searle describing her service as a VAD in India'.
MSS Eur R202, Katherine Mabel Smith-Pearse. Recording of interview about her childhood in India, nursing during World War I and time spent as principal of a school in Raipur.
MSS Eur R136, Dorothy B. Thomas. Recording of interview about her work with Lady Minto's Nursing Service, 1928–34, her experiences in Burma and time spent in Jalpaiguri.
MSS Eur A207, 'Memorabilia and Photographs of Sister Mary Cossey'.

*Rockefeller Foundation Archives, Sleepy Hollow, New York*

Record Group 1.1 (Projects, 1912–2000), Series 464C, Box 10.
Record Group 1.2 (Projects, 1912–2000), Series 464C, Boxes 53, 54.
Record Group 2 (General Correspondence, 1927–89), Series 100, Boxes 3–6, 320, 360, 398. Series 464C, Box 461.
Record Group 5.2 (International Health Board, 1911–1951, Special Reports), Series 464, Box 49.
Record Group 5.3 (International Health Board, 1911–1951, Routine Reports) Series 464C, Box 204.
Record Group 6.1 (Paris Field Office), Series 2.1 (Post-war Correspondence), Box 44.
Record Group 12.1 (Diaries): Anna M. Noll.

*UK National Archives, Kew*

'West Bengal Nursing Council (India), Correspondence 1948–62', DT
18/74.
'Correspondence with Labour Attache, New Delhi, on the Status of Nurses
Organisations in India, following an Enquiry from Miss F. Goodall of
the Royal College of Nursing', LAB 13/1288.
'Immigration/UK/: Trained Nurses: Difficulties Of', c. 1967, FCO 50/84.

*University of Birmingham, Church Missionary Society Collection*

Papers of the Medical Department:

- M/AC2/1, 1946–49.
- M/AC2/2, 1946–49.
- M/AC/3.
- M/AD2, 1944.
- M59/AC1, 1957–59.
- M59/AC2, 1951–53, 1954–55.
- M59/E2/1.
- *Health and Wealth* newsletter, 1953–62. M59/E2/2

West Asia (Group 2) Missions, G2-I-1-L19.

*USA National Archives and Records Administration, College Park, MD*

State Department Records, USAID, Record Group 286, Entry 385, Boxes
157, 159.

*Wellcome Library for the History and Understanding of Medicine,
London*

File of Sir Weldon Dalrymple-Champney, GC/139/H.2/1.
File of Janet Vaughan, India 1944–45, GC/186/6.

## Interviews

Bai, Sulochana (Principal, School of Nursing, SUT Hospital).
Thiruvananthapuram, 3 December 2005.
Bhansali, Shakuntala (Student at CMC Ludhiana, 1952–56). By Telephone,
London to Alton, Hampshire, 23 August 2005.
Chandrakanthi, C. (Dean, College of Nursing, Amrita Institute of Medical
Sciences and Research Centre, Kochi). Thiruvananthapuram, 4 December
2005.
Cherian, Thankamma (Principal, School of Nursing, Cosmopolitan Hos-
pital). Thiruvananthapuram, 22 November 2005.

Conroy, Judy (International Section Manager, Australian Nursing and Midwifery Council). By Telephone, Melbourne to Canberra, 30 August 2006.

Doohan, Jennifer (Royal College of Nursing UK, Project Development Officer). By Telephone, London, 11 August 2006.

Harnar, Ruth (Missionary Nurse and USAID Consultant). By Telephone, Melbourne to Indianapolis, 30 July 2004.

Khurana, G. (President of the Delhi Government Nurses' Union and the All India Government Nurses' Federation). New Delhi, 6 February 2006.

Koshy, Annamma (former Superintendent of Nursing at St Stephen's Hospital, Delhi). Thiruvalla, 9 December 2005.

Kuruvilla, Aleyamma (former Dean of CMC Vellore, TNAI President and CMAI President). Thiruvalla, 9 December 2005.

Jacob, Bella Mary (Manager, Thiruvananthapuram office, Manjooran's Group of Institutes). Thiruvananthapuram, 30 November 2005.

Jacob, Jolly (Principal, Lords School of Nursing). Thiruvananthapuram, 1 December 2005.

Jose, A. Nirmal (Deputy Principal, Lisie Hospital School of Nursing). Ernakulam, 5 December 2005.

Kamalam, Mrs (Principal, GG School of Nursing). Thiruvananthapuram, 29 November 2005.

Khannan, Evelyn (Assistant Secretary, TNAI). New Delhi, 27 January 2006.

Lowe, Daisy (Student at CMC Vellore, 1960–65). By Telephone, London to South Wales, 24 August 2005.

Mathew, Rachel (Principal, School of Nursing, KIMS Hospital). Thiruvananthapuram, 23 November 2005.

Platts, Eileen. (Missionary Nurse at CMC Ludhiana, 1953–88). London, 27 August 2005.

Sr Sylvia (Principal, Little Flower School of Nursing, Jubilee Hospital). Thiruvananthapuram, 25 November 2005.

Soman, C. R. (Founding Chairman of Health Action By People). Thiruvananthapuram, 28 December 2004.

Sreelatha, Dr (Doctor at the Thiruvananthapuram Mental Hospital). Thiruvananthapuram, 11 November 2005.

Subbiah, Nanthini. (Deputy Secretary-General, TNAI). New Delhi, 27 January 2006.

Thampy, P. K. (General Secretary, Kerala Government Nurses' Association). Thiruvananthapuram, 28 December 2004.

Vasantha, Mrs (Superintendent of Nursing at the Thiruvananthapuram Mental Hospital). Thiruvananthapuram, 11 November 2005.

Vijayarakhavan, Dr (Cardiologist at KIMS Hospital). Thiruvananthapuram, 25 November 2005.

Discussions with MSc (nursing) students, College of Nursing, Thiruvananthapuram, January 2005.

## Published Sources

Abana, C. I., 'Report of the Honorary Branch Secretary, Delhi, from August 1945 to June 1946', *NJI*, vol. 38, no. 2, 1947, pp. 82–83.

Abel-Smith, Brian, *A History of the Nursing Profession*, London: Heinemann, 1960.

Abraham, Meera, Religion, *Caste and Gender: Missionaries and Nursing History in South India*, Bangalore: B. I. Publications, 1996.

Abrams, Sarah Elise, 'Seeking Jurisdiction: A Sociological Perspective on Rockefeller Foundation Activities in Nursing in the 1920s', in Anne Marie Rafferty, Jane Robinson and Ruth Elkan (eds), *Nursing History and the Politics of Welfare*, London and New York: Routledge, 1997, pp. 208–25.

Academy for Nursing Studies, Hyderabad, 'Situational Analysis of Public Health Nursing Personnel in India: Based on National Review and Consultation in Six States', Hyderabad: Academy for Nursing Studies, 2005.

Adranvala, T. K., 'President's Address', *NJI*, vol. 42, no. 1, 1951, pp. 6–8.

———, 'Trends in Nursing Education', *Journal of the Christian Medical Association of India*, vol. 32, no. 5, 1957, pp. 255–58.

———, 'Developments in Nursing 1947–57', *NJI*, vol. 49, no. 10, 1958, pp. 326–28, 334.

———, 'Letter to the Editor', *Indian Journal of Public Health*, vol. 8, no. 2, 1964, pp. 78–79.

———, 'A Review of Post-basic and Post-graduate Training of Nurses', *NJI*, vol. 56, no. 9, 1965, pp. 247–48.

———, 'Nursing in India — 1908–1968', *NJI*, vol. 59, no. 11, 1968, pp. 369–71.

———, 'Professional Behaviour: Some Aspects of Nursing Practice', *NJI*, vol. 64, no. 10, 1973, p. 357, 363.

———, 'A Point to Ponder', *NJI*, vol. 66, no. 5, 1975, p. 97.

———, 'Nursing Profession in India', in Usha Sharma and B. M. Sharma (eds), *Encyclopaedia of Women and Education: Volume 3, Women and Professions*, New Delhi: Commonwealth, 2001, pp. 168–79 (originally published c. 1957).

Aggarwal, K. C., 'Research in Nursing II — It's High Time to Act Now', *NJI*, vol. 67, no. 12, 1967, pp. 263–64.

———, 'Some Suggested Structural Changes in Nursing Education', *NJI*, vol. 67, no. 7, 1976, pp. 169–71.

Agnes, Flavia, 'Protecting Women against Violence?: Review of a Decade of Legislation, 1980–1989', in Partha Chatterjee (ed.), *State and Politics in India*, Oxford: Oxford University Press, 1997, pp. 521–65.

Agnihotri, Indu, and Vina Mazumdar, 'Changing Terms of Political Discourse: Women's Movement in India, 1970s–1990s', *Economic and Political Weekly*, vol. 30, no. 28, 1995, pp. 1869–78.

Aiken, Linda H., James Buchan, Julie Sochalski, Barbara Nichols, and Mary Powell, 'Trends in International Nurse Migration', *Health Affairs*, vol. 23, no. 3, 2004, pp. 69–77.

Ali, Maqbool, 'The Role and Training of *Dais* (2)', *NJI*, vol. 50, no. 5, 1959, pp. 168–69.

All India Government Nurses Federation, 'Representation to Honourable Prime Minister, Government of India, in respect of Nursing Profession on behalf of Fourth National Convention on 26th–27th September, 2000, at New Delhi', New Delhi, 2000.

Allen, Belle Jane, *A Crusade of Compassion for the Healing of the Nations*, West Medford, MA: Central Committee of the United Study of Foreign Missions, 1919.

Amrith, Sunil, 'Development and Disease: The United Nations and Public Health, c. 1945–1955', in Martin Daunton and Frank Trentmann (eds), *Worlds of Political Economy: Power and Knowledge, Eighteenth Century to the Present*, Basingstoke and New York: Palgrave Macmillan, 2004, pp. 217–40.

———, 'The United Nations and Public Health in Asia, c. 1940–1960', PhD Dissertation, Christ's College, Cambridge University, 2004.

———, *Decolonizing International Health*, Basingstoke: Palgrave Macmillan, 2006.

———, 'Political Culture of Health in India: A Historical Perspective', *Economic and Political Weekly*, vol. 42, no. 2, 13 January 2007, pp. 114–21.

Anagol, Padma, 'Indian Christian Women and Indigenous Feminism, c. 1850–c. 1920', in Clare Midgely (ed.), *Gender and Imperialism*, Manchester: Manchester University Press, 1998.

Anderson, W., 'Excremental Colonialism: Public Health and the Poetics of Pollution', *Critical Inquiry*, vol. 21, 1995, pp. 640–69.

Andhra Mahila Sabha. 'Role of Voluntary Agencies in the Implementation of Public Health, Medical Care and Family Planning Programmes under Five Year Plans', National Health Seminar, 29–31 December 1965, Andhra Mahila Sabha Nursing Home, Madras.

Andrist, Linda C., 'The History of the Relationship between Feminism and Nursing', in Linda C. Andrist, Patrice K. Nicholas and Karen A. Wolf (eds), *A History of Nursing Ideas*, Sudbury, MA: Jones and Bartlett, 2006, pp. 5–22.

Annan, Kofi, 'Managing Migration Better', *The Hindu*, 29 January 2004, p. 10.

Anonymous, '6th Biennial Conference: Resolutions', *NJI*, vol. 63, no. 12, 1972, pp. 421–22.

——, 'A Career Guide for Nurses', in Narender Nagpal (ed.), *Nursing Perspectives: Indian Nursing Year Book: 1984–85*, Delhi: TNAI, 1985, p. SC 5.

——, 'A Preliminary Blueprint: Central Institute of Nursing', *NJI*, vol. 81, no. 8, 1990, pp. 235–36.

——, 'Abortion Act: Nurses' Rights on Moral Grounds Defended', *NJI*, vol. 62, no. 11, 1971, pp. 352, 374.

——, 'Bombay Presidency Nursing Association: Half-Yearly Examination for Nurses and Midwives, August and September, 1916', *NJI*, vol. 7, no. 9, 1916, p. 194.

——, 'Brain Trust on the Theme: Family Welfare', *NJI*, vol. 63, no. 12, 1972, pp. 414–17.

——, 'Branch Affairs', *NJI*, vol. 66, no. 7, 1975, pp. 179–82.

——, 'Business Session: Problems of Student Nurses', *NJI*, vol. 64, no. 12, 1973, pp. 411–12.

——, 'Calendar', *NJI*, vol. 49, no. 10, 1958, p. 343.

——, 'Candidates for TNAI Elections October 1972 — Bombay', *NJI*, vol. 63, no. 9, 1972, pp. 317–19.

——, 'Colombo Plan Nurses', *NJI*, vol. 44, no. 8, 1953, pp. 204–5.

——, 'Development of Nursing Services under Ninth Five Year Plan', in TNAI, *Indian Nursing Year Book, 1998–1999*, New Delhi: TNAI, 1999.

——, 'Examination Questions Florence Nightingale Memorial Scholarship, 1938', *NJI*, vol. 29, no. 4, 1938, pp. 99–102.

——, 'Extracts from the Minutes of the Conference of the TNAI, Delhi, 1941', *NJI*, vol. 32, no. 4, April 1941, pp. 110–15.

——, 'Govt Ignoring Nurses' new JAC', *Hindustan Times*, 22 January 1987, p. 3.

——, 'Graduate Nurses', *NJI*, vol. 59, no. 6, 1968, pp. 179–81.

——, 'Greetings and Messages', *NJI*, vol. 49, no. 10, 1958, pp. 317–25.

——, 'Health Chief Ignorant of Nurses' Recruitment', *The Times of India*, 23 January 1987, p. 3.

——, 'Hospitals', *The Statesman*, Calcutta, 17 May 1948.

——, 'In Memoriam: Miss Jankibai Sabnis', *NJI*, vol. 42, no. 7, 1950, p. 203.

——, 'International Nurses' Day: Celebrations throughout the Country', *NJI*, vol. 95, no. 11, November 2004, pp. 246–50.

——, 'Judge asks Victim to Consider Marrying Rapist', *The Age*, Melbourne, 5 May 2005, p. 11.

Anonymous, 'KGMCTA Condemns Ongoing Campaign and HC Dismisses Students' Plea', *The Indian Express*, Thiruvananthapuram, 19 November 2005.

———, 'Minutes of the 28th Annual Conference of the Trained Nurses' Association of India (continued from the January issue)', *NJI*, vol. 30, no. 2, 1939, pp. 47–52.

———, 'New Building to House College of Nursing', *NJI*, vol. 62, no. 9, 1971, pp. 295–96.

———, 'News and Notes', *NJI*, vol. 33, no. 8, 1942, pp. 200–209.

———, 'News', *NJI*, vol. 62, no. 3, 1971, pp. 77, 90–91, 93–94.

———, 'News from TNAI Headquarters', *NJI*, vol. 97, no. 1, 2006, p. 3.

———, 'Nursing Dreams: Medical Caregivers to get U.S. Green Card within one year', *Times of India*, 19 July 2005, p. 24.

———, 'No Solution yet to Nurses Strike', *The Times of India*, 22 January 1987, p. 3.

———, 'Nurses' Strike enters 13th day', *Hindustan Times*, 1 February 1987, p. 5.

———, 'Nursing World', *NJI*, vol. 66, no. 1, 1975, pp. 15, 21.

———, 'Obituaries', *NJI*, vol. 66, no. 2, 1975.

———, 'Pay Scales for Nursing Personnel as Recommended by the Fourth Central Pay Commission: Central Government, Union Territories and Armed Forces', *NJI*, vol. 77, no. 8, 1986, pp. 214–15.

———, 'People', *NJI*, vol. 62, no. 6, 1971, p. 205.

———, 'Personal Notes and News', *NJI*, vol. 51, no. 11, 1960, p. 325.

———, 'Plan to recruit Ad hoc Nurses', *Hindustan Times*, 23 January 1987, p. 1.

———, 'Policy of the Trained Nurses' Association of India', *NJI*, vol. 42, no. 1, 1951, p. 41.

———, 'Policy Statement on Strike', *Indian Nursing Year Book: 1998–1999*, New Delhi: TNAI, 2000.

———, 'Précis of Honorary Provincial Secretaries' Reports', *NJI*, vol. 32, no. 4, 1941, pp. 123–32.

———, 'Problems of Nurses in Rajasthan: Memorandum Submitted', *NJI*, vol. 62, no. 3, 1971, pp. 75–76.

———, 'Realities of Nursing', *NJI*, vol. 63, no. 12, 1972, p. 418.

———, 'Reports', *NJI*, vol. 62, no. 1, 1971, pp. 13–14, 29.

———, 'Resolution passed by the Members of the Trained Nurses' Association of India assembled at Conference and forwarded to The Hon. Mr Rajagopalachariar, the Hon. Dr. Rajan and the Surgeon-General with the Government of Madras on November 11th, 1938', *NJI*, vol. 30, no. 2, 1939, pp. 42–43.

———, 'Resolutions: The Trained Nurses' Association of India in Session at Jaipur from September 26 to October 1, 1960, Adopted the Following Resolutions', *NJI*, vol. 51, no. 11, 1960, p. 312.

Anonymous, 'Resolutions', *NJI*, vol. 62, no. 6, 1971, p. 198.

——, 'Rural Health Mission Flagged Off', *Deccan Herald*, 13 April 2005.

——, 'Sexual Assault Reports False, Fabricated, say Students', *The Indian Express*, Thiruvananthapuram, 19 November 2005.

——, 'Sack Notice for 25 Striking Nurses?', *Sunday Observer*, New Delhi, 25 January 1987, p. 5.

——, 'Socio-economic Status of Nurses in India', *NJI*, vol. 63, no. 12, 1972, pp. 405–6.

——, 'Striking Nurses Stage Rally at Nirman Bhavan', *The Times of India*, 28 January 1987, p. 3.

——, 'The Health Survey and Development Committee (Bhore Committee), 1943–46: A Synopsis of the Findings', *Indian Nursing Year Book, 1986–8*, New Delhi: TNAI, 1988.

——, 'The Trained Nurses' Association of India: An Introduction', *Indian Nursing Year Book 1996–97*, New Delhi: TNAI, 1998.

——, 'TNAI attends Dialogue for "Safe Delhi"', *NJI*, vol. 7, no. 2, 2006, p. 27.

——, 'TNAI Council Meets', *NJI*, vol. 62, no. 3, 1971, p. 68.

——, 'TNAI Scholars — 1971', *NJI*, vol. 62, no. 6, 1971, p. 202.

——, 'Victims of Male Aggression', *Hindustan Times*, 11 January 1987, p. 7.

——, 'WHO Fellowships', *NJI*, vol. 42, no. 4, 1951, p. 125.

——, 'Wanted Advertisements', *NJI*, vol. 38, no. 2, 1947.

——, 'Women's Hospitals in India and Their Nursing', *NJI*, vol. 96, no. 4, 2005 (reprinted from April 1911) p. 77.

Anthony, Frank, *Britain's Betrayal in India: The Story of the Anglo-Indian Community*, Bombay: Allied Publishers, 1969.

Aravamudan, Gita, 'Nurses and Nuns of Kerala', in Devaki Jain (ed.), *Indian Women*, Delhi: Publications Division, Ministry of Information and Broadcasting, Government of India, 1975, pp. 251–59.

Arnold, David, *Colonizing the Body: State Medicine and Epidemic Disease in Nineteenth Century India*, Berkeley: University of California Press, 1993.

——, 'Crisis and Contradiction in India's Public Health', in Dorothy Porter (ed.), *The History of Public Health and the Modern State*, Amsterdam, Atlanta: Rodopi, 1994.

——, 'Public Health and Public Power: Medicine and Hegemony in Colonial India', in Dagmar Engels and Shula Marks (eds), *Contesting Colonial Hegemony: State and Society in Africa and India*, London: British Academic Press, 1994, pp. 131–51.

Arora, P., 'Perspectives on Indian Nursing', *NJI*, vol. 47, no. 9, 1976, pp. 223–24.

Arora, Swarnlata, and Germaine Krysan, 'A Look at Nursing and Family Planning', *NJI*, vol. 58, no. 11, 1967, pp. 281–84.

Arunima, G., *There Comes Papa: Colonialism and the Transformation of Matriliny in Kerala, Malabar, c. 1850–1940*, New Delhi: Orient Longman, 2003.

Association of Nursing Superintendents in India (ANSI), *Report of the Association of Nursing Superintendents of India 1907*, Cawnpore: ANSI, 1907.

Bachu, Amaravathy, 'Public Health Nursing: How They Are Different in the United States', *NJI*, vol. 61, no. 11, 1970, pp. 361, 373.

Bagchi, Amiya Kumar and Krishna Soman, *Maladies, Preventives and Curatives: Debates in Public Health in India*, New Delhi: Tulika, 2005.

Balfour, Margaret, 'Indian Nursing — Its Past and Future', *NJI*, vol. 14, no. 2, 1923, pp. 28–35.

Balfour, Margaret and Ruth Young, *The Work of Medical Women in India*, London: Oxford University Press, 1929.

Ball, R., 'Divergent Development, Racialised Rights: Globalized Labour Markets and the Trade of Nurses: the Case of the Philippines', *Women's Studies International Forum*, vol. 27, no. 2, 2004, pp. 119–33.

Baly, Monica, *Florence Nightingale and the Nursing Legacy*, London: Croom Helm, 1986.

Banerjee, Nirmala, 'Analysing Women's Work Under Patriarchy', in Kumkum Sangari and Uma Chakravarti (eds), *From Myths to Markets: Essays on Gender*, New Delhi: Manohar, 2001, pp. 321–40.

Barr, M., 'Editorial', *NJI*, vol. 8, no. 8, 1917.

Barry, Elda M., 'Letter to the Editor', *NJI*, vol. 44, no. 8, 1953, pp. 202–3.

Basu, Srimati, 'Review Essay: Janaki Nair, *Women and Law in Colonial India: A Social History*', *Gender and History*, vol. 11, no. 1, 1999, pp. 173–76.

Bhattacharya, Sanjoy, Mark Harrison and Michael Worboys, *Fractured States: Smallpox, Public Health and Vaccination Policy in British India, 1800–1947*, Hyderabad: Orient Longman, 2005.

Bhullar, G., 'Letter to the Editor', *NJI*, vol. 66, no. 8, 1975, p. 173.

Bischoff, Lillian M., 'This I Believe', *NJI*, vol. 59, no. 11, 1968, pp. 372–73.

Bleakley, Ethel, *Meet the Indian Nurse*, London: Zenith Press, 1949.

Blunt, Alison, *Domicile and Diaspora: Anglo-Indian Women and the Spatial Politics of Home*, Melbourne: Blackwell, 2005.

Borthwick, Meredith, *The Changing Role of Women in Bengal, 1849–1905*, Princeton: Princeton University Press, 1984.

Brush, Barbara and Rukmini Vasupuram, 'Nurses, Nannies and Caring Work: Importation, Visibility and Marketability', *Nursing Inquiry*, no. 13, 2006, pp. 181–85.

Buhler-Wilkerson, Karen, *No Place like Home: A History of Nursing and Home Care in the United States*, Baltimore: Johns Hopkins University Press, 2001.

Burke, Milly, 'Letter to the Editor', *NJI*, vol. 8, no. 1, January 1917, p. 21.

Burrage, Michael, Konrad Jarausch and Hannes Siegrist, 'An Actor-based Framework for the Study of the Professions', in Michael Burrage and Rolf Torstendahl (eds), *Professions in Theory and History: Rethinking the Study of the Professions*, London,: Sage Publications, 1990, pp. 203–25.

Burton, Antoinette, *Burdens of History: British Feminists, Indian Women, and Imperial Culture, 1865–1915*, Chapel Hill and London: University of North Carolina Press, 1994.

Ceniza Choy, Catherine, *Empire of Care: Nursing and Migration in Filipino American History*, Durham and London: Duke University Press, 2003.

Central Bureau of Health Intelligence, Health Information of India 2002, New Delhi: Central Bureau of Health Intelligence, 2004.

Central Treaty Organisation, 'Conference on Nursing Education', 14–25 April 1964, Tehran, Iran.

Chakravarti, Uma, 'Gender, Caste and Labour: The Ideological and Material Structure of Widowhood', in Martha Alter Chen (ed.), *Widows in India: Social Neglect and Public Action*, London: Sage Publications, 1998, pp. 63–92.

Chalkley, A. M., *A Textbook for the Health Worker (ANM): Volume II*, revised edn, New Delhi: New Age International Publishers,1985.

Chakrapani, A. C., 'Minutes of the 49th Conference — TNAI', *NJI*, vol. 51, no. 11, 1960, pp. 305–6, 311.

Charles, S. X., 'Mode of Delivery by Untrained Dais in and around Vellore', *Journal of the Christian Medical Association of India*, vol. 46, no. 2, 1971, pp. 82–87.

Chatterjee, Partha, *The Nation and its Fragments: Colonial and Postcolonial Histories*, Princeton: Princeton University Press, 1993.

———, 'Development Planning and the Indian State', in Partha Chatterjee (ed.), *State and Politics in India*, Oxford: Oxford University Press, 1997, pp. 271–98.

———, 'Introduction: A Political History of Independent India', in Partha Chatterjee (ed.), *State and Politics in India*, Oxford: Oxford University Press, 1997, pp. 1–40.

Chattopadhyay, Kamaladevi, 'The Women's Movement: Then and Now', in Devaki Jain (ed.), *Indian Women*, New Delhi: Publications Division, Ministry of Information and Broadcasting, Government of India, 1975, pp. 27–36.

Chawla, Satish, 'Address to XX TNAI Biennial Conference', *NJI*, vol. 95, no. 1, 2004.

———, 'As Nurses We are One', *NJI*, vol. 96, no. 12, 2005, pp. 270–72.

Chawla, Satish, 'Address to SNA Platinum Jubilee and Biennial Conference', *NJI*, vol. 96, no. 1, 2005, p. 9.

Cherian, A., 'Role of Nursing in India Today', *NJI*, vol. 67, no. 11, 1976, pp. 258–59.

Cheriyan, T., 'Future of Nursing', *Christian Nurse*, no. 230, 1970, p. 17.

Chesney, Mrs., 'An Appeal to Trained Nurses', *NJI*, vol. 13, no. 1, 1922, p. 2.

Chew, Dolores, 'The Search for Kathleen McNally and Other Chimerical Women: Colonial and Post-colonial Gender Representations of Eurasians', in Brinda Bose (ed.), *Translating Desire: The Politics and Gender of Culture in India*, New Delhi: Katha, 2002, pp. 2–29.

Chhuttani, P. N., 'India', in John Z. Bowers and Professor Lord Rosenheim (eds), *Migration of Medical Manpower: Papers from an International Macy Conference*, New York: The Josiah Macy, Jr. Foundation, 1971, pp. 9–20.

Clark, Alice M., 'Training for Leadership', *NJI*, vol. 42, no. 2, 1951, pp. 66–68.

Committee from the Christian Medical Association of India, Burma and Ceylon and the Nurses' Auxiliary (CMAI Committee), 'A Survey of Nursing and Nursing Education in Mission Hospitals and Schools of Nursing in India', Mysore: Wesley Press and Publishing House, 1947, pp. 70–74.

Connolly, Cynthia Anne. 'Beyond Social History: New Approaches to Understanding the State of and the State in Nursing History', *Nursing History Review*, vol. 12, 2004, pp. 5–24.

Coordinating Agency for Health Planning (CAHP), 'Report of a Nursing Survey in India carried out under the Auspices of the Coordinating Agency for Health Planning and the Trained Nurses' Association of India', New Delhi, 1974.

Craig, Margaretta, 'The College of Nursing, New Delhi: Progress Report to the TNAI November 1946', *NJI*, vol. 38, no. 2, 1947, pp. 70–74.

Das, P. P., 'ANM Uniforms', *NJI*, vol. 62, no. 1, 1971.

Davies, Celia, 'A Constant Casualty: Nurse Education in Britain and the USA to 1939', in Celia Davies (ed.), *Rewriting Nursing History*, London: Croom Helm, 1980, pp. 102–22.

———, 'Introduction', in Celia Davies (ed.), *Rewriting Nursing History*, London: Croom Helm, 1980, pp. 11–17.

Davies, Celia, *Gender and the Professional Predicament in Nursing*, Buckingham and Philadelphia: Open University Press, 1995.

Davies, Celia, 'The Sociology of Professions and the Professions of Gender', *Sociology*, vol. 30, 1996, pp. 661–78.

Dhaulta, Jaiwanti P., 'A Report on the Community Nurses' Meet', *NJI*, vol. 78, no. 1, pp. 17–18.

Dingwall, Robert, Anne Marie Rafferty and Charles Webster, *An Introduction to the Social History of Nursing*, London: Routledge, 1988.

Dorabji, Indira, 'Greeting Message', *NJI*, vol. 59, no. 11, 1968, p. 366.

Ehrenreich, B., and A. R. Hochschild, *Global Women: Nannies, Maids and Sex Workers in the New Economy*, London: Granta Books, 2003.

Elisha, D. S., 'Readers' Views: An Appeal to Health Visitors', *NJI*, vol. 73, no. 11, 1982, p. 298.

Engels, Dagmar, 'The Politics of Childbirth: British and Bengali Women in Contest, 1890–1930', in P. Robb (ed.), *Society and Ideology: Essays in South Asian History presented to Professor Kenneth Ballhatchet*, Delhi: Oxford University Press, 1993, pp. 222–46.

Farr, S. E., 'Improvements in the Provincial Nursing Service 1945–1946 of the United Provinces', *NJI*, vol. 38, no. 2, 1947, pp. 56–58.

Fitzgerald, Rosemary, 'A "Peculiar and Exceptional Measure": The Call for Women Medical Missionaries for India in the Later Nineteenth Century', in Robert A. Bickers and Rosemary Seton (eds), *Missionary Encounters: Sources and Issues*, Richmond: Curzon Press, 1996, pp. 174–96.

———, 'Rescue and Redemption: The Rise of Female Medical Missions in Colonial India During the late Nineteenth and early Twentieth Century', in Anne Marie Rafferty, Jane Robinson and Ruth Elkan (eds), *Nursing History and the Politics of Welfare*, London: Routledge, 1997, pp. 64–79.

———, '"Making and Moulding the Nursing of the Indian Empire": Recasting Nurses in Colonial India', in Avril Powell and Siobhan Lambert-Hurley (eds), *Rhetoric and Reality: Gender and the Colonial Experience in South Asia*, New Delhi: Oxford University Press, 2006.

Forbes, Geraldine, 'Managing Midwifery in India', in Dagmar Engels and Shula Marks (eds), *Contesting Colonial Hegemony: State and Society in Africa and India*, London: British Academic Press, 1994, pp. 152–72.

———, 'Medical Careers and Health Care for Indian Women: Patterns of Control', *Women's History Review*, vol. 3, no. 4, 1994, pp. 515–30.

———, *Women in Modern India*, Cambridge: Cambridge University Press, 1998.

———, *Women in Colonial India: Essays on Politics, Medicine and Historiography*, New Delhi: Chronicle Books, 2005.

———, 'Negotiating Modernities: The Public and Private Worlds of Dr Haimabati Sen', in Avril Powell and Siobhan Lambert-Hurley (eds), *Rhetoric and Reality: Gender and the Colonial Experience in South Asia*, New Delhi: Oxford University Press, 2006, pp. 223–46.

Foundation for Research in Community Health, 'Health Status of the Indian People: Supplementary Document to Health for All: An Alternative Strategy', 1987.

French, Francesca, *Miss Brown's Hospital: The Story of the Ludhiana Medical College and Dame Edith Brown, O.B.E. its Founder*, London: Hodder and Stoughton, 1954.

Gamarnikow, Eva, 'Sexual Division of Labour: The Case of Nursing', in Annette Kuhn and AnnMarie Wolpe (eds), *Feminism and Materialism: Women and Modes of Production*, London and Boston: Routledge and Kegan Paul, 1978.

Garvey, Anthony, 'Counting the Costs: The Irish Government is under Fire after a Recent Tragedy Revealed the Extent of the Funding Crisis in the Country's Nursing Services', *Nursing Standard*, vol. 17, no. 46, 2003, p. 12.

George, Sheba, *When Women Come First: Gender and Class in Transnational Migration*, Berkeley: University of California Press, 2005.

Goodrich, Annie, 'Letter to the Editor — Miss Goodrich's Honorary Membership', *NJI*, vol. 5, no. 3, 1914, p. 98.

Gourlay, Jharna, *Florence Nightingale and the Health of the Raj*, Aldershot, UK: Ashgate, 2003.

Government of Bombay, 'The Five-Year Plan for Bombay State (1951–52 to 1955–56)', Bombay: The Directorate of Publicity, Government of Bombay, 1953.

Government of India, 'Report of the Health Survey and Development Committee' (Bhore Report), New Delhi: Health Survey and Development Committee, 1946.

———, 'Development Schemes in the First Five Year Plan', New Delhi: Planning Commission, 1952.

———, 'First Five Year Plan', New Delhi: Planning Commission, 1952.

———, 'Pay Scales for Nursing Personnel as Recommended by the Fourth Central Pay Commission: Central Government, Union Territories and Armed Forces', vol. 77, no. 8, 1986, pp. 214–15.

———, *India: A Reference Annual*, New Delhi: Ministry of Information and Broadcasting, 1953–99.

———, 'Second Five Year Plan', New Delhi: Planning Commission of India, 1956.

———, 'Report of the Health Survey and Planning Committee' (Mudaliar Committee), New Delhi: Ministry of Health, 1961.

———, 'Third Five Year Plan', New Delhi: Planning Commission of India, 1961.

———, 'Fourth Five Year Plan, 1969–74', New Delhi: Planning Commission of India, 1970.

———, 'Draft Fifth Five Year Plan', New Delhi: Planning Commission, 1973–74.

Government of India, 'Draft Five Year Plan 1978–83', New Delhi, Planning Commission, 1978.

———, 'The Approach to the Seventh Five Year Plan 1985–90', New Delhi: Planning Commission of India, 1984.

———, 'Fourth Central Pay Commission Report', New Delhi: Ministry of Urban Development, 1986.

———, 'Health Information of India 2002', New Delhi: Central Bureau of Health Intelligence, 2004.

Government of Kerala, 'Report of the Third Kerala Pay Commission', Trivandrum: Government of Kerala, 1978.

Government of Madras (Education and Public Health Department), 'Order No. 3837 for the Reorganisation of the Provincial Nursing Service', *NJI*, vol. 30, no. 2, 1939, pp. 40–42.

Government of Rajasthan, 'Report of the Rajasthan Pay Commission', Jaipur: Government Central Press, 1981.

Government of Uttar Pradesh, 'Report of the Second U.P. Pay Commission', Allahabad: Government of Uttar Pradesh, 1980.

Grant, John B., *The Health of India*, London: Oxford University Press, 1943.

Griffin, Edris, 'Health Visitors' League', *NJI*, vol. 13, no. 8, 1922, pp. 194–95.

———, 'Health Visitors' Page', *NJI*, vol. 14, no. 2, 1923, pp. 48–49.

Gulati, Leela, 'Asian Women Workers in International Labour Migration: An Overview', in Anuja Agarwal (ed.), *Migrant Women and Work*, New Delhi: Sage Publications, 2006, pp. 46–72.

Haggis, Jane, 'White Women and Colonialism: Towards a Non-recuperative History', in Clare Midgley (ed.), *Gender and Imperialism*, Manchester and New York: Manchester University Press, 1998, pp. 45–78.

Hallam, Julia, 'From Angels to Handmaidens: Changing Constructions of Nursing's Public Image in Post-war Britain', *Nursing Inquiry*, vol. 5, 1998, pp. 32–42.

Harigovindan, Narayani, 'Employment of Women in the Medical Department of the Government of Travancore', Proceedings Volume, XIX Annual Session, South Indian History Congress, 1999.

Harnar, Ruth M., 'Social Forces and Factors Influencing Nursing Education in India', *NJI*, vol. 68, no. 3, 1976, pp. 54–58.

Harrison, Mark, *Public Health in British India: Anglo-Indian Preventive Medicine, 1859–1914*, Cambridge: Cambridge University Press, 1993.

Hart, Chris, *Nurses and Politics: The Impact of Power and Practice*, New York: Palgrave Macmillan, 2004.

Hartley, Diana, 'The First General Secretary Looks Back', *NJI*, vol. 69, no. 10, 1958, p. 336–38.

Hawthorne, Lesleyanne, 'The Globalisation of the Nursing Workforce: Barriers Confronting Overseas Qualified Nurses in Australia', *Nursing Inquiry*, vol. 8, no. 4, 2001, pp. 213–29.

Helmstadter, Carol, 'From the Private to the Public Sphere: The First Generation of Lady Nurses in England', *Nursing History Review*, vol. 9, 2001, pp. 127–40.

Hess, Gary R., 'The Role of American Philanthropic Foundations in India's Road to Globalization During the Cold War Era', in Soma Hewa and Darwin H. Stapleton (eds), *Globalization, Philanthropy and Civil Society: Toward a New Political Culture in the Twenty-First Century*, New York: Springer Science and Business Media, 2005, pp. 51–52.

Holkar, M. N., 'Letter to the Editor', *NJI*, vol. 66, no. 5, 1975, p. 107.

Indian Nursing Council, 'Syllabus and Regulations: Diploma in General Nursing and Midwifery', New Delhi: Indian Nursing Council, 2001.

———, *Guide for School of Nursing in India 2002*, New Delhi: Indian Nursing Council, 2002.

———, 'List of Schools of Nursing Recognised and Permitted to Admit Students for the Academic Year 2005–2006', New Delhi: Indian Nursing Council, 2005.

———, 'List of Colleges of Nursing for Basic B.Sc (N) Programme who are Permitted to Admit Students for the Academic Year 2005–2006', New Delhi: Indian Nursing Council, 2005.

International Council of Nurses, 'Learning to Investigate Nursing Problems', Report of an International Seminar on Research in Nursing, Oberoi Maidens Hotel, New Delhi, 14–28 February 1960.

Jaggi, O. P., *Western Medicine in India: Medical Education and Research*, Lucknow: Atma Ram, 1979.

Jain, Devaki, *Women's Quest for Power: Five Indian Case Studies*, Ghaziabad: Vikas Publishing House, 1980.

———, *Women, Development and the UN: A Sixty-year Quest for Equality and Justice*, Chesham: Indiana University Press, 2005.

Jeffery, Patricia, Roger Jeffery and Andrew Lyon, *Labour Pains and Labour Power: Women and Childbearing in India*, New Delhi: Manohar, 1989.

Jeffery, Roger, 'Allopathic Medicine in India a Case of Deprofessionalisation?', *Society, Science and Medicine*, vol. 11, 1977, pp. 561–73.

———, *The Politics of Health in India*, Berkeley: University of California Press, 1988.

———, 'Toward a Political Economy of Health Care: Comparisons of India and Pakistan', in Monica Das Gupta, Lincoln C. Chen and T. N. Krishnan (eds), *Health, Poverty and Development in India*, Delhi: Oxford University Press, 1996, pp. 270–94.

Jeffrey, Robin, 'Culture and Governments: How Women Made Kerala Literate', *Pacific Affairs*, vol. 60, no. 3, 1987, pp. 447–72.

———, *Politics, Women and Well-Being: How Kerala Became 'a Model'*, Houndmills and London: Macmillan, 1992.

———, 'Legacies of Matriliny: The Place of Women and the "Kerala Model"', *Pacific Affairs*, vol. 77, no. 4, 2004–5, pp. 647–64.

Joglekar, Kamal S., *Hospital Ward Management, Professional Adjustments and Trends in Nursing*, Bombay: Vora Medical Publications, 1990.

John, Mary E., 'Feminisms and Internationalisms: A Response from India', *Gender and History*, vol. 10, no. 3, 1998, pp. 539–48.

Jones, Margaret, 'Heroines of Lonely Outposts or Tools of the Empire? British Nurses in Britain's Model Colony: Ceylon, 1878–1948', *Nursing Inquiry*, vol. 11, no. 3, 2004, pp. 148–60.

Kalisch, Phillip A., and Beatrice J. Kalisch, *The Advance of American Nursing*, Boston: Little, Brown & Company, 1986.

Kamalamma, S., 'The Role of a Public Health Nurse in Family Planning Programme', *NJI*, vol. 59, no. 12, 1968, pp. 392–93, 397.

Kapadia, K. B., and R. K. Julius, 'Nurse Practitioner Programme', *NJI*, vol. 67, no. 7, 1976, pp. 173–74.

Kavadi, Shirish N., *The Rockefeller Foundation and Public Health in Colonial India 1916–1945: A Narrative History*, Pune and Mumbai: Foundation for Research in Community Health, 1999.

Kaviraj, Sudipta, 'Modernity and Politics in India', *Daedalus*, vol. 129, no. 1, 2000, pp. 137–62.

Kermode, Michelle. 'Safer Injections, Fewer Infections: Management of Needles and Sharps and Occupational Blood Exposure in Rural North Indian Health Settings', Unpublished PhD Dissertation, University of Melbourne, 2004.

Khaparde, Saroj, 'Meeting the Needs of the Community', *Social Welfare*, vol. 35, no. 10, 1989, p. 6.

Kilgour, John L., 'Foreign Medical Graduates in the United Kingdom', in John Z. Bowers and Professor Lord Rosenheim (eds), *Migration of Medical Manpower: Papers from an International Macy Conference*, New York: The Josiah Macy, Jr. Foundation, 1971, pp. 1–8.

Kingma, Mireille, *Nurses on the Move: Migration and the Global Health Economy*, New York: Cornell University Press, 2005.

Kisku, A. K., 'Nursing Education Needs Change', *NJI*, vol. 64, no. 12, 1973, pp. 409, 412.

Krishna Raj, Maithreyi, 'Why Women's Studies? Some Feminist Perspectives', *Women's Studies in India: Some Perspectives*, Bombay: Popular Prakashan, 1986, pp. 34–41.

Kumar, Deepak (ed.), *Disease and Medicine in India: A Historical Overview*, New Delhi: Tulika, 2001.

Kurian, Aleyamma, 'Study of the Implementation Phase of a Curriculum Change in Christian Schools of Nursing of South India', Unpublished PhD Dissertation, Teachers College, Columbia University, New York, 1976.

———, 'The "2 + 1" Nursing Curriculum: An Evaluation', *NJI*, vol. 73, no. 10, 1982, pp. 260–61.

Kurien, Prema, *Kaleidoscopic Ethnicity: International Migration and the Reconstruction of Community Identities in India*, New Brunswick, NJ: Rutgers University Press, 2002.

Kurup, C. P. B., 'Nurses' Role in Health Care Policies', *NJI*, vol. 77, no. 11, 1986, pp. 283–85.

Kuruvilla, Aleyamma, 'Letter from Miss A. Kuruvilla', in *College of Nursing, Christian Medical College and Hospital: Golden Jubilee Souvenir 1946–1996*, Vellore: College of Nursing, Christian Medical College, 1996.

Kuruvilla, Joseph, 'Occupational Stress in Nursing', *Social Welfare*, March 1989.

Lakshmi Devi, Kumari, 'United We Stand', *NJI*, vol. 41, no. 10, October 1950, pp. 264–65.

———, 'The Fruits of Freedom', *NJI*, vol. 44, no. 8, 1953, pp. 187–88.

Lal, Maneesha, 'The Politics of Gender and Medicine in Colonial India: The Countess of Dufferin's Fund, 1885–1888', *Bulletin of the History of Medicine*, vol. 68, no. 1, 1994, pp. 29–66.

———, '"The Ignorance of Women is the House of Illness": Gender, Nationalism and Health Reform in Colonial North India', in M. Sutphen and B. Andrews (eds), *Medicine and Colonial Identity*, London: Routledge, 2003, pp. 14–40.

Lang, Sean, 'Saving India Through its Women', *History Today*, vol. 55, no. 9, September 2005, pp. 46–51.

———, 'Drop the Demon *Dai*: Maternal Mortality and the State in Colonial Madras, 1840–1875'. *Social History of Medicine*, vol. 18, 2005, pp. 357–78.

Lazarus, Hilda, 'Countess of Dufferin's Fund: Women's Medical Service News', *Journal of the Association of Medical Women in India*, vol. 32, no. 2, 1944, p. 68.

———, *Our Nursing Services*, Aundh: Aundh Pub. Trust, for the All India Women's Conference, 1945.

Lee, Marilyn B. and Ismat Saeed, 'Oppression and Horizontal Violence: The Case of Nurses in Pakistan', *Nursing Forum*, vol. 36, no. 1, 2001.

Leslie, Julia, and Dominik Wujastyk, 'The Doctor's Assistant: Nursing in Ancient Indian Medical Texts', in Pat Holden and Jenny Littlewood (eds), *Anthropology and Nursing*, London: Routledge, 1991, pp. 25–30.

Loch, Catharine Grace, *Catharine Grace Loch, Royal Red Cross, Senior Lady Superintendent, Queen Alexandra's Military Nursing Service for India: A Memoir (With an Introduction by Field-Marshal The Earl Roberts V.C., K.G., O.M.)*, London: Henry Frowde, 1905.

Lynaugh, Joan E., 'From Chaos to Transformation', in Barbara L. Brush, Joan E. Lynaugh, Geertje Boschma, Anne Marie Rafferty, Meryn Stuart, and Nancy J. Tomes (eds), *Nurses of All Nations: A History of the International Council of Nurses, 1899–1999*, Philadelphia: Lippincott, 1999, pp. 111–42.

Mackenzie, Lorna S., 'Letter to the Editor', *NJI*, vol. 7, no. 10, 1916, pp. 206–7.

Malik, Harji, 'Planning for Nursing Services — A Must: A Report on a Workshop', *NJI*, vol. 59, no. 7, 1968, pp. 206–7, 226.

Mani, Lata, *Contentious Traditions: The Debate on Sati in Colonial India*, Berkeley: University of California Press, 1998.

Manntaraveetil Lakshmy Amma, 'An Account of My Life and My Home-Making', in J. Devika (ed.), *Her-Self: Gender and Early Writings of Malayalee Women*, Kolkata: Stree, 2005, pp. 10–21.

Manocha, Lalita, 'Challenges for Nursing Profession: A Retrospection', in TNAI, *Indian Nursing Year Book 1996–97*, New Delhi: TNAI, 1997, pp. 113–16.

Marks, Shula, *Divided Sisterhood: Race, Class and Gender in the South African Nursing Profession*, London: Macmillan, 1994.

———, 'What is Colonial about Colonial Medicine? And what has Happened to Imperialism and Health?', *Social History of Medicine*, vol. 10, no. 2, 1997.

Marsiljie, Lois M., Vera K. Pitman, Ann Jansma Zwemer, and K. V. Annamma, *A New Textbook for Nurses in India: The Foundations of Nursing*, vol. 1, Madras: B. I. Publications, 1986.

Mathew, George, 'Fair Deal to Nurses', *NJI*, vol. 63, no. 12, 1972, p. 401.

Mayo, Katherine, *Mother India*, London: Butler and Tanner, 1927.

McMenamin, Dorothy, 'Identifying Domiciled Europeans in Colonial India: Poor Whites or Privileged Community?', *New Zealand Journal of Asian Studies*, vol. 3, no. 1, 2001.

Meadows, Sandra, Ros Levenson and Juan Baeza, *The Last Straw: Explaining the Nursing Shortage*, London: King's Fund, 2000.

Mehan, Nirmala, J. P. Gupta, and R. S. Gupta, 'Development of Nursing Education in India', *Health and Population*, vol. 15, nos. 3–4, 1992, pp. 125–32.

Mehta, Jivraj Narayan, 'Medical Services in India (The Sir George Birdwood Memorial Lecture)', *Journal of the Royal Society of Arts*, vol. 113, no. 5112, 1965.

Mejia, A., H. Pizurki and E. Royston, *Physician and Nurse Migration: Analysis and Policy Implications*, World Health Organization, 1979.

Melosh, Barbara, *'The Physician's Hand': Work Culture and Conflict in American Nursing*, Philadelphia: Temple University Press, 1982.

Mill, C. R., 'Some Advantages of Joining the "Trained Nurses' Association of India"', *NJI*, vol. 97, no. 2, 2006 [1910].

Ministry of Health and Family Welfare, 'Annual Reports, 1976–2006', New Delhi: Government of India.

Mohan, N. Shantha, *Status of Nurses in India*, New Delhi: Uppal Publishing House, 1985.

Moore, Judith, *A Zeal for Responsibility: The Struggle for Professional Nursing in Victorian England, 1868–1883*, Athens: University of Georgia Press, 1988.

Mudaliar, A. Lakshmanaswami, *Collected Speeches of Dr. A. Lakshmanaswami Mudaliar, Vice-Chancellor, University of Madras*, Madras: The Dr A. L. Mudaliar 71st Birthday Celebration Committee, 1957.

Mulholland, Helene, 'Plan to Train Indian Nurses as RMNs then bring them to UK', *Nursing Times*, vol. 99, no. 25, p. 4.

Nagpal, Narender, 'Workshop on Trends in Health Care System and its Implications for Nursing', *NJI*, vol. 66, no. 5, 1975, p. 103.

———, 'It's not all Green on the Other Side of the Hedge', *NJI*, vol. 67, no. 7, 1976, pp. 160–62.

———, 'Why Blame the Nurse?', *NJI*, vol. 67, no. 7, 1976, p. 153.

———, 'The Healing Hands', *NJI*, vol. 67, no. 3, 1976, p. 1.

———, 'It's Never Too Late', *NJI*, vol. 67, no. 9, 1976, p. 209.

———, The Joint Conference', *NJI*, vol. 73, no. 9, 1982, p. 229.

———, 'Was the Strike Worthwhile?', *NJI*, vol. 57, no. 3, 1987, p. 57.

———, 'The High Power Committee', *NJI*, vol. 78, no. 10, 1987, p. 253.

———, 'End of an Agitation', *NJI*, vol. 81, no. 3, 1990, p. 73.

———, 'Development of Nursing and Health Care: 1947–2000', in *History and Trends in Nursing in India*, New Delhi: TNAI, 2001.

Nair, K. Rajasekharan, *Evolution of Modern Medicine in Kerala*, Thiruvananthapuram: Published by Mrs T. Indira Nair, Medical College, Trivandrum.

Nair, Sreelekha and Madelaine Healey, 'A Profession on the Margins: Status Issues in Indian Nursing', Occasional Paper, Centre for Women in Developing Societies, 2006.

Nair, Sreelekha and Marie Percot, 'Transcending Boundaries: Indian Nurses in Internal and International Migration', Occasional Paper, Centre for Women in Developing Societies, New Delhi, 2007.

Nandi, Proshanta K. and Charles P. Loomis, 'Professionalization of Nursing in India: Deterring and Facilitating Aspects of Culture', *Journal of Asian and African Studies*, vol. 9, nos. 1–2, 1977, pp. 43–59.

Naraindas, V., 'Family Planning and Public Health', *NJI*, vol. 59, no. 5, 1968, pp. 149, 151.

Nelson, Sioban, *Say Little, Do Much: Nurses, Nuns and Hospitals in the Nineteenth Century*, Philadelphia: University of Pennsylvania Press, 2001.

Noordyk, Wilhelmina, 'Conferences of Other Days', *NJI*, vol. 49, no. 10, 1958, pp. 339–40.

Oishi, Nana, *Women in Motion: Globalization, State Policies and Labor Migration in Asia*, Stanford, California: Stanford University Press, 2005.

Oommen, T. K., *Doctors and Nurses: A Study in Occupational Role Structures*, Delhi: Macmillan, 1978.

Oonnie, C., 'Nursing Students of the 70's', *NJI*, vol. 64, no. 12, 1973, pp. 410–12.

Packard, Randall, 'Malaria Dreams: Postwar Visions of Health and Development in the Third World', *Medical Anthropology*, vol. 17, 1997, pp. 279–96.

———, 'Postcolonial Medicine', in R. Cooter and J. Pickstone (eds), *Medicine in the Twentieth Century*, Amsterdam: Rodopi, 2000.

Percot, Marie, 'Indian Nurses in the Gulf: Two Generations of Female Migration', *South Asia Research*, vol. 26, no. 1, 2006, pp. 41–62.

———, 'Indian Nurses in the Gulf: From Job Opportunity to Life Strategy', in Anuja Agarwal (ed.), *Migrant Women and Work*, New Delhi: Sage Publications, 2006, pp. 155–76.

Philip, M., 'Secretary's Report', *NJI*, vol. 63, no. 12, 1972, pp. 412–13.

Planning Commission of India, *Draft Fifth Five Year Plan 1974–79*, vol. 2, New Delhi: Government of India, 1973–74.

Powar, J. D., 'Nursing Functions and Law in India', *NJI*, vol. 66, no. 1, 1975, p. 4.

Powell, Avril and Siobhan Lambert-Hurley (eds), *Rhetoric and Reality: Gender and the Colonial Experience in South Asia*, New Delhi: Oxford University Press, 2006.

Purohit, V. B., S. G. Nitsure and A. Gunian, 'Nurses' Strike', *NJI*, vol. 61, no. 12, 1970, p. 412.

Qadeer, Imrana, 'The World Development Report 1993: The Brave New World of Primary Health Care', in Mohan Rao (ed.), *Disinvesting in Health: The World Bank's Prescriptions for Health*, New Delhi: Sage Publications, 1999.

Rafferty, Anne Marie, 'Internationalising Nursing Education during the Interwar Period', in Paul Weindling (ed.), *International Health Organisations and Movements, 1918–1939*, Cambridge: Cambridge University Press, 1995, pp. 266–82.

Rafferty, Anne Marie and Geertje Boschma, 'The Essential Idea', in Barbara Brush, Joan E. Lynaugh, Geertje Boschma, Meryn Stuart, Anne Marie Rafferty and Nancy J. Tomes (eds), *Nurses of All Nations: A History of the International Council of Nurses, 1899–1999*, Philadelphia: Lippincott, 1999.

Raghavachari, Ranjana, *Conflicts and Adjustments: Indian Nurses in an Urban Milieu*, New Delhi: Academic Foundation, 1990.

Rai, Shirin M., 'Women and the State in the Third World: Some Issues for Debate', in Shirin M. Rai and Geraldine Lievesley (eds), *Women and the State: International Perspectives*, London: Taylor and Francis, 1996, pp. 5–22.

Rajalakshmi, T. K., 'Birth Control in Disguise', *Frontline*, 11 February 2005, pp. 81–82.

Rajan, Rajeswari Sunder, *Real and Imagined Women: Gender, Culture and Postcolonialism*, London: Routledge, 1993.

———, *The Scandal of the State: Women, Law, and Citizenship in Postcolonial India*, Durham: Duke University Press, 2003.

Rajkumari Amrit Kaur, *Rajkumari Amrit Kaur*, New Delhi: Lok Sabha Secretariat, 1992.

Ramanamma, A., and Usha Bambawale, 'Occupational Attitudes of Nurses: A Sociological Study', *The Journal of Sociological Studies*, January 1984, pp. 82–94.

Ramanna, Mridula, *Western Medicine and Public Health in Colonial Bombay, 1845–1895*, London: Sangam Books, 2002.

Ramasubban, Radhika, *Public Health and Medical Research in India: Their Origins and Development under the Impact of British Colonial Policy*, Stockholm: Swedish International Development Cooperation Agency's Department for Research Cooperation (SAREC), 1982.

———, 'Imperial Health in British India, 1857–1900', in R. McLeod and M. Lewis (eds), *Disease, Medicine and Empire: Perspectives on Western Medicine and the Experience of European Expansion*, London: Routledge, 1988, pp. 38–60.

Ramusack, Barbara, 'Embattled Advocates: The Debate over Birth Control in India, 1920–40', *Journal of Women's History*, vol. 1, no. 2, 1989, pp. 34–64.

———, 'Cultural Missionaries, Maternal Imperialists, Feminist Allies: British Women Activists in India, 1865–1945', *Women's Studies International Forum*, vol. 13, no. 4, 1990, pp. 309–21.

Rao, Kasturi Sundar, *An Introduction to Community Health Nursing (with Special Reference to India)*, Chennai: B. I. Publications, 1997.

Ray, Bharati (ed.), *From the Seams of History: Essays on Indian Women*, Delhi: Oxford University Press, 1995.

Regunathan, Sudhamahi, 'Nurses don't Wear Short Frocks and Kiss Doctors', *The Times of India*, 20 January 1996, p. 11.

Rist, Gilbert, *The History of Development: From Western Origins to Global Faith*, London: Zed Books, 1997.

Rosenberg, Charles E., *The Care of Strangers: The Rise of America's Hospital System*, Baltimore and London: The John Hopkins University Press, 1987.

Roy, Anupama and Sadhna Arya, 'When Poor Women Migrate: Unravelling Issues and Concerns', in Anupama Roy and Sadhna Arya (eds), *Poverty, Gender and Migration*, London: Sage Publications, 2006, pp. 19–48.

Roy, W. T., 'Hostages to Fortune (A Socio-political Study of the Anglo-Indian Remnant in India)', *Plural Societies*, no. 2, 1974, pp. 55–63.

Sakaria, T. T., and A. K. Gupta, 'Plight of Nurses', *Hindustan Times*, 25 January 1987.

Samuel, S. A., *Guide for School of Nursing in India*, New Delhi: Indian Nursing Council, 2002.

Sangari, Kumkum and Sudesh Vaid (eds), *Recasting Women, Essays in Colonial History*, New Delhi: Kali for Women, 1989.

Sapra, U., 'Punjab Nurses', *NJI*, vol. 63, no. 10, 1972, p. 363.

Saradamoni, Kunjulekshmi, *Matriliny Transformed: Family, Law and Ideology in Twentieth Century Travancore*, New Delhi: Sage Publications, 1999.

Saramma K. U., 'The Sad Plight of Nurses', *NJI*, vol. 62, no. 1, 1971, p. 29.

Saramma K. V., Letter to the Editor, *NJI*, vol. 66, no. 5, 1975, p. 107.

Sarkar, Tanika, *Hindu Wife, Hindu Nation: Community, Religion and Cultural Nationalism*, Delhi: Permanent Black, 2001.

Satyamurthy, T. V., 'Impact of Centre-State Relations on Indian Politics: An Interpretative Reckoning 1947–1987', in Partha Chatterjee (ed.), *State and Politics in India*, Oxford: Oxford University Press, 1997, p. 232–70.

Schlotfeldt, Rozella M., 'Structuring Nursing Knowledge: A Priority for Creating Nursing's Future', in Linda C. Andrist, Patrice K. Nicholas and Karen A. Wolf (eds), *A History of Nursing Ideas*, Sudbury, MA: Jones and Bartlett, 2006, pp. 287–91.

Schroeder, Yvonne, 'Post-Basic Nursing Education: Principles of Administration as Applied to Advanced Programmes in Nursing Education', vol. 1, London: International Council of Nurses, 1957.

Sengupta, Maya, 'Letter to the Editor', *NJI*, vol. 66, no. 4, 1975, p. 79.

Shiva Kumar, A. K., 'Budgeting for Health: Some Considerations', *Economic and Political Weekly*, vol. 40, no. 14, 2 April 2005, pp. 1391–96.

Singer, Milton, 'Introduction: The Modernization of Occupational Cultures in South Asia', in Milton Singer (ed.), *Entrepreneurship and Modernization of Occupational Cultures in South Asia*, Durham, NC: Duke University, 1973, pp. 1–15.

Singh, R. N., 'In Memoriam', *NJI*, vol. 66, no. 4, 1975.

St Stephen's Hospital, 'St Stephen's Hospital Souvenir: Issued on the Occasion of the Foundation Stone Laying Ceremony of the New Building by Shri V. V. Giri, President of India, On Sunday the 13th February', Delhi, 1972.

Stephens, T., 'TNAI in Uttar Pradesh', *NJI*, vol. 73, no. 8, 1982, pp. 216–18.

———, 'Point–Counter-Point: Socio-Economic Background of Nurses in a Hospital Organization', *NJI*, vol. 81, no. 7, 1990.

Stuart, Meryn and Geertje Boschma, 'Seeking Stability in the Midst of Change', in B. L. Brush and J. E. Lynaugh (eds), *Nurses of All Nations*, Philadelphia: Lippincott, 1999, pp. 71–110.

Summers, Anne, *Angels and Citizens: British Women as Military Nurses 1854–1914*, London and New York: Routledge and Kegan Paul, 1988.

Takahashi, Aya, *The Development of the Japanese Nursing Profession: Adopting and Adapting Western Influences*, London: Routledge Curzon, 2004.

Thacker, M., 'Editorial', *NJI*, vol. 13, no. 4, 1922, p. 74.

———, 'Annual Conference', *NJI*, vol. 14, no. 1, 1923, p. 100.

Thapan, Meenakshi, 'Series Introduction', in A. Agrawal (ed.), *Migrant Women and Work*, New Delhi/Thousand Oaks/London: Sage Publications, 2006, p. 9.

The Marchioness of Linlithgow, 'The School of Nursing Administration, New Delhi', *NJI*, vol. 31, no. 2, 1943, pp. 71–72.

Thomas, K., 'Report of the Health Visitors' League', *NJI*, vol. 51, no. 11, 1960, p. 311.

Thresyamma, C. P., *Fundamentals of Nursing: Procedure Manual for General Nursing and Midwifery Course*, New Delhi: Jaypee Brothers, 2002.

Tilak, Sindhu, 'Letter to the Editor', *NJI*, vol. 66, no. 3, 1975, p. 58.

———, 'Readers' Views: Nursing and the Role of the TNAI', *NJI*, vol. 73, no. 12, 1982, p. 314.

Tomkinson, E. M., 'The Work of the "Association for Moral and Social Hygiene"', *NJI*, vol. 30, no. 2, 1939, pp. 52–57.

Tooley, Sarah A., *The History of Nursing in the British Empire*, London: S. H. Bousfield & Co., 1906.

Trained Nurses' Association of India, *Indian Nursing Year Book 1986–87*, New Delhi, 1987.

———, *Indian Nursing Year Book 1990–92*, New Delhi, 1992.

———, *Indian Nursing Year Book 1996–97*, New Delhi, 1997.

———, *Indian Nursing Year Book 1998–1999*, New Delhi, 1999.

———, *Indian Nursing Year Book 2000–2001*, New Delhi, 2001.

———, *Indian Nursing Year Book 2002–2004*, New Delhi, 2004.

———, 'Resolution passed by the Members of the Trained Nurses' Association of India assembled at Conference and forwarded to The Hon. Mr Rajagopalachariar, The Hon. Dr Rajan and the Surgeon-General with the Government of Madras on November 11th, 1938', *NJI*, vol. 30, no. 2, 1939, pp. 42–43.

Vaughan, Megan, *Curing Their Ills: Colonial Power and African Illness*, Cambridge: Polity Press, 1991.

Varkey, Simmy M., 'Immigration of Nurses: Problems, Prospects and Challenges', *NJI*, vol. 97, no. 7, 2006, pp. 258–60.

Venkataachalam, Radha and Krishna G. Seshadri, 'Think Health, Think India: A Few Fast Measures will see the Corporate Indian Healthcare Industry Continue to Rise', *Business India*, 12–25 April 2004, Health Supplement, pp. 93–94.

Virani, Pinki, *Aruna's Story: The True Account of a Rape and its Aftermath*, New York and New Delhi: Viking, 1998.

Walsh, Judith E., *Domesticity in Colonial India: What Women Learned When Men Gave Them Advice*, Lanham: Rowman and Littlefield, 2004.

Wasi, Muriel, 'Trends and Priorities: Training for Leadership', in Muriel Wasi (ed.), *The Educated Woman in Indian Society*, Bombay and New Delhi: Tata McGraw Hill, 1971, pp. 163–75.

Watts, Ethel A., *The Handbook of the Trained Nurses' Association of India*, Madras: Trained Nurses' Association of India, 1931.

———, 'The Years That Have Passed', *NJI*, vol. 49, no. 10, 1958, pp. 333–34.

White, Catherine E., 'Letter to the Editor', *NJI*, vol. 42, no. 4, 1951, p. 100.

Wilkinson, Alice, *A Brief History of Nursing in India and Pakistan*, Delhi: TNAI, 1958.

Witz, Anne, 'The Challenge of Nursing', in Jonathan Gabe, David Kelleher and Gareth Williams (eds), *Challenging Medicine*, London: Routledge, 1994, pp. 23–45.

Wolf, Karen A., The Slow March to Professional Practice', in Linda C. Andrist, Patrice K. Nicholas and Karen A. Wolf (eds), *A History of Nursing Ideas*, Sudbury, MA: Jones and Bartlett, 2006, pp. 305–18.

World Health Organization (WHO), 'Postbasic Nursing Education Programmes for Foreign Students: Report of a Conference, Geneva, 5–14 October 1959', World Health Organization Technical Reports Series 199, Geneva: WHO, 1960.

———, 'WHO Expert Committee on Nursing: Fifth Report', Geneva: WHO, 1966.

———, 'Efforts Under Way to Stem "Brain Drain of Doctors and Nurses"', *Bulletin of the World Health Organization*, vol. 83, no. 2, 2005, p. 85.

Young, Ken, 'Globalization and the Changing Management of Migrating Service Workers in the Asia-Pacific', in Kevin Hewison and Ken Young (eds), *Transnational Migration and Work in Asia*, Abingdon and New York: Routledge, 2006, pp. 15–36.

Yrjala, Ann, *Public Health and Rockefeller Wealth: Alliance Strategies in the Early Formation of Finnish Public Health Nursing*, Tavastg: Abo Akademi University Press, 2005.

Zachariah, Alice, 'News from the States: Andhra Pradesh', *NJI*, vol. 50, no. 8, 1959, pp. 273–74.

———, 'Wanted, a Criteria', *NJI*, vol. 62, no. 2, 1971, p. 63.

———, 'A Tribute to a Departed Friend', *NJI*, vol. 66, no. 5, 1975, p. 107.

Zachariah, K.C., E. T. Mathew and S. Irudaya Rajan, *Dynamics of Migration in Kerala: Dimensions, Differentials and Consequences*, Hyderabad: Orient Longman, 2003.

Zwemer, Ann, 'Letter to the Editor: Volunteer Service in Hospitals', *NJI*, vol. 62, no. 7, 1971, p. 237.

## Internet Sources

Academy for Nursing Studies, Hyderabad, 'Situational Analysis of Public Health Nursing Personnel in India: Based on National Review and Consultation in Six States', Conducted for Training Division, Ministry of Health and Family Welfare, Government of India, with support from UNFPA India (the UN Population Fund), 2005, http://www.whoindia. org/Linkfiles/HSD_Resources_Situation_Analysis_of_Public_Health_ Nursing_Personnel.pdf (accessed 3 January 2007).

Amrita Institute of Medical Sciences School of Nursing, http://www.aims. amrita.edu/school-of-nursing/nursing-home.php (accessed 12 March 2013).

Anonymous, 'Rebirth for Aruna, say Joyous Mumbai Hospital Staff', *Deccan Herald*, 7 March 2011, http://www.deccanherald.com/content/143798/ rebirth-aruna-say-joyous-mumbai.html (accessed 25 February 2012).

———, 'On Rape Judgment Day, Court to Victim: He wants to Marry you', *Express India*, 3 May 2005, http://cities.expressindia.com/fullstory. php?newsid=127644 (accessed 6 May 2005).

———, 'Nursing Admissions: Male Aspirants' Quota "Meagre"', *The Hindu*, 18 August 2005, http://www.hindu.com/2005/08/18/stories/2005081 821070300.htm (accessed 30 January 2006).

———, 'Nurses, Technicians join Anti-OPD Chorus', *Chandigarh Tribune*, Online Edition, 28 November 2002, http://www.tribuneindia. com/2002/20021129/cth3.htm (accessed 26 July 2006).

———, 'Nurses go West', *The Times of India*, 19 January 2005, City Supplement, Mumbai, http://timesofindia.indiatimes.com/articleshow/995616. cms (accessed 15 January 2005).

———, 'Nurses who don't even know how to Pick a Vein', *The Hindu*, 15 October 2004, http://www.hindu.com/2004/10/15/stories/200410151 4410300.htm (accessed 3 August 2006).

———, 'Delhi Rape Case: JMS Stages Angry Demo against Hospital', *People's Democracy*, vol. 27, no. 39, 28 September 2003, http://pd. cpim.org/2003/0928/09282003_delhipercent20jms.htm (accessed 9 July 2005).

———, 'Directive to Complete Probe in Rape Case', *The Hindu*, Kochi edition, 10 January 2006, http://www.thehindu.com/2006/01/10/stories/ 2006011007090500.htm (accessed 12 January 2006).

Anonymous, 'Delhi Hospital Ward Boy gets Life Sentence for Rape', *Outlook India*, 4 May 2005, http://www.outlookindia.com/pti_news. asp?id=295969 (accessed 6 May 2005).

———, 'Florence Nightingale Anniversary: Nurses Air their Grievances', *The Tribune*, Chandigarh, 13 May 2004, http://www.tribuneindia.com/ 2004/20040513/ncr3.htm (accessed 14 April 2012).

———, 'India Exporting Nurses to UK and US', *The Guardian*, 23 September 2004, available at the India Resource Center website, http://www. indiaresource.org/news/2004/1037.html (accessed 1 September 2006).

———, 'Shanti Mukund Rape Victim declines Convict's Marriage Proposal', *Hindustan Times*, 4 May 2005, http://www.hindustantimes.com/news/ 181_1347603,000600010001.htm (accessed 12 May 2005).

———, 'Supporting UK nurses — band 5 nurses to be taken off the Home Office shortage occupation list', UK Department of Health Press Release, 3 July 2006, http://www.gnn.gov.uk/environment/fullDetail.asp?Rele aseID=211686&NewsAreaID=2&NavigatedFromDepartment=False (accessed 24 July 2006).

Beary, Habib, 'Indian Nurses' American Dream', BBC News Online: International Version, 1 September 2003, http://news.bbc.co.uk/2/hi/ health/3191525.stm (accessed 15 December 2005).

Buchan, James, 'International Recruitment of Nurses: United Kingdom Case Study', London: Royal College of Nursing, 2002, http://www. rcn.org.uk/publications/pdf/irn-case-study-booklet.pdf (accessed 22 May 2006).

———, 'Here to Stay? International nurses in the UK', London: Royal College of Nursing, 2003, http://www.rcn.org.uk/publications/pdf/heretostay-irns.pdf (accessed 20 July 2006).

Buchan, James and Delanyo Dovlo, 'International Recruitment of Health Workers to the UK: A Report for DFID', February 2004, http://www. equinetafrica.org/bibl/docs/BUChres310108.pdf (accessed 27 May 2013).

Buchan, James and Ian Seccombe, 'Worlds Apart? The UK and International Nurses', London: Royal College of Nursing, April 2006, http://www. rcn.org.uk (accessed 25 August 2006).

Center for Nursing Advocacy, 'Go West, Young Nurse?', 2005, http:// www.nursingadvocacy.org/news/archives/2005/jan.html (accessed 26 July 2006).

———, 'Could Shortage-Driven Migration change Nursing's Gender Gap?, http://www.nursingadvocacy.org/news/2005aug/23_new_kerala.html (accessed 5 June 2006).

Commission on Graduates of Foreign Nursing Schools (CGFNS) website, http://www.cgfns.org (accessed 7 August 2006).

Commonwealth Secretariat, 'Companion Document to the Commonwealth Code of Practice for the International Recruitment of Health Workers', London, 2003, http://www.thecommonwealth.org/Internal/34044/ codes_of_practice/ (accessed 26 July 2006).

Das, Joy and Moumita Ghosh, 'The Main Attraction: Hefty Salaries', *The Hindu*, 22 November 2004, Education Plus, Karnataka, http://www. hinduonnet.com/edu/2004/11/22/stories/2004112200250400.htm (accessed 19 January 2006).

Dasgupta, Debarshi, 'Nursing High Hopes', *The Hindu*, 31 July 2003, http://www.thehindu.com/thehindu/mp/2003/07/31/stories/2003073 100250100.htm (accessed 15 November 2004).

Dogra, Sapna, 'Delhi Nurses' Union seeks Rs.10 Lakh Compensation for Rape Victim', *Express Healthcare Management*, 1–15 October 2003, http://www.expresshealthcaremgmt.com/20031015/hospinews02.shtml (accessed 27 November 2006).

———, 'Delhi has a Long Way to Go in Ensuring Security of Nurses', *Express Healthcare Management*, 16–31 January 2004, http://www.express healthcaremgmt.com/20040131/nursingspecial02.shtml (accessed 27 November 2006).

Doraisamy, Vani, 'Global Demand for Trained Indian Nurses Skyrocketing', *The Hindu*, Chennai, 20 September 2005, http://www.hindu.com/ 2005/09/20/stories/2005092015530500.htm (accessed 10 August 2006).

Falaknaaz, Syed, 'India Faces Acute Shortage of Teaching Staff in Nursing Colleges', *Express Healthcare Management*, 1–15 December 2003, http://www.expresshealthcaremgmt.com/20031215/focus01.shtml (accessed 20 February 2005).

Government of India, 'Fifth Five Year Plan', New Delhi: Planning Commission of India, 1976, http://planningcommission.nic.in/plans/planrel/ fiveyr/welcome.html (accessed 10 June 2006).

———, 'Sixth Five Year Plan', New Delhi: Planning Commission of India, 1981?, http://planningcommission.nic.in/plans/planrel/fiveyr/default. html (accessed 24 October 2006).

———, 'Seventh Five Year Plan', vol. 2, New Delhi: Planning Commission of India, 1985, http://planningcommission.nic.in/plans/planrel/fiveyr/ default.html (accessed 24 October 2006).

———, 'Eighth Five Year Plan', vol. 2, New Delhi: Planning Commission of India, 1992, http://planningcommission.nic.in/plans/planrel/fiveyr/ default.html (accessed 25 October 2006).

———, 'Ninth Five Year Plan', vol. 2, New Delhi: Planning Commission of India, 1997, http://planningcommission.nic.in/plans/planrel/fiveyr/ default.html (accessed 25 October 2006).

Government of India, 'Tenth Five Year Plan (2002–2007)', New Delhi: Planning Commission of India, 2002, http://planningcommission.nic. in/plans/planrel/ fiveyr/default.html (accessed 25 October 2006).

————, 'National Rural Health Mission', New Delhi: Ministry of Health and Family Welfare, 2005, http://mohfw.nic.in/nrhm.html (accessed 14 November 2006).

Gupta, Anu, Bharti Roy Choudhury and Indira Balachandran, 'Women's Beliefs about Disease and Health', 1997, http://www.hsph.harvard.edu/ grhf/SAsia/suchana/1299/rh402.html (accessed 30 January 2007).

International Council of Nurses, 'Nurse:Patient Ratios', ICN *Nursing Matters* Fact Sheet, 2003, http://www.icn.ch/matters_rnptratio_print.htm (accessed 21 September 2006).

Jacob, Satish, 'Delhi's Nurses want Strike to Spread', BBC News Online, 10 May 1998, http://newsrss.bbc.co.uk/2/low/world/s/w_asia/90516. stm (accessed 12 April 2012).

Jolly, Susie, Emma Bell and Lata Narayanswamy, 'Gender and Migration in Asia: Overview and Annotated Bibliography', BRIDGE, Institute of Development Studies, University of Sussex, http://www.bridge.ids.ac.uk/ reports_gend_sect.htm (accessed 26 March 2006).

Kalita, Purba, 'Nursing System in Poor Health', *The Times of India*, 9 September 2003, http://timesofindia.indiatimes.com/cms.dll/html/ uncomp/articleshow?msid=174084 (accessed 3 March 2004).

Khadria, Binod, 'International Nurse Recruitment in India', *Health Services Research*, vol. 42, no. 3, Part II, 2007, p. 6, http://www.blackwell-synergy.com/doi/abs/10.1111/j.1475-6773.2007.00718.x (accessed 14 April 2012).

Limb, Julia, 'Foreign Nurses Exploited, Union says', 19 October 2005, The World Today, ABC Radio, http://www.abc.net.au/worldtoday/content/ 2005/s1485986.htm (accessed 26 July 2006).

Malone, Beverly, 'Government Targeting of Overseas Nurses Beggars Belief, says RCN', 3 July 2006, http://www.rcn.org.uk/news/mediadisplay.php? ID=2067&area=Press (accessed 20 July 2006).

McVeigh, Tracy, 'Nurse Exodus leaves Kenya in Crisis', *The Observer*, 21 May 2006, http://observer.guardian.co.uk/world/story/0,,1779773,00. html (accessed 15 August 2006).

Ministry of Health and Family Welfare, 'Annual Report 2001–2002', New Delhi: Government of India, 2002?, http://mohfw.nic.in/reports/Annual percent20Reportpercent202000-01.pdf/Partpercent20-I-6.pdf (accessed 6 May 2004).

Ministry of Overseas Indian Affairs, http://moia.gov.in (accessed 3 August 2006).

————, 'State Nodal Officers for Matter Related to Overseas Indians', Ministry of Overseas Indian Affairs, http://moia.gov.in/showinfo1. asp?linkid=315 (accessed 3 August 2006).

Ministry of Overseas Indian Affairs, *Annual Report 2006*, New Delhi: Government of India, 2006, http://moia.gov.in/showsublinklevel2. asp?sublink2id=187 (accessed 3 August 2006).

Naeem Mohaimen, 'The Other NRIs Come to India', *The Subcontinental*, 22 January 2004, available at the India Resource Center website, http://www.indiaresource.org/news/2004/1005.html (accessed 22 August 2006).

National Health Service, 'Indian Nurses Programme: Guidance for Trusts', Leeds, 2005, http://www.nhsemployers.org/workforce/workforce-540. cfm (accessed 24 July 2006).

———, 'International Nursing Recruitment', Leeds, 2006, http://www. nhsemployers.org/workforce/workforce-527.cfm (accessed 20 July 2006).

Rai, Usha, 'Forging a Bond in a Government Hospital', *The Tribune*, Chandigarh, 16 December 2003, http://www.tribuneindia.com/2003/ 20031216/edit.htm#7 (accessed 22 August 2006).

Rosen, Rana, 'Male Nurses from Rajasthan', *Medill News Service*, on Immigration Here & There Project website, http://www.immigration hereandthere.org/2006/06/male_nurses_from_rajasthan.php (accessed 12 December 2006).

———, 'From East to West', *Outlook*, 24 July 2006, YaleGlobal Online, website of the Yale Center for the Study of Globalization, http://yale global.yale.edu./index.jsp (accessed 27 July 2006).

Royal College of Nursing, 'Success with Internationally Recruited Nurses: RCN Good Practice Guidance for Employers in Recruiting and Retaining', London, 2005, http://www.rcn.org.uk/publications/pdf/success_ with_irns.pdf (accessed 20 July 2006).

———, 'Working Well Initiative: Internationally Recruited Nurses: Good Practice Guidance for Health Care Employers and RCN Negotiators', London, July 2002, http://www.rcn.org.uk/publications/pdf/irn-insides-001-788.pdf (accessed 20 July 2006).

Sainath, P., 'Commerce and Crisis Hit Wayanad Students', *The Hindu*, 30 January 2005, India Together website, http://www.indiatogether. org/2005/jan/psa-student.htm (accessed 4 June 2005).

Yusufzai, Ashfaq, 'Pakistan: Nurses Get Little Training or Respect', The Center for Nursing Advocacy, 4 June 2006, http://www.nursingadvocacy. org/news/2006/jun04_pakistan.html (accessed 9 September 2006).

# About the Author

MADELAINE HEALEY has a PhD from La Trobe University, Melbourne, Australia. Her research interests include Indian public health care system, the role of women professionals therein and migration of Indian nurses. She has written a range of articles highlighting the neglected role of trained nurses, both in the Indian public health care system and in Indian women's history. She is also an independent researcher, with commercial research experience in health care in the UK.

# Index

Milton Keynes UK
Ingram Content Group UK Ltd.
UKHW022051141024
449569UK00031B/1594